In Search of Madness

In Search of MADNESS

Schizophrenia and Neuroscience

R. Walter Heinrichs

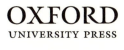

OXFORD

UNIVERSITY PRESS

2001

OXFORD
UNIVERSITY PRESS

Oxford   New York
Athens   Auckland   Bangkok   Bogotá   Buenos Aires   Calcutta
Cape Town   Chennai   Dar es Salaam   Delhi   Florence   Hong Kong   Istanbul
Karachi   Kuala Lumpur   Madrid   Melbourne   Mexico City   Mumbai
Nairobi   Paris   São Paulo   Shanghai   Singapore   Taipei   Tokyo   Toronto   Warsaw

and associated companies in
Berlin   Ibadan

Copyright © 2001 by Oxford University Press, Inc.

Published by Oxford University Press, Inc.
198 Madison Avenue, New York, New York 10016

Oxford is a registered trademark of Oxford University Press.

Library of Congress Cataloging-in-Publication Data
Heinrichs, R. Walter, 1952–
In search of madness : schizophrenia and neuroscience / R. Walter Heinrichs.
p.   cm.
Includes bibliographical references and index.
ISBN 0-19-512219-4
1. Schizophrenia.   I. Title.
RC514.H434   2001
616.89'82—dc21   00-062335

1 3 5 7 9 8 6 4 2

Printed in the United States of America
on acid-free paper

To Peter and Marika

May you know only the madness of passion and never the illness that is described in these pages.

PREFACE

Schizophrenia: a harsh-sounding name for a harsh illness. I first encountered its puzzling nature as a young psychologist when I moved from a general to a psychiatric hospital. Neurological and surgical patients, not schizophrenia patients, had been the focus of my work at the general hospital. Like most neuropsychologists I found the effects of frontal brain damage especially challenging. I worked intensively in rehabilitation with several patients, trying to teach them to overcome the heavy inertia of their mental life. My efforts were largely unsuccessful, but the experience taught me about the frontal brain and its executive role in behavior. Schizophrenia seemed altogether different, an illness of excess rather than deficiency. For every similarity that it had with frontal brain disease there was a striking dissimilarity. But then I moved to the psychiatric hospital. Imagine my surprise in finding schizophrenia ascribed in part to the frontal lobes. Yet it was the beginning of my fascination with the illness as a brain disease. I went on to search for deficits in cognitive brain function that might underlie delusions, hallucinations, and incoherence. I found many deficits in many patients. However, not all patients had the same deficits, and some had none at all. And the symptoms of madness seemed to carry on independently of these deficits. It was as if the schizophrenic mind had a life of its own even as it emerged from the same organ that produced normal thought and feeling. I decided to study the illness and its science comprehensively and in detail and to report the findings of my study. This book is the outcome of that decision.

My labors—and labors they were—began in a tiny office at the Royal Edinburgh Hospital during my sabbatical in 1994–95. I thank Eve Johnstone, Professor of Psychiatry at the University of Edinburgh, for her benign neglect and for use of the library. I thank Ian Deary of the psychology department at Edinburgh, his wife Anne, and the entire Deary family for their warm hospitality and stimulating conversation. As writing progressed, several colleagues read chapter drafts and provided helpful comments. They included Richard Bentall, Vinod Goel, Irving Gottesman, Ronan O'Carroll, and Philip Seeman. Special thanks goes to Professor Gottesman, who reviewed the entire manuscript. Ray Fancher provided me with insight into the nature of book writing and Robert Rosenthal gave me insight into effect sizes. In addition, a number of graduate students contributed to the clinical research and quantitative synthesis reported in the book. They include Allison Bury, Danielle Case, Lara Davidson, Stephanie McDermid, Lesley Ruttan, Teri Sota, Carey Sturgeon, and Konstantine Zakzanis. Several classes of students enrolled in my Advanced Research in Psychology course endured early versions of the book. The Ontario Mental Health Foundation supported my clinical research into schizophrenia at Queen Street Mental Health Center in Toronto. York University helped me finish the book by providing assistance in the form of a Faculty of Arts Research Grant. Sylvia Maat, Mary Maleki, Raj Maharaj, and Barbara Thurston helped me print and duplicate the manuscript. Finally, I thank Joan Bossert and the editorial and production staff at Oxford for their guidance and professional support. "Five Long Years," as the old John Lee Hooker song goes. But now it is done. I hope that anyone with an open mind and a genuine interest in schizophrenia will enjoy reading it.

R. Walter Heinrichs

March 2000
Toronto, Ontario, Canada

CONTENTS

In Search of Madness

1

● ●

ILLNESS AND
EVIDENCE

Empty your mind, for a moment, of stereotypes about schizophrenia. Never mind the staring lunatic; forget the ruined panhandler. Let the misunderstood visionary and the creative eccentric stand aside. Resist the amusement, but accept the discomfort, of a witness of madness. And ignore temporarily the pull of science that transforms, too smoothly, human suffering into chemistry. Focus instead on the experience of a woman with mental illness. Ruth is a real person, but her name has been changed. This is her madness, drawn from interview notes and from her own words:

> Around my neck, and hanging down from each shoulder there is something like a creature. It comes at night. I know it's there because I can feel weight. It coils around me yet remains invisible. An invisible burden. It feels like an enormous leech on my body and it touches me in familiar ways and in intimate places. It reeks of animal smells. It has a strong vagina smell that rises from its sliding body. It is incredibly powerful and irresistible. I can't resist it.

Listen to her story, obtained from hospital records. The sensation of a huge leech or creature was so upsetting that Ruth began to think about death a lot. At times these thoughts evolved into a conviction that death might come any day. She found it hard to sleep or concentrate on daily life activities. It was the creature and the fear of death it inspired that led her to the hospital. Ruth complained to the nurses of feeling rundown, tired, and unable to get up in the morning, and she was admitted to the ward. The creature remained a secret.

3

Ruth found a place in a corner of the ward's lounge where she smoked, talked to herself, smiled, and remained isolated. During interviews with a psychiatrist she denied hearing any voices and denied seeing anything unusual. Her medication was changed to include antidepressant as well as antipsychotic drugs. Then after a few weeks she was discharged. The ideas about dying had diminished, and she seemed happier, "brighter," to the nursing staff. The hospital stay had lasted 6 weeks. Twenty-one months later Ruth was back, convinced of impending death; she was admitted to the same hospital and given a diagnosis of schizophrenia.

Where do the roots of madness lie? Are they apparent, for all to see, in a person's past? Ruth was born in a city in Canada and had no major childhood medical problems. She did well in school, with marks in the seventies, until her fourth year of high school. Her parents' backgrounds were unremarkable. Her father was a salesman, her mother worked as a cleaner. Both parents had very limited education, but they worked hard to provide basic necessities. There is no evidence of serious psychiatric problems in either one.

This is hardly a background conducive to madness—no appalling childhood of abuse and monstrous evil, no years of torture at the hands of perverted parents, no moral failure, no criminality. The backgrounds of people who develop schizophrenia can be surprising in their sheer ordinariness. However, there is more. Ruth was 17 years old when concentration and memory problems began to occur, making it hard for her to complete academic assignments. By the age of 19 she had dropped out of high school and had a stormy, unhappy marriage that ended when her husband left the relationship. Shortly after this piercing rejection she was hospitalized for the first time. Is this an obvious clue? Not really. Rejection does not cause madness. If emotional pain and distress were sufficient to cause schizophrenia, everyone would be touched with psychosis at some point in their lives. Did rejection contribute to the illness in some way or make it worse? Perhaps. But there are no easy answers to the schizophrenia puzzle.

Consider another person with mental illness, a man named William, as he describes his psychotic experience:

The most hilarious aspect of the hospital is the shower. Why would they ask God to have a shower? This makes me laugh. I have heard the voices of great men in history and seen the rainbow of hope. I am willing to take on da Vinci and beat him, but the rhythm of the building is hypnotic and it unbalances me. If only they would do EEG and IQ tests I could prove that I am God. My beard has grown to fulfill the prophecy of a King of Kings, and I know that my powers will be lost on my 33rd birthday. I anticipate my crucifixion. But I will search for the devil and kill him. Perhaps if I kill my brother I will be the only son in the Father's eye. Yes, I must go and look for my brother the devil.

William was hospitalized almost continuously for 7 years, broken by periods when he discharged himself against medical advice. Treatment included electroconvulsive therapy as well as antipsychotic medication, but these had little apparent effect. Police often returned him to hospital. On one occasion his landlord instigated a complaint because William had vomited, defecated, and urinated throughout the apartment. When the police arrived he was running around naked and speaking nonsense. William became involved increasingly in using street drugs as well as alcohol, and he was charged with assault on several occasions. The diagnosis was schizophrenia.

Look into his life history. The family was large, with nine children. William's mother was hospitalized with schizophrenia and suicide attempts during his adolescence. His father was a general factory laborer and seems to have led a normal life. William had no learning problems or failed grades in school, but he left after 9 years of education to work. As early as age 12 he had trouble with the police and was involved with gangs and placed on probation. At 18 he was convicted on drug charges and spent a year in prison. His first psychiatric hospital admission occurred at the age of 26 years, and this began a long sequence of admissions and discharges throughout his adult life. A computerized tomography (CT) brain scan was carried out after this first admission. The scan was normal, as was most of the neurological examination. However, the exam did find that William had abnormal reflexes on both sides of his body, implying atrophy of frontal brain areas. Moreover, electroencephalography (EEG) testing suggested possible epilepsy with a seizure focus in the right cerebral hemisphere of the brain.

In contrast with Ruth's history, William's background includes abundant evidence of familial mental illness, childhood maladjustment, drug abuse, antisocial behavior, and later, "soft" signs of brain damage. There is no shortage of potential clues to the etiology of an illness. Yet are these just the characteristics of a turbulent life, or are they vital factors in the development of schizophrenia? Did they cause the illness, aggravate its expression, or just exist independently? How is it possible to account for the absence of such characteristics in Ruth's background if both patients have the same disorder?

Consider James, one more person with schizophrenia.

At some point, the parasite had bitten into the inner brain—my inner brain. Now the instructions are, increasingly, to bite off my penis, slash my face, jump in front of a car. If these actions are not carried out, I will be forced to comply. I am helpless and worthless. The parasite is a source and a voice, in the depths of my brain, in the flesh of my leg and hands, in the curve of my back, with terrible control over what I am allowed to think and do. The voice has made my life into a life of torture. Death is preferable to this. The voice is right.

James was hospitalized after separating from his wife. Nursing staff described him as irritable; he talked to himself and paced restlessly around the ward. He showed very little emotion and was guarded. Antipsychotic medication made the "voice" go away. However, he became convinced that hospital staff members were going to castrate him, and he discharged himself. His symptoms returned, but James was not hospitalized again for 11 years.

In this case, there is again no family history of mental illness. James's father was a businessman; his mother stayed at home, and the family moved frequently. There were no life-threatening complications during James's birth, but the delivery was difficult and required forceps after 36 hours of labor. As an infant his development was physically normal, but he was slow to talk. He was diagnosed with a learning disability as early as the age of 2. At the age of 5 or 6 James had a serious concussion and lost consciousness for about 2 hours. This was the result of an accidental fall. In addition, his mother observed that as a child James was unresponsive to affection. He constricted his body when cuddled and seldom smiled or displayed positive emotion. He also earned poor grades, mostly Ds, in school and was held back because of learning difficulties. Eventually James finished high school at age 26 and later held down a number of sales jobs. His father usually arranged the jobs for him, but they were short-term, and James was fired often for poor performance. He was diagnosed with schizophrenia at the age of 33. There is no sign of drug or alcohol abuse and no record of criminal activity or antisocial behavior.

In a very general sense, the two men with schizophrenia both experienced childhood adjustment problems. However, these problems were very different in kind. James was emotionally withdrawn and unresponsive, never aggressive; had early language and learning difficulties; and suffered a serious head injury. William had a psychotic parent, whereas James had average parents. During adolescence William abused drugs, and James avoided them.

If all three schizophrenia patients are considered jointly, other more subtle contrasts emerge. Their symptoms differ. Ruth experienced hallucinations that involved touch (tactile hallucinations) and smell (olfactory hallucinations). She never heard voices (auditory hallucinations), saw apparitions (visual hallucinations), or felt persecuted (paranoid delusions). She never felt special or unusually powerful (grandiose delusions). William, on the other hand, had delusions of power and divinity with both auditory and visual hallucinations. His speech was hard to follow, and his emotional responses were unusual or inappropriate to the social situation. He never reported tactile and olfactory hallucinations, however, and showed few of the "negative" symptoms of the illness, like apathy or withdrawal, that resemble depression. Finally, James had exclusively auditory hallucinations and persecutory delusions and did not show signs of grandiosity or incoherent speech. His emotional life and behavior seem somewhere between the other two patients—James was unexpressive perhaps and unsociable but not depressed.

Schizophrenia is an inconsistent illness. It is full of clues, false leads, and blind alleys, suggestive patterns of evidence that some, but not all, patients share. Indeed, people who share a diagnosis of schizophrenia often share little else. As in these brief case descriptions, most patients with the illness differ from each other in terms of symptoms, family background, and childhood. They also differ from each other in a wide variety of biological features. Researchers and clinicians refer to this dissimilarity within groups of schizophrenia patients as *heterogeneity*. Heterogeneity has been recognized as a pervasive feature of schizophrenia since the pioneering descriptions of the illness in the early years of this century. It is part of what makes schizophrenia such a puzzle to scientists, such a challenge to mental health practitioners, and such a trial to a patient's relatives and friends (see Torrey, 1995).

But there is much more to consider than heterogeneity. A substantial proportion of people with schizophrenia, perhaps half or slightly more, recover to some degree (see Buchanan & Carpenter, 2000; Möller & Von Zerssen, 1995). In fact, the long-term picture for people with the illness is better than it has ever been in the past. Yet this is also an illness that associates with pessimism. There is no cure and no means of prevention. Symptoms can only be managed, with medication, sometimes at the cost of unpleasant side effects. Moreover, the illness has social consequences. Many schizophrenia patients are stigmatized and shunned. Bereft of work and life skills, they are seen wandering the city, frozen in strange postures on street corners, begging in the park, railing at unseen adversaries on the sidewalk. They are unwelcome in general hospital emergency wards and unwelcome as neighbors in the community. All too often people with schizophrenia end their lives in tragedy—crushed by traffic on the expressway or neglected in doorways. And for some, death comes as the price of madness itself. A patient obeys the insistent voices that promise omnipotence and is betrayed by gravity, sailing into space supported only by convictions of power. Another leaps to intercept a subway train with a fatally subjective strength. Of course most people know that schizophrenia is a serious condition that manifests itself in disturbed thoughts and feelings. But who could imagine thoughts and feelings like these? Who could imagine a belief so compelling, a fear so relentless, a voice so persuasive, a pleasure so remote, a despair so final, a madness so complete?

If this is not enough to convey the seriousness of the illness, a host of statistics can be summoned to underscore the suffering, prevalence, and social burden of schizophrenia. In North America and Europe there is about a 1% risk that a person will develop the illness at some point in his or her life (Jablensky, 1995). Schizophrenia exists throughout the world but occurs disproportionately in younger people during the third decade and strikes men and women in equal numbers (Hafner & an der Heiden, 1999; Sartorius et al. 1986). Yet men seem to develop the disorder at an earlier age than women (Norquist & Narrow, 2000;

Stromgren, 1987). It occurs more often in lower socioeconomic classes, although this relation is not clearly causal (Saugstad, 1989). A person with schizophrenia is also prone to a variety of other medical conditions, more likely to commit suicide, and less likely to complete secondary or postsecondary education or to remain employed (Müijen & Hadley, 1995). Patients with schizophrenia often suffer from other psychiatric disorders as well, especially depression, and they are vulnerable to alcoholism and drug abuse (Kendler, Gallagher, Abelson & Kessler, 1996). Schizophrenia patients occupy up to one-quarter of hospital beds in the United States (Davies & Drummond, 1990), and they represent a significant proportion of homeless people (Buchanan & Carpenter, 2000).

Accordingly, for many, this is a disabling condition. Welfare, unemployment, sheltered workshops, dependence on family members—these are the likely concomitants of prolonged schizophrenic illness. It does not kill a person directly. But the illness hollows the passion and the pleasure out of life. At best, a kind of truce may grow between the vitality that struggles to emerge and the restrained but unconquered illness. The symptoms grow familiar, if not benign, or the illness may remit and recede. Madness becomes quiet and bides its time, hiding in the underground of life, suppressed by chemistry, never forgotten.

The Science of Schizophrenia

Over the last two decades, with the rapid development of the neurosciences, the hope and even confidence has arisen that schizophrenia will soon be understood, perhaps defeated, or at least rendered less disabling and less burdensome on the individual and on society. It is hoped that knowledge about the structure and function of the brain can be applied to schizophrenia and yield major breakthroughs in science and treatment. Increased funds have been provided for schizophrenia research in many countries, while new specialty journals disseminate the burgeoning scientific findings on the illness. The International Congress of Schizophrenia Research meets every 2 years, with increasing numbers of submissions. Newspapers carry stories about incipient advances in the neurobiology and genetics of serious mental illness. In 1989 the U.S. Congress declared the coming decade the "Decade of the Brain." Distinguished scientists and physicians began to suggest that the end of the decade would see definitive understanding of schizophrenia (e.g., Gottesman, 1991, pp. xii, 246; Mesulam, 1990). At the end of the millenium the end of madness would be in sight, if not in our grasp.

There is certainly no shortage of research on the illness. My students and I used a computer search of the published scientific literature to count the number of articles on schizophrenia over the last 3 decades. Figure 1.1 displays the results of this search. There was a time, in the early 1960s, when talented young

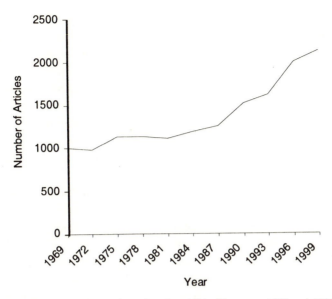

Figure 1.1. Scientific articles on schizophrenia published between 1969 and 1999. The large increase in publication during the late 1980s coincides with the growing availability of brain-scanning technology. (Source: Medline.)

researchers were not attracted to schizophrenia and the number of articles could be measured in the hundreds. The number grew slowly through the 1970s and early 1980s. Then major technical advances in brain imaging occurred and these techniques became available to researchers. Hence, productivity increased sharply during the late 1980s and 1990s to a current average of about 2,000 articles per year—a 100% increase over 30 years. However, is proximity to the truth about schizophrenia growing in step with this large quantitative growth in scientific publishing?

My aim in this book is to test the view that definitive understanding of schizophrenia is in sight by examining the strength and consistency of evidence in a number of important research areas. The science of schizophrenia is a search for abnormalities that distinguish and cause the illness. Across the diversity of neuroscience, where is evidence strong and compelling, where is it weak and disappointing? Is schizophrenia yielding its secrets to the steady application of technology and time and effort? And is the heterogeneity illustrated in the clinical vignettes of Ruth, William and James just some peculiarity of individual cases, or does it extend into neuroscience research as a major challenge in its own right? To pursue these questions I have selected a wide spectrum of research areas to explore. It is unlikely that many scientists would disagree with what I have included, but some may argue that other areas should also be covered. What I provide is a broad representative sampling and evaluation of schizophrenia science but not an exhaustive one. The sampling is extensive, and intensive, but not absolute in scope. Here is a synopsis of what lies ahead.

I consider symptoms first because they form the basis for diagnosis. Diagnosis, in turn, is the foundation of any science of disease. Of special interest in chapter 2, "The Nature of Symptoms," is the "positive" triad of hallucinations, delusions, and thought disorder. These are some of the strangest and most perplexing phenomena in human psychology—what do we know about them? The mental processes that underlie symptoms have been studied by a small number of psychologists. I will explain their work and evaluate the strength and consistency of the evidence.

"The Mark of Madness" (chapter 3) focuses on the topic of "markers" of schizophrenia. A disease marker is an objective characteristic, behavioral or biological in nature, that can reliably identify who has or will have a disease—even in the absence of obvious symptoms. A successful marker would remedy the great problems associated with an exclusively symptom and history-based diagnostic scheme like the one used for schizophrenia. A marker would have wide applications to research areas like genetics and to the early identification of people at risk for the illness. This was a very popular area of research during the 1980s and early 1990s, especially the study of abnormal eye movements and evoked potentials—are they the long-awaited markers for schizophrenia? This chapter describes the various cognitive and psychophysiological indices that are regarded as potential markers and reports on evidence relevant to each one.

"Executive Incompetence" (chapter 4) broaches directly, for the first time in the book, the question of what defective brain regions may contribute to schizophrenia. Of special interest are the various cognitive abilities termed "executive" functions that associate with the prefrontal part of the brain. These functions are a major scientific puzzle on their own, quite apart from any involvement with schizophrenia. I review what is known about the frontal lobes and consider evidence that bears on the idea that a defective frontal brain is a necessary component of schizophrenia. Does the answer to the riddle of how the brain produces madness begin here, or does frontal brain research provide only weak and inconsistent evidence?

The review of the executive brain is complemented by a consideration of the temporal lobes and the brain's semantic system in chapter 5, "The Biology of Meaning." Together, the frontal and temporal lobes, along with the basal ganglia, are the most intensively studied regions of the brain in relation to schizophrenia. I describe the behavioral and biological characteristics of the temporal lobes, with a focus on the left temporal area. How strong and consistent is the evidence that temporal lobe abnormalities are one of the causes of schizophrenia?

"Neurochemical Tempest" (chapter 6) begins with what may be the most widely acknowledged scientific fact about schizophrenia: most patients' symptoms improve in response to dopamine-blocking antipsychotic medication. This discovery launched the study of neurotransmitter abnormalities in the illness. I describe the elements of neurochemistry implicated in schizophrenia with particular attention to dopamine, serotonin, and glutamate. Are the abnormalities that have been discovered of sufficient magnitude to distinguish schizophrenic and healthy people, and how consistent is the evidence?

"The Strangeness of Children" (chapter 7) is concerned with life before the illness strikes. I search for biological and behavioral antecedents of schizophrenia that may reflect an early brain lesion or a genetic predisposition to develop the illness. Studies that seek the answer to schizophrenia in the evolving nervous system or in early problems in maturation are extremely difficult to conduct. Yet the idea that the illness is an aberration of neurodevelopment is probably the most generally held belief in contemporary research. Does the evidence justify this belief? What about the social environment of the developing child? As with other chapters, I provide a tutorial at the beginning on the basic knowledge needed to appreciate the research findings and then present and weigh the evidence itself.

Having completed the core of my empirical review of content areas, I then focus on current theoretical ideas about schizophrenia and how they explain the illness. There has never been a shortage of imaginative speculation about the origins and nature of madness. However, theories of schizophrenia are seldom evaluated critically in terms of their ability to solve the root scientific problems of the illness. These problems include neurogenesis—what goes wrong in the brain to cause the illness? They include the puzzle of symptom formation—how do delusions, hallucinations, thought disorder, and negative symptoms arise? They include the problem of etiology and how genetic and environmental influences combine to cause schizophrenia. Finally, the root problems include the timing of the illness—why it emerges in young adult life, and the problem of heterogeneity and why patients are so different from each other in so many ways. I have selected the most comprehensive and influential ideas and assessed their success in resolving these problems.

In the final chapter, "The End of the Beginning," I use the compiled evidence to provide an overview and synthesis of schizophrenia and neuroscience. I consider whether the long-awaited breakthrough is in the making—and it is just a matter of time and the continued application of the assumption that schizophrenia is one neurological condition—or whether a major reconstruction of assumptions and ideas about the illness is needed. I consider the possibility that neuroscience must change in fundamental ways if it wants to crack the schizophrenia puzzle.

Although my analysis is broad, not all research topics could be included in the depth they deserve. Perhaps the most obvious omission is a chapter devoted exclusively to the genetics of schizophrenia. In part, this omission reflects the fact that the bulk of earlier evidence in population genetics has been well summarized for general readers and researchers by experts like Gottesman (1991) and Zuckerman (1999; pp. 349–362). A second reason for not including an in-depth treatment of genetics is that the most exciting recent developments in this field undoubtedly derive from the use of genetic linkage strategies, the search for candidate genes, and the techniques of molecular biology. Molecular biology and neurogenetics have enormous potential for clarifying the etiology of the illness. If genes that play a role in the illness are identified along with the products of these genes and their neurological effects, then it may be possible to track schizophrenia from molecules to mind. But that is a potential future rather than an existing body of evidence. I am concerned here primarily with evaluating what is known about the illness as a disorder of brain and mind. On the other hand, genetic considerations are everywhere in schizophrenia research. So I do provide a basic summary and include genetic perspectives in chapter 3, chapter 7, and chapter 8. For recent discussions and critiques of genetic research on schizophrenia I recommend articles and books by Faraone, Tsuang, and Tsuang (1999), Moises and Gottesman (2000); Pogue-Geile and Gottesman (1999), Kendler, (2000), and Zuckerman (1999, pp. 349–362).

I was also selective in other ways. The book focuses on ideas and evidence that have received sustained scientific attention, or what Meehl (1990a) calls ideas with "track records." It is the accumulation of evidence over time and across different investigators that comprises the real knowledge base for schizophrenia. And the book is concerned primarily with science, with understanding, and not with clinical issues in diagnosis, treatment, and rehabilitation. I have not lost sight of the fact that, like all illnesses, schizophrenia is an expression of human suffering and not just an intellectual puzzle. But a puzzle it is, and that is the topic of this book.

Finally, I have a reader and an audience in mind—this book is meant for students and researchers who want a comprehensive synthesis of the neuroscience evidence on schizophrenia. Yet it is also meant for anyone who just wants to learn more about the illness, anyone willing to think and work through some moderately challenging material, anyone who has been moved by madness in some way and is willing to be moved again by reading this book.

Rules of Evidence

I have indicated a concern with evidential strength and consistency in describing the research topics that form the basis for my review. However, little has been said about how to calibrate these aspects of evidence—the tools that are needed to assess the knowledge base in schizophrenia science. The rest of this chapter is devoted to the nature of evidence and how it will be weighed.

The traditional way of assessing research literature is remarkably imprecise. Studies are described one at a time, or grouped in some thematic or technical way, in an attempt to summarize, integrate, and make sense of the findings. The aggregation of statistically significant results, or the absence of such results, defines the state of knowledge in a field of research. This assessing, integrating, synthesizing activity is an important function for research reviews, and I provide it myself in the chapters that follow. Nevertheless, there are serious drawbacks to traditional literature reviews, and it is inadvisable to rely exclusively on them in evaluating a field as complex and challenging as the study of schizophrenia. Indeed, conventional ways of evaluating the scientific status of a field are vulnerable to criticism on several grounds (see Hedges & Olkin, 1985; Wolf, 1986).

In most reviews of research, findings are included or excluded, praised or disparaged, on the basis of the reviewer's subjective impressions or bias. One study that supports the reviewer's point of view is given great weight and another study that contradicts it is downplayed. Scientists, like everyone else, are prone to bias and subject to the influence of personal values when engaged in an exercise of judgment and criticism. However, the most serious problem with traditional literature reviews is their failure to provide explicit information on evidential strength and consistency. Of course, there is an implicit standard of evidence, the test of statistical significance, without which studies are seldom published. Yet information regarding statistical significance is not information regarding the magnitude of evidence. In fact, statistical significance testing may serve to obscure rather than to illuminate the strength of a researcher's findings.

Generations of undergraduate students in biological and social science have learned, often painfully, that statistical tests signify whether or not an investigation has identified something important that cannot be attributed to the vagaries of chance and coincidence. But these tests furnish only an impression of evidence and do not actually say anything about its strength (Bakan, 1966; Cohen, 1994). As an illustration, suppose that some aspect of brain chemistry is measured in a group of patients with schizophrenia and in a group of healthy people. The measurements are averaged, and a statistical test is run to see if the difference between groups is "significant." Say that the difference turns out to be significant statistically in the usual form of a probability value like 5%. In other words, there is only a 5% chance of incorrectly rejecting the idea that there are no differences between the schizophrenia and control groups. Such a result sounds impressive, if convoluted. But it tells the investigator almost nothing about *how different* the two groups really are in terms of brain chemistry. It says nothing about what proportion of patients are truly "abnormal." If the patients and healthy people have different group averages but still overlap by, say, 50%, in their individual measurements, then this aspect of neurochemistry cannot be an essential feature of schizophrenia. Too many healthy people will have the same brain chemistry as the patients. No matter what the outcome of a statistical test, the degree of separation between groups tells the real story of how strong or weak the findings are. Paradoxically, information on group separation is exactly what is required and exactly what is missing in most traditional research reviews.

Inferential statistics and significance testing are relatively recent developments (e.g. Fisher, 1947) in science. If they are the basis of evidence, how did earlier scientists ever get along without them? And they did. In biology, for example, the cell theory developed in the nineteenth century proposed that all living organisms were composed of units called cells. These units were held to be the structural and functional foundation of life. Early microscopes allowed the theory to be tested and confirmed the occurrence of cells in all observable life forms. Moreover, the evidence was consistent across investigators as different scientists around the world repeated the same observations with the same results (Ebert, Loewy, Miller, & Schneiderman, 1973, pp.18–20). The strength of evidence was enormous, but no statistical tests were available—or needed.

In practice, scientists know that statistical significance cannot be equated with evidential strength. Many also know that really powerful findings, where control and patient groups do not overlap even slightly on the measurement of interest, make statistical tests unnecessary. Moreover, as Cohen (1994) reminds researchers, generalizable knowledge has more to do with replication—repeating, reproducing, the finding—than with inferential statistics. Nonetheless, statistical significance continues to underpin criteria for publication in many fields of behavioral and biological science (see Meehl, 1978, 1986). It is natural to wonder if discoveries that approach the magnitude of cell theory and other advances in the sciences are being made in relation to schizophrenia, and if not, to what extent research is falling short and in what area. But answering such questions requires a yardstick for evidence that actually does the job.

Effect Sizes as Evidence

Smith and Glass (1977) and Cohen (1988) have suggested a helpful index of evidence in the form of the *effect size*. An effect size refers to the magnitude of difference between one group of people and another on some measurement of importance. A common effect size is Cohen's d, where the average of one group is subtracted from the average of another group, usually a control group. This difference is divided by the pooled standard deviation, a statistic that reflects the amount of dispersion or variability that exists around the group averages. Thus research results can be expressed in units or degrees of group separation. The effect size d directly mirrors the magnitude of difference between groups of healthy and ill people and makes evidential strength explicit.

Consider an example from physical medicine, the outcome of coronary bypass surgery versus standard medication in reducing angina—chest pain—from heart disease. Lynn and Donovan (1980) calculated an effect size of $d = .80$

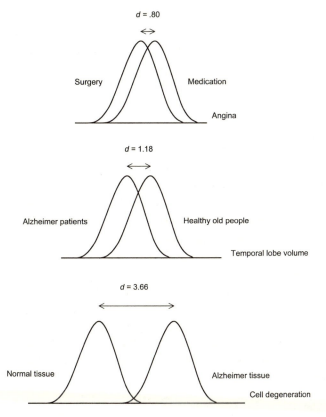

Figure 1.2. Effect size results for three different comparisons. The top pair of overlapping distributions shows angina severity in cardiac patients receiving standard medication or bypass surgery (Lynn & Donovan, 1980). The medication group is displaced to the higher end of the severity scale. However, the joint group overlap is still almost 53%. The middle pair of distributions compares temporal lobe brain volumes measured with magnetic resonance imaging in patients with Alzheimer's disease and in healthy old people (Zakzanis, 1998). The joint overlap is about 39%, which is a "large" effect, but the group difference is still too small to base the diagnosis of dementia on brain-scan results. The lower pair of distributions overlaps by only about 3%. This comparison reflects group differences in microscopic nerve cell degeneration measured in post-mortem brain tissue (Ball & Lo, 1977). The degeneration is much more extensive in Alzheimer's disease than in normal aging and represents a neuropathological marker for dementia.

using angina ratings among patients who underwent each treatment. I have represented this effect size in the form of two idealized normal distributions in figure 1.2. Notice that the distribution of patients receiving surgery is displaced to the left of the group that received only medication. This displacement occurs along a continuum that reflects an increasing severity of angina. To be precise, the medication and surgical angina averages differ by .80 pooled standard deviation units—the effect size. Overall, there is clearly a positive effect of surgery on chest pain compared with medication alone. However, there is also considerable overlap between the two distributions. In other words, some patients who had surgery experience the same degree of chest pain as some patients who did not. Cohen (1988) has provided tables that allow this degree of overlap to be expressed as a percentage. Hence, an effect size of $d = .80$ corresponds to a joint distribution overlap of about 53%. Roughly half of the treated and untreated patients are indistinguishable in terms of angina symptoms. So does the surgery work or not? There is a demonstrable group effect, whereby on average, surgical patients are better off than medicated patients are. However, surgery is no guarantee of symptom relief for everyone 100% of the time.

It turns out that many medical and psychological treatments judged helpful have effect sizes that separate only partially groups of treated and untreated patients (Lipsey & Wilson, 1993). Yet these treatments have practical significance in that they offer the possibility of relief to an ill person. Thus evidential strength is partly a function of the specific theoretical or practical problem under study. Clinical practitioners do not require absolute discrimination or the complete absence of group overlap. They require evidence that, on balance, receiving the treatment increases the likelihood that the average patient will be better off. Comparatively modest effect sizes are sufficient to satisfy this requirement. On the other hand, it would be a mistake to assume that such modesty suffices in all research situations.

Causality and Evidence

The calibration of evidence becomes especially important whenever data that bear on etiology or causal mechanisms and processes are reviewed and evaluated. This kind of evidence must be very powerful to support a theory that purports to explain the causes of a disease or holds that certain features or characteristics are primary traits of an illness. Such high expectations for evidence contrast with the kind of results needed in research on treatment effectiveness, where modest effect sizes may be all that is required.

To gain a perspective on this issue, consider a compilation of brain scanning studies of patients with Alzheimer's disease collected by Zakzanis (1998). The studies surveyed all used brain imaging to measure brain tissue volumes in Alzheimer's patients and healthy old people. Degenerative changes in the temporal lobes of the brain have long been regarded as a primary aspect of the pathology of Alzheimer's dementia (see Iqbal & Wisniewski, 1983, pp. 48–56). Therefore, Alzheimer's patients should show evidence of degeneration in the form of smaller temporal lobe volumes, when compared with healthy elderly subjects. Comparison of average temporal lobe volumes in these groups yields an effect size of $d = 1.18$. This corresponds to about two-thirds separation of healthy old people and dementia patients and yields the distribution overlap shown in figure 1.2. It is a large effect but not large enough for all purposes. For example, it is not large enough to support an argument that brain scanning is a highly accurate way of diagnosing the presence of Alzheimer's disease. Too many (39%) dementia patients and healthy old people have similar temporal lobe volumes. The effect size is also not large enough to say that temporal lobe shrinkage is a primary aspect or marker of brain pathology in Alzheimer's disease. Statements about causality and primary disease features require extremely powerful evidence, with virtually no overlap between healthy and sick people.

Now consider an earlier study by Ball and Lo (1977). These researchers used analyses of brain tissue obtained from deceased Alzheimer's patients and compared them with normal tissue. Microscopic cellular changes were observed in the hippocampus, a structure in the temporal lobe that is essential for memory formation. The results correspond to an effect size of $d = 3.66$. Using Cohen's (1988) idealized distributions, this translates into almost no group overlap, as shown in the lowest graph of figure 1.2. In the actual data none of the normal brains had degenerative changes to the degree seen in the Alzheimer's brains. The result makes sense because degeneration in hippocampal cells is a key feature of dementia. It must be close to the cause of the disorder, even if it is not the final word in Alzheimer's pathology. Thus, it seems reasonable to expect extremely large effect sizes if these effects index primary disease features or attributes. Smaller effects are expected for disease features that have weaker links with primary causes or pathologies, and these smaller effects may or may not be involved in all cases of an illness.

Inadvertently, researchers probably spend most of their time studying processes and effects that turn out to be peripheral and weakly related to the topic of interest. Such is the nature of science, with its many dead ends, wrong ideas, and dashed hopes. Knowing the strength of evidence is crucial in determining whether an effect or characteristic is a blind alley, a partial answer, or a major discovery that sheds light on an illness. Reporting research results in the form of effect sizes allows the evidence in question to be laid bare and not obscured, inflated, or dismissed by the vagaries of testing for statistical significance.

Meta-analysis and Cumulative Evidence

In traditional literature reviews, an informal running tally is often kept of significant and nonsignificant studies on a given topic. This enumeration has been called the "box-score" or "vote count" approach to evidence (Light & Smith, 1971). Five studies report significant results in support of the hypothesis, and two studies did not find significant results. Therefore, the hypothesis "wins" by a ratio of 5:2. Aside from the uncertain relation between statistical "wins" and evidential strength, this rough-and-ready tally provides no precise estimate of cumulative evidence or consistency. The studies that fail to find significant results may have failed for procedural reasons. Studies with nonsignificant results may have included insufficient numbers of people in their samples. They may have used inferior instruments—or superior instruments. And in the case of schizophrenia, researchers are also dealing with a disorder that is heterogeneous. Hence, inconsistencies between studies may reflect something fundamental about the illness instead of procedural flaws or differences. This issue of consistency is too important to be left to box-score tallies and the subjective impressions of the reviewer. A better way of compiling study outcomes and results is needed.

When a large number of studies are carried out on the same dependent measure or variable, the results can be expressed in effect sizes and compiled into a superordinate study, or meta-analysis (Hedges & Olkin, 1985; Smith & Glass, 1977; Wolf, 1986). A listing of individual study outcomes calculated as effect sizes immediately conveys the consistency of findings in the field as a whole. Various more precise indices can be used to calibrate this degree of consistency. Not surprisingly, meta-analysis is gradually replacing the traditional narrative review as the preferred way of synthesizing evidence. It offers tools for the assessment of evidence in terms of magnitude and consistency that are superior to traditional significance testing and "box-score" tallies. Nonetheless, these new techniques have their own limitations, and they must be used with caution. There is no point in repeating the mistakes of statistical testing through excessive and inappropriate use of yet another quantitative technique.

Therefore, consider the most common criticisms of meta-analysis. A frequent complaint has been called the "apples and oranges" argument. This criticism holds that most studies differ too much in design features and dependent variables to justify a synthesis. Studies do not all measure exactly the same thing, so they should not be combined into a meta-analysis. Thus in Smith and Glass's (1977) classic meta-analysis of the effects of psychotherapy, somewhat different therapeutic approaches were combined into one category. This may have done violence to important differences by collapsing psychotherapeutic apples and oranges into a generic category. In schizophrenia research the apples and oranges mistake could be made by, say, combining studies of different brain regions into a single meta-analysis. It makes little sense to lump two studies that measure frontal brain volume in with two studies that measure temporal lobe brain volume. However, in these situations, no "lumping" need occur. A straightforward listing of individual studies along with the brain region measured and associated effect size may suffice to expose the evidence. Such an effect size display is still preferable to box-score tallies or significance results as a means of making the evidence apparent. It is also important not to get too carried away with the apples and oranges problem. After all, no two investigations are ever exactly alike, and when taken to its extreme the apples and oranges argument prevents any kind of generalization. There are instances where combining many different studies and results does make sense. Eclectic combinations can provide a very general perspective on the average strength of evidence across many specific fields of research. And this kind of general overview, a panorama of evidence, may sometimes reveal broad trends in knowledge that would otherwise never be noticed.

Another cautionary point concerns what an effect size from a single study cannot do. Namely, it is not an inferential statistic. It does not allow the investigator to generalize and make an inference about all schizophrenia patients. A study effect size is simply a descriptive statement that pertains to the particular patients and control participants used in that one study. But there is a remedy. As individual effect sizes accumulate over many studies and are combined into a meta-analysis, this aggregation becomes a sample on its own—a sample of effect sizes. In these cases confidence intervals can be calculated that turn the average effect into an inferential statistic in its own right. That is, the average effect can be expressed along with a range of values, a kind of margin of error, within which the effect will occur with a specified probability, like 95% of the time. Similar bounds are placed around the results of opinion polls, so that a result is considered accurate within a range of percentage points "19 times out of 20"—in other words, 95% of the time. A confidence interval that includes zero means that the average effect could be zero as well. When this happens, there is no escape. The body of evidence can only be considered weak and unreliable. Hence, if all or virtually all studies on a given topic are included in a meta-analysis, the average effect size and its confidence interval are powerful general statements about the quality of evidence that researchers have collected.

In view of these considerations, I have adopted a meta-analytic approach to the neuroscience of schizophrenia for this book. Each chapter that reviews research findings begins with a background tutorial and an introduction to key issues and then builds to a meta-analytic summary of the evidence. However, I did not adopt rigid expectations for evidential strength. In the case of putative neurological causes of the illness, extremely strong effects are a reasonable expectation. Yet this expectation may not be justified in each research area. Hence, I report and discuss effect sizes in relation to their strength and consistency and whether they are sufficient to support the idea that prompted the study in the first place. I also decided to concentrate on articles published from 1980 through the end of 1999. The most influential diagnostic system for schizophrenia, *DSM-III* (*Diagnostic and Statistical Manual of Mental Disorders*, 3rd ed., American Psychiatric Association, 1980), was introduced at the beginning of this period, leading to greater uniformity in diagnosis than what is found in earlier years. In addition, many of the new functional and structural brain-imaging techniques like positron emission and nuclear magnetic resonance first became available around 1980. Earlier writing and research are described for historical and theoretical purposes, but the meta-analytic reviews in this book are limited to work from the last 20 years.

Conclusion

It is a long psychological distance from the story of how schizophrenia manifests itself in individual lives to the analysis of how the illness can be captured by statistical concepts and research data. Nonetheless, this distance is worth traveling. Good evidential tools are necessary because the study of individual patients shows that schizophrenia is an illness rich in clues and possibilities. It is an illness that inspires speculation and prompts explanation. The result is a bounty of suggestive ideas and over 2000 published research articles per year. The vast majority of these articles report statistically significant findings—differences between patients and healthy people that may or may not advance our understanding of schizophrenia. The tools of meta-analysis provide a way of sorting through the mass of evidence with an eye toward two key questions. First, how strong is the evidence in support of a given research idea? Second, is the evidence consistent across studies, or do different studies examining similar questions yield contradictory results? Now consider these tools and questions and the symptoms that are the first clues in the search for madness.

oped a hierarchy that distinguished "fundamental" from "accessory" symptoms. In constructing this hierarchy he departed from Kraepelin's evenhanded observations and descriptions and placed great emphasis on some symptoms while diminishing the importance of others. Bleuler regarded many of the symptoms described by Kraepelin, including hallucinations and delusions, as accessory rather than as fundamental to the illness.

According to Bleuler, fundamental symptoms included disturbances of "association" and their influence on thought. Schizophrenia was distinguished by erratic thinking where conventional associations among ideas were altered. A patient was asked to describe a walk in the park and wrote: "The mountains which are outlined in the swellings of the oxygen are beautiful." Ideas and words were altered to serve idiosyncratic, usually illogical, functions. A patient whose daughter converted to Catholicism wrote a letter explaining the nature of a rosary as "a prayer multiplier, and this in turn is a prayer for multiplying and as such is nothing else but a prayer mill, and is therefore a mill-prayer machine which is again a prayer-mill machine" and continued in this way for several pages. In schizophrenic thought, ideas seemed chained together with unrelated meanings, personal associations, phonetic similarities, and abrupt departures from standard usage (Bleuler, 1950, pp. 19, 28).

Like Kraepelin, Bleuler distinguished cognitive symptoms, including the associative disturbances, from emotional symptoms, or disturbances of "affectivity." Bleuler agreed that patients appeared to be indifferent to friends, family, work, recreation, pain, and pleasure. During a hospital fire he noted that some patients remained on a burning ward, seemingly unconcerned by the danger. On another occasion, Bleuler observed a woman asking, without any outward emotion or sign of distress, the ward doctor not to kill her. He also noted the apparent inappropriateness of many emotional reactions, terming this "parathymia." One man with parathymia danced around the hospital floor humming popular songs, but in a heartbreaking tone of voice with an upset facial expression. A female patient approached staff members with a friendly expression and tone of voice, only to say: "I really would like to slap your face, people like you are usually called sons of bitches." At other times, emotional behavior seemed to involve a basic kind of ambivalence, not just inappropriate or contradictory emotions. One patient was intensely anxious and afraid of being shot by the ward attendants but could be seen frequently begging an attendant to shoot her. In many people with schizophrenia this apparent ambivalence extended to "will" or purposive behaviors. A man appeared to want to eat his meal yet not want to eat. He sat in front of his plate, brought the spoon to his mouth, and then returned the spoon to the plate. This behavior was repeated many times without anything actually being eaten. Ambivalence could be seen in the intellectual sphere as well, so that the speech and writing of patients often contained logical contradictions. "I am a human being like yourself" maintained one man, "even though I am not a human being" (Bleuler, 1950, pp. 52–54).

Bleuler argued that there was a final type of fundamental symptom, involving autism, or detachment from reality. Patients with schizophrenia appeared to live in a world of their own and failed to react to influences from "the outside." Many ignored their surroundings, avoided eye contact, covered their heads with clothing, or stared at blank walls. At the same time, many people with the illness harbored an inner life of fantasy that was accepted as reality. Paradoxically, conventional reality was viewed with skepticism. Bleuler describes being approached by a patient who insisted that "they say . . . you are the doctor, but I don't know it . . . you are really Minister N." It was common for patients to maintain both an autistic and a conventional kind of reality. However, it was usually convention that seemed strange to the patients. They often complained that objects and people were no longer what they were supposed to be. One woman who was discharged from hospital found community life incomprehensible. It was like "running around in an open grave, so strange did the world appear" (Bleuler, 1950, pp. 66–68).

Patients who were autistic also had attention-related symptoms like distractibility and poor concentration, along with motivational problems, including loss of drive and initiative in everyday activity. Yet this withdrawal was paired, oddly, with impulsive tendencies. Internal perceptions and preoccupations could lead to sudden, ill-conceived decisions, despite the patient's apparent disinterest in everyday life.

When autism combined with dissociation and ambivalence the combination made the schizophrenia patient appear demented to the observer. Hence the illness was confused originally with global intellectual decline. Bleuler felt that schizophrenia did not represent a true intellectual deterioration or dementia. Instead, the illness involved a subordination of the intellect to the fundamental symptoms and to their devastating effect on mental life.

Developments since Bleuler and Kraepelin

The psychiatric pioneers discussed similar kinds of "psychic" symptoms in relation to their schizophrenia patients. To be sure, differences are also evident in the importance and theoretical interpretation assigned to individual symptoms. Despite shifts in emphasis within and between the legacies of Bleuler and Kraepelin, the same kinds of behaviors are included in contemporary accounts and analyses of schizophrenic symptoms. No new symptoms have been discovered or elicited. The only changes have been attempts to subcategorize and differentiate some aspects of the illness from others (see Schneider, 1959). Thus "positive" symptoms have been distinguished from "negative" symptoms (Strauss, Carpenter, & Bartko, 1974). Positive symptoms include delusions and hallucinations. They seem to be abnormal additions to mental life, whereas negative symptoms are deficits, or losses, like reduced motivation, impoverished speech, or emotional withdrawal. Nevertheless, schizophrenic illness is as recognizable in the writings of the pioneers as it is in contemporary textbooks of psychiatry or in the current diagnostic and statistical manual (*DSM-IV*, 1994).

Symptoms and Diagnosis

Symptoms play a major role in diagnosis—deciding who actually has schizophrenia and who has some other disorder. In the *DSM-IV* (1994) diagnostic criteria, five kinds of symptoms are identified as characteristic of schizophrenia. They include the delusions and hallucinations described by earlier psychiatrists, along with disorganized speech. Disorganized speech, a more objective term for Kraepelin's (1919) notion of incoherence, overlaps with Bleuler's (1950) concept of associative symptoms. The fourth symptom-related criterion, grossly disorganized or catatonic behavior, involves odd movements and postures seen in some patients. Kraepelin described aspects of catatonia in considerable detail, but both Bleuler (1950) and Schneider (1959) regarded it as accessory rather than as fundamental to schizophrenia. Finally, the fifth criterion, negative symptoms, comprises disturbances described as symptoms of "affectivity" or emotion by the pioneers. These symptoms include emotional indifference, autistic withdrawal, and loss of drive and initiative.

Although schizophrenia, like all diseases, is defined by its symptoms, *DSM-IV* (1994) places several qualifications on the relation of symptoms to diagnosis. First, no single symptom is obligatory. If delusions are sufficiently "bizarre" they may satisfy the symptom criterion on their own. Similarly, if hallucinations comprise voices commenting on behavior, this too may "qualify" as a primary diagnostic symptom. However, patients can also meet the symptom criterion without ever showing evidence of delusions or hallucinations. There is no uniform, invariant presenting symptom or set of symptoms for schizophrenia but an aggregation of qualitatively different characteristics. Any one of the five kinds of symptoms may, or may not, indicate the presence of the illness, depending on the cooccurrence of other symptoms or, in the case of delusions and hallucinations, depending on the features of the symptom itself (e.g., bizarreness).

Another qualification on the relation between symptoms and the disease entity of schizophrenia is the stipulation that social and occupational dysfunction must coexist with symptoms. In other words, evidence is required that the symptoms are actually disabling to the person in some way. It is not enough to have crazy thoughts; they must be tied to a general deterioration in daily life. Moreover, a person must demonstrate symptoms for at least a month to be considered a candidate for schizophrenia. Finally, even when these criteria are all met, several disorders that can resemble schizophrenia, like depression and mood disorder, must be ruled out or distinguished.

Each of the three patients described in the introductory chapter meet the symptom criterion for schizophrenia. Ruth, the woman who could smell and feel a creature around her neck, clearly had tactile and olfactory hallucinations. She did not hear voices commenting on her behavior—the symptom referred to in *DSM-IV* (1994) as having special diagnostic value. However, Ruth also had negative symptoms comprising withdrawal and affective "flattening." Accordingly, she "qualified" for the symptom criterion by having at least two *kinds* of symptoms. In contrast, both of the men had delusions that could be considered "bizarre" in the *DSM-IV* (1994) context. William was convinced of his own divinity; James felt controlled by an alien parasite. Hence they met the symptom criterion for schizophrenia just on the basis of one positive symptom.

The diagnostic process becomes more complicated when negative and mood-related symptoms figure prominently in the patient's psychological life. Ruth's behavior was withdrawn and "flat" from an emotional standpoint. But she also described thoughts of approaching death, suicide, hopelessness and self-deprecation. These are often symptoms of severe depression, and they raise the possibility of a major mood disorder with psychotic features rather than schizophrenia as the root of her problems. In support of this point, the hospital records show that she was treated with antidepressant medication for "depressive features" at several points in her history.

Strictly speaking, a patient cannot receive simultaneously a diagnosis of schizophrenia and a diagnosis of major mood disorder. Still, there are conditions like schizoaffective disorder, which involves the symptom criterion for schizophrenia coupled with symptoms of a major mood disorder. Differential diagnosis in the case of coexisting mood and psychotic symptoms centers on whether delusions or hallucinations are secondary, reflecting what is basically an emotional disorder, or primary, reflecting probable schizophrenia—a challenging discrimination to make in some cases.

One way to make the distinction is to decide whether symptoms are "congruent" with the patient's depressed mood or "bizarre" and seemingly detached from the patient's prevailing emotional state. Thus a severely depressed person might "hear" voices accusing him or her of being worthless garbage. Such people may become delusional and believe that they are the cause of all evil in the world and deserve to be punished. But these mood-congruent psychotic symptoms are probably products of the mood state and not symptoms of schizophrenia. Additional considerations that assist differential diagnosis include whether the full spectrum of depressive features, including weight changes, loss of interest and pleasure, sleep alterations, and fatigue, are present (see *DSM-IV*, 1994).

In practice it can be hard to differentiate types of psychotic experience without considerable experience on the diagnostician's part. Are hallucinations of feeling and smelling a creature mood-congruent or not? Ruth described her creature hallucination as a burden that weighed her down and made her think about death. This could be interpreted as mood-congruent. On the other hand, she did not have hallucinations that were deprecating, or negativistic, involving guilt, self-hatred, or related depressive themes. In difficult cases like this one, careful interviewing and examination of hospital records can sometimes reveal that in the past the positive psychotic symptoms persisted even when the mood symptoms were in remission. Alternatively, the patient may never have experienced depression without the presence of psychotic symptoms. In such a case a schizophrenic disorder probably underlies the patient's behavior, although depressive features may also exist. In Ruth's situation, clinical notes and observations from previous hospitalizations eventually led to the diagnosis of schizophrenia rather than to depression with psychotic features.

Each of the patients described in chapter 1 also showed the necessary signs of a decline in personal, social, and occupational functioning that must accompany the symptoms of true schizophrenia. Ruth neglected her physical care and was unable to live successfully in supported housing. William, with delusions of divinity, was unable to cope with living in an apartment by himself and was charged with assault at one point. James, who felt controlled by a parasite, experienced marital breakdown in tandem with his symptoms and became unemployed. Finally, exclusionary criteria, like the timing of drug and alcohol abuse, or physical illness, relative to the psychotic symptoms, are important. For example, William had a history of street drug abuse that stretched into early adult years. This had to be ruled out as a cause of his psychotic episode.

Hence schizophrenia is an illness wherein symptoms are necessary but not sufficient for diagnosis. A thorough history and the exclusion of conditions that resemble schizophrenia are essential aspects of the diagnostic process. Nonetheless, symptoms are of critical importance in identifying the illness. A careful reading of the *DSM-IV* section on schizophrenia offers no objective signs, or laboratory findings, to support a diagnosis of the illness. Accordingly, much of the burden of diagnostic proof rests with a patient's symptom picture.

The Mind of Madness

There is more to symptoms than their importance in the pragmatics of diagnosis. They also reveal the private mental life of a person with a terrifying disorder. This inner life is of interest and importance in its own right. To study the symptoms of schizophrenia is to study the human mind, misshapen and beleaguered by illness perhaps, but the mind nonetheless. Why do people with schizophrenia claim to see, hear, smell, and touch things that do not exist? How is it possible for someone to develop a belief in their own divinity or to interpret random events as causally, symbolically, and personally connected?

Symptoms and Clinical Tests of Cognitive Ability

One view holds that schizophrenic symptoms are abnormal products of cognitive processes like thinking and reasoning, perception and attention that have been altered by the disease process. Hence patients with schizophrenia and, more specifically, those with particular symptoms like delusions or hallucinations should have measurable cognitive defects.

There are basically two ways of trying to test this idea. The first, easiest, and most popular way is to apply standard clinical tests of cognitive ability to patients with schizophrenia and to correlate the results with the severity of specific symptoms. These clinical tests comprise a great variety of different tasks. Some require solving visual puzzles and problems or remembering lists of words or stories; others involve naming a series of common objects, generating words that begin with specified letters, or matching the relative positions of lines in space and others may require copying geometric shapes and patterns (see Lezak, 1995). Normal cognition is built from these basic component skills that allow experience to be organized, preserved, and provided with meaning. Surely it would seem that the bizarre thoughts and perceptions of the person with schizophrenia are rooted in some basic abnormality of cognitive functioning.

Yet it is one of the many puzzles of schizophrenia research that cognitive phenomena as extreme and dramatic as delusions and hallucinations are seldom related strongly to standard measures of cognitive ability. To be sure, certain kinds of symptoms, including thought disorder and negative symptoms like impoverished speech and withdrawal, correlate moderately with cognitive test scores. But the two most distinctive positive symptoms of schizophrenia seem to exist independently of standard cognitive performance.

The cognitive puzzle is illustrated by the work of Liddle and associates on three basic symptom clusters that describe schizophrenia (Liddle & Morris, 1991; Liddle, 1994). One cluster, termed "psychomotor poverty," consists of characteristics like decreased speech and movement. The severity of psychomotor poverty correlates moderately with patients' ability to generate words rapidly and to scan visual displays accurately. A second cluster, thought disorder and bizarre emotional behavior, correlates moderately with the same cognitive tests, as well as with tasks measuring mental flexibility. However, the "reality distortion" factor, consisting of delusions and hallucinations, is not related to *any* of the cognitive tests. Several other investigators have confirmed the same pattern of results (Bilder, Mukherjee, Rieder, & Pandurangi, 1985; Chen, Wilkins, & McKenna, 1994; Franke, Maier, Hain, & Klingler, 1992; Van der Does, Dingemans, Linszen, Nugter, & Scholte, 1993). Occasional exceptions like Green and

Walker's (1986a) finding of a modest relation between positive symptoms and distractibility have proven hard to reproduce. The consensus seems to be that transitory positive symptoms may correlate with cognitive tests if the symptoms interfere with the patient's attention to the test, but persisting positive symptoms exist independently of cognitive ability.

To illustrate the lack of concordance between delusions and hallucinations and cognitive impairment on standard tests, consider the three patients described in chapter 1. Consider as well one of the most common clinical tests of spatial cognition and planning, the Complex Figure Test (see Lezak, 1995, pp. 569–578; Osterrieth, 1944). The ability to draw an accurate copy of a design like the one shown in the upper left of figure 2.1 can be affected by general mental ability (Chiulli, Yeo, Haaland, & Garry, 1989), academic achievement (Rosselli and Ardila, 1991), and most severely, by various forms of brain damage (Lezak, 1995, pp. 576–578). Proceeding clockwise, the first two copies show how neurological patients with focal lesions in right and left sides of the brain perform on the task. The next three, the copying efforts of Ruth, William, and James, would be considered to be within normal limits. The patients may have cognitively based symptoms, but this test does not reveal any severe underlying cognitive impairment. Moreover, although the patients' symptoms differ from each other, there is little difference in their cognitive-constructional ability.

None of this is to say that patients with schizophrenia are *never* impaired on copying tasks, and therein lies another aspect of the puzzle. Figure 2.2 shows several additional copying results from different schizophrenia patients. There certainly are some impaired performances in the patient population. However, impairment is not a feature of the illness as a whole and does not appear to be related to the presence or absence of positive symptoms or to distinctions between different kinds of positive symptoms (e.g., delusions versus hallucinations). Indeed, what figures 2.1 and 2.2 really demonstrate is the diversity, or heterogeneity, of cognitive ability that can exist in schizophrenia, as well as the apparent independence of this ability from positive symptoms.

Perhaps positive symptoms do not relate to cognitive abilities because standard tests fail to tap the cognitive processes that are involved in symptom formation. After all, the formation of, say, delusions, may not involve processes like visual planning and drawing, rapid word generation, memory for word lists, abstract categorization, or other skills typically measured by the clinical neuropsychologist. Standard tests and positive symptoms may both involve cognitive processes, but very different kinds of cognitive processes.

Symptoms and Cognitive Neuropsychology

The second major way of trying to find the cognitive basis of symptoms involves tasks designed specifically to index schizophrenic thinking. There may be

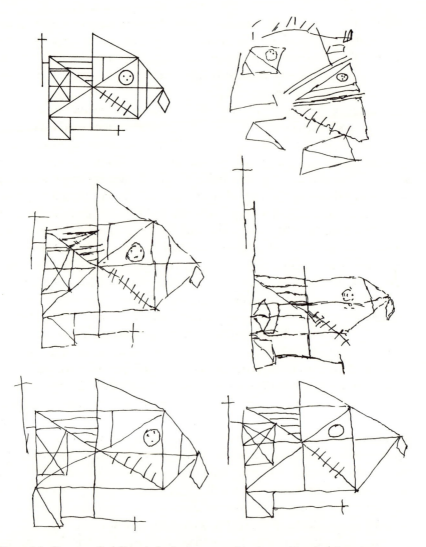

Figure 2.1. Drawing disabilities in brain damage and in three schizophrenia patients. Attempts to copy Osterrieth's (1944) complex figure (upper left) reveal a severe spatial disturbance in the case of a man with a right cerebral hemisphere stroke (upper right). Proceeding clockwise, left hemisphere damage appears to produce loss of detail, but the shape is preserved. Ruth (lower right), a female schizophrenia patient, has a normal copy apart from a few minor errors, as do William and James, two male patients with the illness.

no point in applying standard tests that were designed with neurological patients in mind to patients with schizophrenia. For example, as figure 2.1 illustrates, copying and visual planning defects are common consequences of strokes in the right cerebral hemisphere of the brain (see Lezak, 1995, pp. 576–578). Therefore, it makes sense to study spatial construction in right brain cerebrovascular disease. However, schizophrenia reveals itself most directly in qual-

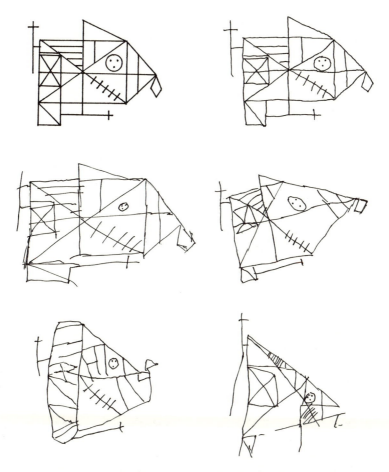

Figure 2.2. The range of cognitive-constructional ability in schizophrenia. Five copies of Osterrieth's (1944) figure (upper left) by schizophrenia patients range from very accurate to severely impaired copy attempts. This aspect of cognition is often impaired in the illness, but impairment seems to occur independently of positive symptoms.

itatively different kinds of cognitive symptoms: peculiar rather than impaired interpretations of the visual world, bizarre memories rather than absent memories, unwarranted inference rather than weakened inference. Researchers may be correct in hypothesizing that more basic cognitive abnormalities underlie symptoms. But they may be incorrect in the choice of ideas and tools used to search for these abnormalities. Focal brain damage as seen in classical neurology may be a poor model for a disorder like schizophrenia. Instead, researchers should cast theoretical ideas about the mental events underlying schizophrenic symptoms into new kinds of cognitive tasks, creating new kinds of tools. The findings and models of current cognitive science and neuroscience can then be used to describe and explain the processes that mediate psychotic mental life (see Cutting, 1985; David and Cutting, 1994, pp. 1–11). This rationale under-pins the cognitive neuropsychological approach to delusions, hallucinations, and thought disorder that has grown and gained ascendancy in recent years.

The Delusional World

Delusions—implausible, rigidly maintained, often fantastic beliefs—are prob-ably the most common, peculiar, and dramatic symptoms of schizophrenia (An-dreasen, 1991). Moreover, recall that if delusions are sufficiently "bizarre," they can, in isolation, satisfy the symptom criterion for schizophrenia in *DSM-IV* (1994). Thus delusions are of preeminent importance in the illness, and under-standing them in cognitive terms should be a priority for a science of symp-toms. What psychological processes might underlie delusions?

The Defective Filter

One of the oldest psychological explanations for delusional thinking involves the concept of a mental filter or screening device. This filter controls the entry of information, thoughts, memories, and perceptions into awareness. The con-trol function may be oriented toward the external environment of sights, sounds, and sensations or towards the inner world of personal feeling, thinking, and memory. Psychotic symptoms, including delusions, are the products of a defective filter.

In the psychoanalytic tradition (Fenichel, 1945), the defective filter takes the form of a weak ego that is no longer capable of distinguishing fantasies, wishes, and fears from reality. The ego of the schizophrenia patient has "regressed" to a childlike state and hence the ensuing symptoms resemble the self-absorption and "narcissistic daydreams" of early childhood. A child might well imagine possessing special powers or being victimized by sinister creatures hidden in closets or under beds. Thus delusions like beliefs in personal divinity are day-dreams, echoes of childhood, that the patient cannot filter out or discriminate from reality. Delusions of penetration or control by external forces are fearful fantasies with unrestricted access to consciousness; fantasies that root, in the Freudian view, in sexual wishes and impulses.

More recently, the internal filter concept has been reworked from the stand-point of cognitive neuropsychology. Frith (1979) argued that a great deal of in-formation processing never reaches consciousness. It is edited out because of in-appropriateness, irrelevance, implausibility, and inaccuracy. This selective editing is disrupted in schizophrenia. The patient becomes aware of multiple meanings of events, contradictory meanings, symbolic associations, and preliminary infer-ences that ordinarily remain suppressed.

Information from the external environment can also be subject to the vagaries of a defective awareness filter. Thus some versions of the filter concept stipulate defective or anomalous sensory experience rather than unedited reasoning as the cause of symptoms. The patient thinks normally but has an unusual experience, "hears" a "voice," feels strange physical sensations, sees more vividly, and develops a delusion as an attempt to explain the experience: "I must be special" or "these feelings are not my own" (see Maher, 1974). Reasoning is preserved, but sights, sounds, smells and touch are distorted, unselective, and inadequately screened.

Accordingly, filter defects may occur at several points in the flow of mental life. They may occur "early" during information processing, when sensory data like sights and sounds are first perceived, or they may occur "late," when sensory data are analyzed and interpreted. In addition, it is possible to conceive of a defective filter in terms of current information in the environment or in terms of old information stored in memory. Thus personal data may connect in a misleading way with unrelated facts in long-term memory and survive the filtering process that normally deletes such connections. More than one kind of filter, sensory or cognitive, current or past, and therefore more than one kind of defect may exist in the delusional mind.

If schizophrenia involves an aberrant perceptual filter, or abnormal sensory experience, patients should be prone to perceptual misjudgments, distortions, and inaccuracies. However, the issue is not decided easily. For example, a substantial body of research suggests that most patients perceive and process standard words and speech in a normal manner (Carpenter, 1976; Cohen, 1978; Done & Frith, 1984; Levin, Yurgelun-Todd, & Craft, 1989; Rochester, Harris, & Seeman, 1973). On the other hand, there is more recent evidence of sensory impairments and perceptual disorder that are consistent with the idea of a defective filter in schizophrenia (Butler and Braff, 1991; Perry, Geyer, & Braff, 1999). For example, many patients with the illness are inaccurate in making simple judgments of spatial orientations of line segments (Heinrichs & Zakzanis, 1998). Unfortunately, such evidence of perceptual deficit has not been found to exist selectively in delusional patients.

The sensory filter hypothesis also predicts that delusions are by-products of hallucinations and similar bizarre experiences. It is the experience of implausible sights, sounds, smells, and feelings—hallucinations—that prompts delusional explanations. The two symptoms should, therefore, occur together at very high frequencies. And to be sure, hallucinations and delusions are often grouped jointly as "positive" symptoms, and they do tend to emerge on the same cluster or factor in factor analytic studies of symptoms (e.g., Liddle, 1987; Liddle & Morris, 1991). Nevertheless, they can be dissociated in individual patients, giving rise to the diagnosis of "delusional disorder" without hallucinations in *DSM-IV* (1994). In addition, hallucinations and delusions often vary independently of each other over time. Addington and Addington (1991) found no significant association between delusions and hallucinations during an initial assessment, although this changed to a moderate correlation after 6 months (see also Hustig and Hafner, 1990). Accordingly, it seems that a person can experience a hallucination without constructing a delusion to explain it, and, conversely, delusional thinking can take place without reference to hallucinations.

Sensory and cognitive filter interpretations of delusions have been superseded to a large extent by metacognitive approaches. These approaches posit the existence of an executive, monitoring, or perspective-taking function that regulates cognition and behavior. The regulatory function can include paying attention to one kind of information over another. It may also include the control of intended actions. Instead of a leaky filter, unable to keep the chaos of the cognitive unconscious or of the outside world at bay, metacognitive views offer the concept of prejudicial or unsupervised decision making.

Metacognition and Delusions

The metacognitive approach is exemplified by the work of Frith (1987, 1992, 1994; Frith and Done, 1988). Two key concepts in his research are "action-monitoring" and "theory of mind." Frith argues that in normal mental life our intentions and actions are monitored and "tagged" so that we recognize them as self-generated. Hence most people experience what they think and do as familiar and personal. In schizophrenia, intentions are translated into action, but the source of the intention is lost. The mind stops monitoring itself. Thus a delusion like the belief that an external force is controlling thoughts is a direct consequence of a failure to recognize internal, self-generated intentions. The sense of familiarity, of authorship, is lost, because the mental monitor has broken down. At the same time, many patients are unable to represent or imagine the actions or intentions of other people. They lack a "theory of mind." Persecutory delusions may form because the paranoid patient cannot imagine someone else's perspective or psychological experience. Instead, idiosyncratic and ultimately sinister speculations are manufactured about the motives and intentions that govern the social world. In a sense, the person with paranoia suffers not from an overactive but from a deficient social imagination.

The idea of action-monitoring suggests that delusional patients should have performance difficulties when deprived of corrective feedback from the environment. If a person with delusions has to rely exclusively on mental representations of his or her own behavior to accomplish a task, he or she should fail. Frith and Done (1989) studied monitoring in schizophrenia by giving delusional patients a kind of video game wherein participants had to "shoot" targets on a display. In the first condition, all aspects of the task were observable, and everyone could use this information to improve performance. As long as this situation persisted there were no performance differences between delusional and nondelusional research participants. However, in the second condition the display was obscured for a period of time after a "shot" was made. In the absence of external information, participants were forced to rely more on internal sources of information to guide performance. During this time, the delusional patients made many more errors than the comparison groups. Error rates equalized again once the occlusion period was over and the shooting display could be observed. Thus, patients with delusions of alien control seem to have a selective difficulty monitoring their own performance. Perhaps the same difficulty exists with respect to monitoring their most private and personal thoughts, leading to the sudden emergence of ideas that seem unfamiliar and foreign, with no apparent authorship.

Frith and his associates (Corcoran, Cahill & Frith, 1997; Frith, 1992, 1994; Frith & Corcoran, 1996) also argue that different metacognitive processes underlie different kinds of delusions. Thus, for example, James, the man described in the first chapter, experienced a delusion of being controlled by a parasite. This might reflect a breakdown in representing and monitoring personal intentions. James lost track of the origins of his own thoughts. But his conviction that the hospital staff were scheming to have him castrated involves something else—a breakdown in representing or imagining the intentions and experience of *other* people. James lacks a "theory of mind" and is unable to "mentalize" and put himself in the place of another person. The result is delusions of persecution.

The theory of mind idea was tested in several experiments, one of which reported data specifically on patients with delusions of persecution, reference, or misidentification (Corcoran, Cahill, & Frith, 1997). Patients and control research participants were given cartoons to interpret, some of which required imagining another person's experience. For example, one cartoon showed a man apparently running in fright from a small crab that dangled from the pole of a fisherman, who in turn evinces surprise at the frightened man's behavior. Unbeknownst to the fisherman, however, a huge shark is rearing itself immediately behind the dock where the fisherman is standing and in full view of the terrified observer. When asked to interpret cartoons like this, patients with paranoid delusions found them hard to understand and explained them poorly in comparison with control subjects. In other words, they could not put themselves in the place of the cartoon figures and imagine the contrasting perspectives that each figure had on the depicted action. Researchers argue that this inability to infer the mental states of other people is the cognitive basis of paranoid delusions.

In addition to defective action-monitoring and impairments in "mentalizing," there is evidence that decision-making is abnormal in patients with persecutory delusions. Some findings suggest that patients with delusions form an abnormally small number of correct hypotheses when faced with a problem-solving situation (Young & Bentall, 1995). Other work suggests the existence of a bias that favors premature judgments about events—judgments based on very little information. For example, Garety, Hemsley, and Wessely (1991; see also Garety & Hemsley, 1994) gave delusional patients a task that required assigning probabilities to events. The "events" in question were beads drawn from jars containing one of two colors. Patients were allowed to make numerous draws to arrive at a decision about the probability of the next bead's color. This provided the opportunity to index how much information delusional patients need in order to make a probability decision. Results showed that they request less information than the amount requested by normal control subjects. Yet in another condition the patients were also more likely than the healthy people to change their predictions after a single disconfirming event. Thus delusional patients seem to have a decision-making bias that leads them to "jump to conclusions" on the basis of minimal information. This bias occurs in terms of both adopting and rejecting beliefs about events (see also Huq, Garety, & Hemsley, 1988). Moreover, premature decision-making seems to occur with meaningful material as well with neutral material like colored beads. Thus Dudley, John, Young, and Over (1997) and Young and Bentall (1997) found that delusional patients were premature in their decisions when personality characteristics rather than colored beads were the stimulus materials.

Perhaps delusions arise because the person with schizophrenia is both impulsive in decision-making and insensitive to the influence of past experience when interpreting new events (Gray, 1998; Gray, Feldon, Rawlins, Hemsley, & Smith, 1991; Hemsley, 1994). Thus a coincidence, like a patient's age matching the estimated age of Christ at crucifixion, may be impulsively misinterpreted as a causal relationship. The influence of past experience that normally helps to determine the plausibility of current experience is attenuated, giving rise to premature and unwarranted inferences—delusions. On the other hand, the research by Garety et al. (1991) implies that beliefs are also changed readily in the illness, an implication that does not jibe with the rigid conviction, the persistence, of many delusions.

Further evidence for biased information processing in delusional patients comes from the work of Bentall and his associates (Bentall, 1994; Kaney & Bentall, 1992; Kaney, Wolfenden, Dewey, & Bentall, 1992; Kinderman, 1994; Kinderman & Bentall, 1996). These researchers argue that the person with persecutory delusions is particularly sensitive to negative or threatening information about himself or herself and the world and tends to externalize the causes of negative events. Moreover, in the delusional mind, memory is biased in such a manner that negative or threatening material is remembered better than neutral material. Thus, threat-related words are often repeated during memory recall (Bentall, Kaney, & Bowen-Jones, 1995; Kaney et al., 1992). Similarly, patients with delusions are abnormally prone to believe that negative events happened to them in the past and will happen again in the future (Kaney, Bowen-Jones, Dewey, & Bentall, 1997). Recent work (Kinderman & Bentall, 1997) has shown that delusional subjects are especially likely to blame negative events on other people. The delusional mind seems both drawn and repelled by negative events and information. Negative material is more accessible to awareness and more salient than positive material yet also more likely to be attributed to external sources or to other people. Kaney and Bentall (1992) argue that this "self-serving" bias is partly a defense against poor self-esteem, a personality trait that may be an inherent feature of patients with persecutory delusions.

Evaluation and Synthesis of Evidence in Studies of Delusions

What about the strength or consistency of the recent research on ideas like action-monitoring and theory of mind? Recall from chapter 1 that Cohen's d is obtained by dividing the difference between two group averages, obtained from, say, schizophrenia patients and healthy participants, by the pooled standard deviation of the groups. As d increases from 0 to .5 to 1.0, and so on, the degree of group separation also increases, with corresponding decreases in distribution overlap from 100% to 67% to 45%, respectively. By the time a d of 3.0 is achieved, only about 7% overlap between schizophrenia and healthy distributions remains—an extremely powerful finding. Now consider the application of this metric of evidence to the study of delusions.

To assess how well the recent research on the psychology of delusions fares in terms of its evidential strength, I looked for studies that provided useable statistics and patient–healthy control comparisons. Unfortunately, there are few suitable studies on topics like action-monitoring and theory of mind. The study by Corcoran, Cahill, and Frith (1997) is especially valuable in this regard. Expressed as an effect size, the difference in "mentalizing" ability between schizophrenia patients and healthy people corresponds to a d of 1.2. Perhaps 62% of the patients and control participants are completely distinguishable from each other on the basis of this ability. In many research contexts such an effect would be considered "large" (Cohen, 1988). With a d of this size, not *every* delusional patient in the study differs from *every* healthy person in terms of theory of mind skills. But the finding is substantial, certainly encouraging. It is unfortunate that no published studies have reproduced it.

In contrast, there are enough usable studies on topics like premature decision-making and biased cognition to compile the individual study results into an average effect that represents each research literature. Table 2.1 shows these average ds, along with associated margins of error and the number of contributing studies. The six studies of premature decision-making in patients with persecu-

Table 2.1 Abnormal cognition and the positive symptoms of schizophrenia

Cognitive Process	Mean d	Confidence Interval	N
Studies of persecutory delusions			
Premature decision-making	.88	.74–1.02	6
Negative cognitive bias	1.24	1.10–1.38	9
Studies of auditory hallucinations			
Externalizing attributions	1.40	.99–1.81	3
Inaccurate speech tracking and monitoring	.91	.57–1.25	4
Studies of thought disorder			
Defective monitoring	1.64	.20–3.08	2
Semantic hyperpriming	.75	−.79–2.29	6
Impaired theory of mind	1.60	1.38–1.82	2

Note: The table shows effect sizes (Cohen's *d*) in absolute values, corrected for sample size and averaged over studies in a research domain. All *d*s are based on differences between schizophrenia patients and healthy participants. N = number of contributing studies; Confidence Interval = 95% confidence interval for the mean *d*. The true population mean value is likely to fall in the indicated range. Confidence intervals that include zero reflect highly unstable findings.

tory delusions yield an average effect size of d = .88 and a margin of error of .14 on either side of this average. Using Cohen's (1988) estimates, this effect size yields an overlap of about 50% between patients and control participants. Hence roughly half of delusional patients and healthy people can be distinguished from each other in terms of the amount of information they require before making a decision. Conversely, about half of the delusional patients probably respond normally to decision tasks.

The average effect for the nine studies of biased cognition in table 2.1 is substantially larger at d = 1.24, with a margin of error of .14. This is a fairly powerful effect, with perhaps two-thirds of the patients and control subjects completely distinguished in terms of their cognitive biases. Moreover, as implied by the modest margin of error, the effect sizes are relatively consistent across studies.

Hence, although not all patients with persecutory delusions show impulsive decision-making or a self-serving bias, at least half probably do, and there are sufficient replications and partial replications in the published literature to justify considerable confidence in the results. The main weakness of these bodies of evidence is the small number of research subjects used in the studies. This applies especially to the decision-making studies, which are based on a total of only 156 patients and control participants.

In summary, recent work on the psychology of delusions holds that this common symptom of schizophrenia arises when the mind makes judgments too quickly on the basis of too little evidence. Delusions also arise when interpretations of experience are biased so that negative events are more available to awareness than positive events and more attributable to external than to personal causes. In addition, there are promising ideas, like Frith's (1992) concepts of action-monitoring and theory of mind, that require more empirical attention. These cognitive inclinations—to lose track of intentions, to judge prematurely, to seek and then disown the negative in life—these are the mental building blocks of delusions.

Yet, on a more critical note, current ideas about the cognitive basis of symptoms like paranoia and alien control do not penetrate very deeply into the delusional mind. Inevitably, notions like self-serving bias or premature decision-making, beg the chicken-or-egg question of ultimate causation: What in turn governs the cognitive processes that underlie these abnormalities? Why do patients have cognitive biases in the first place, and are such biases producers or products of delusions? Furthermore, to what extent does the research on delusional cognition offer new insight? Perhaps research concepts like "sensitivity to negative events" and "externalizing tendencies" simply recast paranoid delusions into the language of social cognition without adding much that is new. Nonetheless, researchers have stripped some of the mystery from delusions and related them to testable cognitive theory. If the strange mental landscape of the delusional mind has not been mapped, it has, perhaps, been partially explored and described, with encouraging prospects for further more sustained study (see Garety & Freeman, 1999).

Counterfeit Experience

In many ways the psychological study of hallucinations has developed in parallel with the study of delusions. Early views held that psychic energy flowed into the sensory system during states of ego relaxation, like sleep, or during states of ego weakness, like psychosis, to produce spurious sights and sounds—dreams and hallucinations (Freud, 1900; Fenichel, 1945). More recently, theorists influenced by cognitive psychology have maintained that "hearing voices" really means that patients are hearing their own internal thought processes and attributing them incorrectly to external sources (e.g., Collicut & Hemsley, 1981). Such faulty attributions are ordinarily edited out of the cognitive system, but in schizophrenia the editing or filtering function fails, and the errors enter awareness.

As a case in point, there is evidence of "silent" activity in the speech musculature of patients who experience auditory hallucinations (Green & Kinsbourne, 1990). Perhaps this physiological activity corresponds to internal speech, and patients fail to recognize it as their own. Such patients may experience their speech as a kind of alien "voice"—an auditory hallucination (see David, 1994, pp. 293–295). However, it is unclear whether silent "speech" is really abnormal because the available data are based on small numbers of patients with no healthy people for comparison. Moreover, covert speech activity does not explain hallucinations in visual, tactile, or olfactory modalities. For example,

Ruth, the female patient in the introductory chapter, had intense hallucinations that she could feel and smell a leech or sluglike creature hanging around her neck. She never reported hearing voices. On the other hand, perhaps covert physiological events analogous to speech activity take place in olfactory and other sensory modalities. In any case, the concept that hallucinations are the result of a misattribution of the patient's own sensory experience is central to contemporary psychological research on hallucinations (Bentall, 1990).

Hallucinations and Source Monitoring

There is evidence that hallucinating patients are poor at recognizing their own thoughts. For example, Heilbrun (1980) studied the ability of hallucinating and nonhallucinating patients to identify their own responses to questions after a delay of 1 week. The two patient groups did not differ in general recall or cognitive abilities. However, the hallucinating patients recognized fewer of their own statements. In a similar vein, Bentall, Baker, and Havers (1991), Morrison and Haddock (1997), and Baker and Morrison (1998) presented research participants with a situation wherein answers to a cognitive task were either generated by the participants or generated by the experimenter. Participants later had to indicate the source of the answers. Hallucinating schizophrenia patients made many faulty attributions whereby their own answers were assigned to an external source. This occurred most often when they had to make source attributions about answers that had a low probability of being true (Bentall et al., 1991) or when self-generated thoughts had emotional content (Morrison & Haddock, 1997). Thus a failure to discriminate internal and external sources of information may be one psychological mechanism underlying the formation of hallucinations.

Vivid Sensory Experience, Suggestibility, and Hallucinations

An alternative or complement to defective source monitoring is the idea that unusually vivid, or inaccurate, sensory and imagery processes exist in hallucinating patients. Schizophrenia changes and distorts the way a person sees, hears, feels, and smells the world. Heilbrun, Blum, and Haas (1983) showed that hallucinating patients make more errors than nonhallucinating patients in locating sounds in the environment. However, David and Cutting (1993) reported more rapid picture identification in hallucinating patients than in healthy controls. Overall, the idea that altered sensory and perceptual experience underpins hallucinations has not received consistent empirical support (but see Havermans et al., 1999; Starker & Jolin, 1982).

The corollary notion that hallucination-prone people are somehow more suggestible, or willing to believe that an event is real on the basis of minimal information, has also received partial support. For example, Bentall and Slade (1985) played recorded tapes of random ("white") noise for hallucinating and nonhallucinating patients. In some tape segments the researchers introduced a voice speaking the word "who." Patients were required to identify segments where the word was spoken. Both groups were equally able to detect the actual word. However, hallucinating patients were more likely to believe that a word had been spoken when the tape comprised only noise. The researchers argued that hallucinating patients are more willing to believe that a stimulus is present in ambiguous situations. Similarly, Young, Bentall, Slade, and Dewey (1987) had hallucinating and nonhallucinating patients listen to white noise and also listen to suggestions that the noise was a song. However, a song was never actually played. Three of the ten hallucinating patients claimed to have heard the song. Haddock, Wolfenden, Lowens, Tarrier, and Bentall (1995) also obtained a small suggestibility effect when hallucinating patients were compared with healthy participants instead of with other patients. The researchers examined the influence of suggestion instructions on misperceiving a repeated word as a new or different word and obtained a very small effect size ($d = .18$). Such results imply at most a mild tendency toward suggestibility in hallucinating patients.

Auditory Hallucinations and Language Processing

Hoffman (1999; Hoffman & Rapaport, 1994) has challenged the view that hallucinations are primarily a product of pathological suggestibility. Instead, defective language processing is held to be responsible for auditory hallucinations like hearing voices speaking or commenting on behavior. This alternate view is based in part on the reported correlation between hallucinations and language-related variables like subtle speech muscle activity or defective language production (Green & Kinsbourne, 1990; Hoffman, 1986). There are also associations between active hallucinatory experience and concurrent regional brain activity in language zones of the cerebral cortex (e.g. Cleghorn et al., 1990). Hence, hearing voices that do not really exist may reflect a malfunction of the mind's ability to generate language in a normal way.

In Hoffman and Rapaport's 1994 study, the suggestibility hypothesis developed by Bentall (1990) was contrasted with the idea that auditory hallucinations are products of defective language processing. Three groups of people—healthy controls, hallucinating patients, and nonhallucinating patients—were compared on a task that required listening to a recording of someone reading a passage from a book. The task was made complex and ambiguous by a superimposed second voice reading unrelated material. This superimposition was done in varying degrees to yield three conditions of increasing psycholinguistic "babble." Participants had to "shadow" or repeat what they heard from the passages.

The authors recorded each person's accuracy in repeating the target passages and also the number of "implausible" responses—incorrect and unlikely attempts at repeating the material. It was argued that accuracy indexed language discrimination and processing skills. In contrast, guessing indexed suggestibility and inclination to fabricate in the presence of noise-contaminated information.

The experimental results revealed that accuracy declined for all subject groups as the "babble" conditions increased in intensity—not a surprising finding. However, the hallucinating patients were substantially ($d = 1.18$) less accurate in repeating the passages than both healthy participants and nonhallucinating patients. At the same time, guessing responses also increased over levels of "babble," but there were no differences between healthy and patient groups. Hence there is nothing to suggest that hallucinating patients generate specious responses to ambiguous information. They simply process language inaccurately. The authors interpreted their results as support for a psycholinguistic defect as the root of auditory hallucinations.

One of the problems in both the suggestibility and psycholinguistic approaches is the use of small patient samples. Another problem is the inclusion of nonschizophrenic psychiatric patients in the hallucination groups. Including patients with schizoaffective disorder and mania in samples of hallucinating schizophrenia patients is defended on the grounds that symptoms (i.e., hallucinations) rather than diagnoses (i.e., schizophrenia) are under study. Nonetheless, different disorders may cause similar symptoms for different reasons.

A further potential interpretive problem is that other cognitive processes may mediate symptoms and therefore research results. For example, an attention-based explanation might account for results like those obtained by Hoffman and Rappaport (1994). Perhaps hallucination-prone patients just find it harder to attend and concentrate on any kind of effortful auditory task, language-based or not. Perhaps they are even distracted by their own auditory hallucinations during the listening exercise. It is noteworthy in this regard that distractibility is one of the few cognitive correlates of positive symptoms (Green & Walker, 1986a). However, Hoffman's group recently replicated their finding of impaired speech perception in hallucinating patients with a larger sample. They also showed that hallucinating patients are not more distractible than other patients, just more impaired at language processing (Hoffman, Rapaport, Mazure, & Quinlan, 1999). This provides important support for the link between speech perception and auditory hallucinations. Still, verification by other researchers is required for a really convincing demonstration of this link and for evidence that attention is not involved. Thus, on the one hand, Haddock, Slade, Prasaad, and Bentall (1996) found that distraction had no effect and hallucinating patients were just generally more error prone than healthy participants in their immediate recall of words. On the other hand, Ishigaki and Tanno (1999) have cast doubt on the assertion that patients with and without hallucinations perform identically on attention tasks.

Studies by Leudar, Thomas, and Johnston (1992,1994) combine some of the above ideas and emphasize defective *monitoring* of speech activity as a basis for auditory hallucinations. It may not be the case that schizophrenia involves abnormal language processing or attention per se. Instead, the illness impairs the ability to detect and self-correct linguistic errors—errors that occur to some degree in healthy people as well. But how separable are monitoring, language perception, and attention? The nature of these processes and hallucinatory experience in schizophrenia needs to be clarified.

Evaluation and Synthesis of Research on Hallucinations

The source-monitoring, suggestibility, and psycholinguistic approaches have produced a small number of findings with respect to auditory hallucinatory experience. These findings suggest that hallucinating patients respond abnormally to conditions of informational uncertainty and may be unable to detect or correct their abnormal responses. This distinguishes them not only from mentally healthy subjects but also from other psychiatric patients, including many with schizophrenia who do not experience hallucinations. Unfortunately, some studies use nonhallucinating psychiatric patients instead of healthy participants as controls, and some report findings as nonparametric statistics that are not amenable to effect size conversions. Nonetheless, to provide at least a rough index of evidential strength in this area, I collected the studies that used both schizophrenia patients and healthy control subjects; their averaged effect sizes are shown in table 2.1.

Three studies provide fairly strong support for the idea that auditory hallucinations spring from a tendency to attribute information to external sources (average effect $d = 1.40$). An effect like this implies that roughly two-thirds of the hallucinating patients and control participants are distinguishable in terms of their source attributions. The results for the linguistic-processing account of hallucinations are also encouraging (average $d = .91$) and imply that at least half of symptomatic patients are distinguishable from control participants in how they monitor and process language. However, findings for suggestibility in relation to hallucinations are scarce, with only one patient–healthy control comparison (Haddock et al., 1995; $d = .18$), underscoring the need for additional work in this area.

Still, these cognitive studies of hallucinating patients imply the bare outlines of an explanation for Ruth's experience of smelling and feeling a creature hanging around her neck. First, she is incorrectly attributing her normal sensations to an external source. It is her own body that she is feeling and smelling.

However, the disease process has impaired her ability to discriminate bodily sensations from external sensory data. Hence she comes to believe that an external source is responsible for her unpleasant physical sensations. She fabricates a theory in the form of a "creature."

But such an account of hallucinations leaves many unanswered questions. Perhaps the nature of the schizophrenic disease process differs in important ways from processes elicited in psychological experiments. Do patients, on their own, habitually externalize the sources of experience? Are they fundamentally confused—poor discriminators of such sources? And if so, does poor discrimination lead inexorably to the experience of "creatures," "voices," or other "forces?" Similarly, if patients hallucinate in response to ambiguity or complex language processing, how does this occur when the ambiguity or language task is not imposed on the patient by a researcher? Does schizophrenia create a kind of unremitting world of "white noise" or linguistic "babble?" Or perhaps everyday experience is already replete with informational uncertainty and noise, even for mentally healthy people. The person with schizophrenia simply responds to this ambient uncertainty with extreme and inaccurate attributions.

In view of the importance of both delusions and hallucinations in schizophrenia and in the diagnostic criteria of *DSM-IV* (1994), it is surprising that only delusions have generated systematic psychological research. Most hypotheses in the study of hallucinations are backed by one or two experiments with few replications. Consider, then, a third positive symptom, thought disorder, and how it has been studied by cognitive science.

Crazy Thoughts

Thought disorder—incoherent, illogical thinking manifested in speech or writing —is usually regarded as the third major kind of "positive" symptom. The patient engages in "crazy talk" and does not make sense. Thought disorder is less prevalent in schizophrenia than either hallucinations or delusions (Jablensky et al., 1992; Landmark, Merskey, Cernovsky, & Helmes, 1990; World Health Organization [WHO], 1973). However, it frequently emerges on a separate factor in multivariate studies of symptoms (Arndt, Alliger, & Andreasen, 1991; Liddle & Morris, 1991). Moreover, unlike delusions and hallucinations, thought disorder has some objective qualities that can be measured in patients' speech. Several clinical rating scales and experimental paradigms exist that evaluate the severity and nature of thought disorder (e.g., Scale for the Assessment of Positive Symptoms [SAPS]; Andreasen, 1984; Positive and Negative Syndrome Scale [PANSS]; Kay, Fiszbein, & Opler, 1987). The experimental studies show that thought-disordered patients have unusual speech patterns. For example, ambiguous grammar and word usages abound in speech samples obtained from "open topic" interviews with thought-disordered patients (Harvey, 1983; Docherty, Schnur, & Harvey, 1988; Docherty, Evans, Sledge, Seibyl, & Krystal, 1994).

Only one of the three patients described in chapter 1 showed evidence of thought disorder: William, the man with grandiose delusions of power and divinity. However, his speech was never recorded verbatim for analysis. Therefore, consider instead Harrow, Lanin-Kettering, and Miller's (1989) example of disordered speech in a patient who was asked to explain the proverb "Don't swap horses when crossing a stream." The patient responded: "That's wish-bell. Double vision. It's like walking across a person's eye and reflecting personality. It works on you, like dying and going to the spiritual world, but landing in the Vella world" (Harrow et al., 1989, p. 609). Here is what is known about this symptom.

Defective Cognition in Thought Disorder

Several cognitive processes have been studied in relation to thought disorder, including the "theory of mind" notion developed by Frith (1992) to explain paranoid delusions. For example, Sarfati and associates (Sarfati & Hardy-Bayle, 1999; Sarfati, Hardy-Bayle, Brunet, & Widlocher, 1999) elicited interpretations of comic strips and found that most patients with thought disorder are inaccurate in the way they attribute intentions to other people. Schizophrenia patients with thought disorder, like those with persecutory delusions, may lack a theory of mind.

In addition, aspects of attention, short-term memory span, and vulnerability to distraction seem to be abnormal in patients with thought disorder (Serper, 1993; Pandurangi, Sax, Pelonero, & Goldberg, 1994). Harvey and associates (e.g., Harvey, Earle-Boyer, & Levinson, 1986; Harvey, Earle-Boyer, Wielgus, & Levinson, 1986) have shown repeatedly that the number of digits that a patient can recall from a series, with or without the presence of distracting stimuli, is related to thought disorder. Presumably, vulnerability to distraction breaks down the coherence and logical flow of normal speech and thought. However, some studies (e.g., Harvey, Earle-Boyer, & Levinson, 1988) have found that digit span without concomitant distraction still correlates with thought disorder and there is evidence that schizophrenia brings with it a reduced ability to recall the first few items on any list of verbal items (Manschreck, Maher, Rosenthal, & Berner, 1991). Unfortunately, none of the early digit span studies compare thought-disordered patients with healthy people directly. Instead, they rely on correlation between digit span and the severity of thought disorder within the schizophrenia sample. Hence it is not possible to say whether digit span is abnormal *and* related to thought disorder in the illness. However, more recent studies sometimes report results from healthy people and thought-disordered patients using tasks that are similar to digit span (e.g., letter–number span; Goldberg et al., 1998). Accordingly, there is suggestive research that effective memory span, the number of information "chunks" that can be held in awareness, may be a key function that contributes to the severity of thought and speech disorder. But whether the span itself is abnormal and tied specifically to thought disorder in schizophrenia is harder to judge from this literature.

Harvey and associates have also shown that schizophrenia patients with thought disorder have difficulty discriminating between different aspects of their own thoughts and speech. The "reality" monitoring task used by Harvey (1985) to study this idea involves presenting thought-disordered and control participants with words that they either speak aloud or simply read silently (see also Johnson & Raye, 1981). Participants are later given all of the words again in a list and asked to indicate those that were actually spoken out loud and those that were only read and thought about. It turns out that thought-disordered patients with schizophrenia make many errors on this task.

Both digit span distractibility and reality monitoring are powerful predictors of the way thought disorder manifests itself in speech. Thus Harvey and Serper (1990) demonstrated the ability of digit span and reality monitoring to predict speech disorder detected in actual speech samples. Digit span emerged as the more powerful predictor. Taken together, these cognitive tasks account for about 73% of the variance in thought and speech disorder severity in schizophrenia samples. However, the bulk of these studies do not compare directly patient and healthy control group performance.

A recent exception to the lack of patient–control comparisons is Kuperberg, McGuire, and David's (1998) extension of the monitoring concept to include "on-line" monitoring of language. In this paradigm, participants are given target words to detect, some of which are embedded in linguistically abnormal contexts. For example, the target word "car" might be presented in a sentence that says: "He ate the *car* quickly." Most people are distracted by violations in sentence context and respond more slowly to the target word as a result. The intriguing and powerful finding ($d = 2.67$) is that thought-disordered schizophrenia patients seem less effected by the presence of abnormal context. That is, the patients respond relatively more quickly than control subjects to the target words when anomalous context is present. It is as if thought disorder creates a kind of insensitivity to normal speech. Perhaps thought-disordered patients are poor monitors of language, as well as being poor monitors of "reality," an idea that echoes the work of Hoffman and Rapaport (1994) and Leudar et al. (1994) on speech tracking and hallucinations.

The relation of thought disorder severity to tasks like digit span distractibility again raises the possibility that a dysfunction of attention underpins some symptoms of schizophrenia. It is even possible that disturbances in reality monitoring and language perception are themselves consequences of basic defects in how attention is allocated to different sources of information. Evidence in this vein comes from a study of selective attention by Wielgus and Harvey (1988). Two auditory messages were presented on headphones in a dichotic-listening paradigm. Schizophrenia patients were asked to attend to, or "shadow," one message and to ignore the other message. Shadowing performance, in terms of errors in repeating the target message, was related to the severity of thought disorder. The authors argued that thought disorder must involve a breakdown in the ability to attend selectively to ongoing streams of information (see also Pandurangi et al., 1994). Perhaps this breakdown in selective attention is broad in scope and includes inattention to the patient's own behavior and internal processes. Seen in this light, the various forms of cognitive monitoring studied in relation to positive symptoms all comprise a kind of selective attention. The normal mind tracks and discriminates information sources continuously to ensure the integrity and coherence of language, thought, and behavior. When this tracking ceases, the symptoms of schizophrenia develop.

Semantic Hyperpriming: A Mental Mechanism of Thought Disorder?

The study of attention-related processes in thought disorder has been supplemented with interest in the topic of semantic priming (Kwapil, Hegley, Chapman, & Chapman 1990; Manschrek et al., 1988; Spitzer et al., 1994). The basic paradigm involves a word recognition or lexical decision task. In lexical decision tasks a person has to decide if an array of letters is a word (e.g., gge versus egg). The speed with which real words are detected can be increased by preceding or "priming" the letter array with a word that has a meaningful or semantic relationship to the target word (e.g., hen-egg). This facilitative effect exists in the normal mind but it is abnormally enhanced in some thought-disordered patients (e.g., Manschrek et al., 1988; Spitzer, Braun, Hermle, & Maier, 1993). Moreover, priming seems to exist within normal bounds in many patients who are not thought disordered (Ober, Vinogradov, & Shenaut, 1995; Vinogradov, Ober, & Shenaut, 1992; but see Henik, Nissimov, Priel, & Umansky, 1995). Some evidence even suggests that seemingly unrelated words can prime targets indirectly through association with a third word (e.g., lion-(tiger)-stripes; see Spitzer et al., 1993). This indirect priming is also enhanced in some thought-disordered patients.

In contrast, phonological, or acoustic, priming tends to inhibit word recognition. That is, priming a letter array with a word that sounds like a target word (e.g. beg-egg) actually slows down the recognition process in healthy people. Phonological similarity inhibits and semantic similarity facilitates word detection in healthy people. However, thought-disordered schizophrenia patients may show less phonological inhibition than healthy people do and less than non-thought-disordered patients (Spitzer et al., 1994).

Hence the incoherent, disjointed, nonsensical quality of schizophrenic language and thought may derive in part from this "hyperpriming." The schizophrenic mind is distinguished by excessive semantic activation of interrelated or indirectly related words that have no strong collective relation to an overriding thought or concept like a sentence or narrative theme. At the same time, phonetic similarities, or "clang" associations, intrude into language because of a failure of phonological inhibition. The concepts of abnormally enhanced semantic priming and uninhibited phonetic associations provide a way of understanding some of the cognitive causes of thought disorder.

Evaluation and Synthesis of Thought Disorder Research

Overall, thought disorder has received more sustained empirical attention than hallucinations from cognitive researchers. However, the number of studies using healthy control group comparisons is still relatively small, and most of these focus on the phenomenon of priming. Table 2.1 summarizes the available studies that used thought-disordered schizophrenia patients and healthy control subjects. The table of average effect sizes shows that only the semantic hyperpriming phenomenon has managed to inspire several replication or partial replication attempts, although the few monitoring and theory of mind findings are impressive in the size of their effects. Taken together, the average semantic hyperpriming effect is a moderate one at $d = .75$. This effect size implies that very roughly half of patients and healthy people are completely distinguishable on the basis of their priming responses. However, the dispersion and confidence interval statistics tell a rather different story. On the one hand there is the study of priming by Spitzer et al. (1993) that produced effects large enough ($d = 4.86$) to separate 98% of the patient and control subjects under study. On the other hand, two recent replication attempts by independent research groups (Besche et al., 1997, $d = -.37$; Aloia et al., 1998, $d = -1.76$) found that thought-disordered patients showed *less* priming than healthy subjects (hypopriming). The heterogeneity of effects is reflected in the confidence interval for the average priming effect, which suggests a margin of error that runs between $d = -.79$ and $d = 2.29$. Hence hyperpriming is something that all thought-disordered patients show in one study and something that much smaller proportions show in other studies. Indeed, it may be reversed in some samples, in light of recent work. The idea of abnormally enhanced connections between words is appealing in relation to thought disorder, and Spitzer and associates (Spitzer, 1997; Weisbrod, Maier, Harig, Himmelsbach, & Spitzer, 1998) continue to support the idea. But consistent replication by independent researchers is needed before the value of hyperpriming can be endorsed.

In summary, thought disorder may be the most objective and understandable of the positive symptoms. Several processes have been implicated as powerful predictors of thought and speech disorder in schizophrenia. The most promising include digit span distractibility, reality monitoring, and abnormal semantic priming. The extent to which these processes are interrelated is not known, but some studies suggest connections between distractibility and reality monitoring.

In addition, the causal sequence of cognitive abnormalities and symptoms is always hard to demonstrate. Is thought disorder a consequence or a cause of distractibility? Moreover, there is a lack of studies comparing thought-disordered patients with healthy people. Nonetheless, this symptom comes closest to being a psychopathological sign, and considerable progress has been made in casting light on its psychological basis.

General Summary and Conclusions

I have concentrated on understanding positive symptoms in this chapter. Negative symptoms are just as important, especially from the standpoint of the patients themselves and their adjustment to the illness. Still, the positive symptoms are more striking, more puzzling, and harder to explain. They are the most anomalous features of schizophrenia, whereas negative symptoms, like withdrawal, disinterest, and apathy, may, in part, represent a person's attempt to cope with the illness that rages inside (see Carpenter, Heinrichs, & Wagman, 1988). The madness of schizophrenia seems closer to the positive symptoms. Indeed the delusions, hallucinations, and disordered thought of the "precocious dementia" that Kraepelin (1896, 1919) described a century ago are among the most mysterious and bizarre forms of human psychological experience. Many of these symptoms do not relate in an obvious or convincing way to traditional ideas of cognitive deficit and brain damage. Standard clinical tests reveal deficits in some patients, but these deficits seem to have lives of their own and occur independently of positive symptoms like delusions and hallucinations. Paradoxically, symptoms are themselves cognitive events, yet they are hard to capture with conventional cognitive measurements.

Fortunately, a few researchers have shed light on the mental processes that mediate positive symptoms. The range of processes includes several forms of altered cognitive monitoring, the mind failing to supervise itself, plus a possible breakdown in attention. In addition, abnormally enhanced sensitivity to word meanings and relationships and a kind of impulsive tendency to construct meanings or make decisions too quickly appear to be involved in positive symptoms. Finally, some symptoms probably arise in conjunction with a bias in understanding the social world, a bias that places a negative value on the actions and motives of other people.

In the case of delusions, the evidence is sufficiently strong to suggest that specific mental features associate with pathologically implausible beliefs. The strength of the evidence is reflected in the effect sizes and in schizophrenia–control distribution overlap figures. Roughly half of the delusional patients are completely distinguished from healthy people on the basis of their premature or impulsive decision-making. This discrimination increases to about two-thirds if negatively biased social cognition is used as the basis for comparison. The evidence with respect to biased cognition in particular is impressively consistent, with few anomalous large or small effect sizes. Therefore, it would be fair to say that the strongest and most consistent evidence in the cognitive literature on positive symptoms is found in relation to delusions. Moreover, there are several additional ideas that may bear fruit in the future if they receive more research attention. These ideas include Frith's (1992) concepts of action-monitoring and theory of mind, which are represented by too few normal control group–patient comparisons to allow for evaluation.

Yet the average effect sizes also imply that many delusional patients are indistinguishable from healthy people on measures of bias and decision-making. But is it reasonable to expect effect sizes that are large enough to separate groups completely in this literature? Probably not. It is likely that considerable "noise" and error exist whenever symptoms are studied. Symptomatic patients do not make the most attentive and engaged research subjects for cognitive experiments. It is also hard to recruit drug-free patients who have active symptoms. Those receiving medication who still retain their symptoms may be unusual and unrepresentative of the patient population. Then there is the inherent difficulty of trying to measure or infer the mental events that precede or cause positive symptoms. All in all, the magnitude of evidence in the study of delusions is encouraging and surprisingly consistent, given the challenges of this field.

The same cannot be said for the study of hallucinations. The number of patient–healthy control comparisons is very small. Here too there are promising ideas, like the concept of source monitoring that derives from Heilbrun's (1980) work and the notion that defective monitoring of language is tied to auditory hallucinations (see Hoffman & Rapaport, 1994). The hypothesis that hallucinations are linked with reduced perceptual thresholds or "suggestibility" (Bentall & Slade, 1985) deserves more attention, although recent work is not encouraging (Haddock et al., 1995). The concept of defective source monitoring may be the most powerful finding in the literature in this area. Hallucinations might be traceable to a basic loss in discrimination skills, skills that ordinarily let the mind sort experience on the basis of its personal or extrapersonal origins. Or it may be that discrimination skills remain, but the mind no longer integrates the contexts of experience into the flow of everyday psychological life. These questions of monitoring, context perception, and the personal and impersonal are encountered everywhere in the study of schizophrenic symptoms. But which processes apply specifically to hallucinations? There are many more questions than answers in the literature on this puzzling symptom.

Heterogeneity raises its head in the case of thought disorder, which is a symptom with objective correlates in terms of speech abnormalities. However, this heterogeneity seems to derive partly from a handful of studies on the topic of semantic hyperpriming. In view of recent work in this area, it is possible that methodological differences between studies, rather than fundamental differences between schizophrenia patients, are responsible for the heterogeneity (see Henik et al., 1995). There is also an extensive and suggestive literature, based on Harvey's (1985) measures of attention and "reality" monitoring, that should be applied to schizophrenia–healthy control group comparisons. It may be that this most objective of positive symptoms is also the most understandable symptom in the long run.

But in some ways researchers have barely illuminated the question of how a man like William becomes convinced of his own divinity; how a woman like Ruth smells her own body but thinks the smell comes from an animal; or why James feels controlled by a parasite. Concepts such as impulsive, biased thinking and unmonitored experience may partly explain positive symptoms. Yet these concepts hint at deeper unknowns and furnish only glimpses of what lies behind or beneath the psychological life of symptoms.

Accordingly, a nagging worry remains about basing the diagnosis and therefore study of an illness so disproportionately on the subjective world of symptoms. To assuage this worry, researchers have attempted to find illness traits that approximate more closely the concept of a sign, an objective symptom. They have even sought psychological and biological traits that might exist prior to the onset of symptoms: objective features of a person that identify the presence, latent or manifest, of schizophrenic illness. The story of these attempts comprises the next chapter.

3
· ·

THE MARK OF
MADNESS

It is hard to define an illness that escapes persistently into the private, shadowed world of symptoms. It is hard to have confidence in diagnoses that rely heavily on one person's judgments about another person's inner world. How can we know with scientific precision what another person feels and thinks? How can anyone be certain that mental life has evolved into madness? Yet researchers and clinicians face the daunting task of identifying who has schizophrenia. Therefore the distinction is made between symptoms and *markers*.

A symptom is a disturbance of mind or body that is linked in some way with disease and abnormal biology. But an illness defined by symptoms is inevitably an illness defined by uncertainty and guesswork. In contrast, markers are objective biological signposts of illness. A marker forms an explicit and relentless parallel to underlying pathology and disease, even if the disease is eventual and hidden rather than immediate and apparent. It is hoped that markers exist for schizophrenia and that they will allow the illness to be detected with accuracy and tracked to its source.

The concept of a disease marker has been imported into schizophrenia research from neurology and genetics. Microscopic abnormalities called neurofibrillary tangles, seen in the brain tissue of a deceased person, confirm the diagnosis of Alzheimer's disease (Walton, 1985, pp. 658–659). They are neuropathological markers. In multiple sclerosis, destructive lesions of the fatty insulation around nerve fibers in the brain and spinal cord are observed (Walton, 1985, pp. 307–308). These lesions are also markers. At a different level of analy-

54

sis, Huntington's disease is linked to a location on chromosome 4 by a genetic marker that takes the form of a specific pattern of DNA (deoxyribonucleic acid) peculiar to people with the disease. The DNA pattern "marks" the location of the Huntington's gene (Gusella et al., 1983).

In schizophrenia research the marker concept has been elaborated to include behavior as well as neuropathology and genetics. Thus a marker may be any indicator, psychological or physical, of a disease or of vulnerability to a disease (Buchsbaum & Haier, 1983; Iacono, 1985, 1998; Szymanski, Kane, & Lieberman, 1991). Any person who has the marker also has the disease or is liable to develop the disease in the future. Therefore, a genuine marker must be prevalent and occur at very high frequencies in those people with the diagnosis. Conversely, a marker must occur at very low frequencies in people who have other disorders, or in healthy people. Once these primary requirements of accurate identification and prevalence are met, it is possible to imagine several kinds of markers: episode, vulnerability, and genetic.

A marker that occurs only during an acute psychotic crisis is termed an *episode* marker. This is much like the concept of a sign in medicine. Schizophrenia is an illness without highly prevalent objective signs. On the other hand, a marker that occurs independently of acute illness episodes and is therefore stable over time may qualify as a trait or *vulnerability* marker. A trait is an enduring physical or behavioral feature of a person. Thus eye and hair color are physical traits. Behavioral and cognitive traits are more controversial, but intelligence is a defensible example of a cognitive trait (see Lindemann & Matarazzo, 1984, pp. 77–99; Matarazzo, 1990). An important feature of a vulnerability marker is its presence long before illness actually strikes. The marker reflects a person's intrinsic biological predisposition to develop the disease. Almost any aspect of human psychology or biology is a potential vulnerability marker.

Vulnerability criteria are hard to meet, but there are still more requirements that can be placed on a marker candidate, thereby qualifying it as a *genetic* marker. If a characteristic or trait meets requirements for a vulnerability marker, and it occurs in patients' close relatives, especially those who develop schizophrenia themselves, a genetic contribution to the characteristic may be indicated. The case for a marker being genetic in origin is strengthened further if it can be shown that the trait is heritable, passed from generation to generation, in the general population. It is natural to think of physical traits in genetic terms. But many cognitive traits like intelligence, memory, and academic aptitude also appear to be influenced, if not determined by, genetic factors (Plomin, Owen, & McGuffin, 1994).

A really useful candidate marker must be relatively specific to the illness under study. If a marker occurs frequently in schizophrenia but is common in mental retardation, depression, and dementia, it loses "specificity" for schizophrenia. Such an undiscriminating marker may simply "mark" any kind of mental disorder. Intelligence is an example of a very nonspecific cognitive trait. Intelligence test scores are effected by a large range of disorders, from Down's syndrome (see Willerman & Cohen, 1990, pp. 594–596) to epilepsy (Whitehouse, Lerner, & Hedera, 1993, pp. 627–628).

It is evident that a behavioral or biological variable must negotiate many hurdles to achieve true marker status—hurdles that are not required of symptoms. However, the search for markers seems imperative in light of the possible benefits. For example, a marker would provide an objective means of making a diagnosis of schizophrenia. An episode marker could confirm or refute a *DSM-IV* (1994) diagnosis. A vulnerability marker would allow at-risk individuals to be identified many years before illness's onset, and attempts at prevention could be made. From a scientific standpoint, early identification of preschizophrenic people would allow the disease process to be studied before the masking effects of acute symptoms and medication take place. A genetic marker would allow the disorder to be traced through families and generations so that, perhaps, the nature of the transmission of illness could be understood (see Gottesman, 1991). Moreover, a disease marker with specificity could provide clues as to the neurobiological mechanisms of the disease itself. The defective neural and physiological systems that give rise to the trait may also give rise to schizophrenia. For all these reasons, the search for illness markers has been actively pursued over the last 2 decades. Here are some of the candidates that this search has yielded so far.

Candidate Markers of Schizophrenia

In the gray area between the subjective world of symptoms and the biology of the disease process lies the family of behavioral disturbances that are potential illness markers for schizophrenia. These disturbances all relate to the idea that attending and concentrating, sustaining mental effort over time, and selecting and processing information from the perceptual world are compromised in the illness.

There is nothing new in proposing a link between attention-related processes and schizophrenia. Bleuler (1950) and Kraepelin (1919) discussed disturbances of attention, like distractibility, as symptoms of dementia praecox. Some contemporary researchers (e.g., Andreasen, 1982; Andreasen & Flaum, 1991) continue to view attention-related disturbances as a negative symptom, whereas others exclude them from symptom inventories (e.g., Kay, Fiszbein, & Opler, 1987). Attention is also seen as a more basic neurocognitive process that underpins symptoms like thought disorder (Harvey & Serper, 1990; Serper, 1993) and the maintenance of hallucinations over time (Heilbrun, Diller, Fleming, &

Slade, 1986). To complicate matters further, attention can be measured in more than one way. It can be inferred from behavior in the way that a symptom is inferred, by observing and questioning the patient, or it can be measured directly with objective tests of cognitive performance. Thus attention is spun erratically into the psychological fabric of schizophrenia: at once a symptom but not a symptom, subjective and objective, all at the same time.

Attention indirectly derives a further quality of objectivity from its loose relation to several indicators of physiological activity. Such indicators include movements of the eyes when a person tracks or follows closely a visual point or stimulus (Levy, Holzman, Matthysse, & Mendell, 1994). Other indicators include electrical brain wave changes that occur in response to sensory events like sounds or flashes of light (Polich & Kok, 1995), as well as event-related alterations in the electrical conductivity of the skin (Dawson, Nuechterlein, Schell, Gitlin, & Ventura, 1994; Erlenmeyer-Kimling, 1987). These physiological measures have been coupled with tasks that require alertness, vigilance, selectivity, mental shifts, concentration, or prolonged mental effort. Hence the physiological indicators and associated tasks afford another way of tapping attention-related processes (see Lezak, 1995, pp. 39–40). And all of these measures and tasks, along with simpler cognitive tests of attention, have been proposed as potential markers for schizophrenia.

Of primary importance in evaluating attention-related disease markers is their ability to discriminate schizophrenia patients from healthy people. It makes little sense to assess trait and genetic criteria like temporal stability or familial prevalence until the ability of a task to identify who has the illness is known. How accurate should a candidate task be in identifying people with schizophrenia?

Research in behavior genetics creates very high expectations for marker accuracy. For example, the Martin-Bell syndrome of facial abnormalities and mental retardation has a genetic marker in males: the fragmentation of the X chromosome. Jacobs and Sherman (1985) examined 524 males with the syndrome and found that only two failed to show the "fragile" chromosome site. This is a marker prevalence of 99.6%. Moreover, several thousand normal males as well as those with other syndromes were free of the marker. Therefore, the marker is both highly sensitive and specific to the Martin-Bell syndrome. Will behavioral markers for schizophrenia do as well?

Assessing the discriminating power of behavioral markers involves a special difficulty. And it is a difficulty that does not occur with many traditional biological markers like color blindness, abnormal blood chemistry, or altered chromosomes: namely, behavioral tasks, even those with a physiological component like brain electrical activity during an attention task, reflect quantitative differences between people rather than qualitative differences.

The Nature of Quantitative Markers

Characteristics of a person that are qualitative include gender, eye color, blood type, and many aspects of health status: presence or absence of the AIDS virus, pregnancy, cancer cells, or tissue injury. These characteristics lend themselves to simple "yes/no" enumeration and to prevalence figures in the form of percentages that are based on samples of sick and healthy people. In contrast, quantitative differences between people are differences in degree, not in kind. Thus age, height, weight, and many psychological features, including intelligence and other cognitive abilities, vary among people on a continuous dimension. This dimension has no clear or obvious boundaries to separate what is normal from what is abnormal. Of course, it is possible to impose boundaries and to say that everyone over or under a certain age, weight, height, or intelligence is "normal" or "abnormal." Yet these are contrived categories and boundaries, and who falls into them depends on what inclusion rules have been adopted by a particular investigator.

Researchers studying behavioral markers of schizophrenia have to be able to make a categorical decision about each patient in their sample. Is the marker present or not? A common strategy is to say that if a patient scores two standard deviations below the control group average then the score will be defined as "abnormal." This definition is clearly arbitrary to some degree. There is nothing special about a value of two standard deviation units. If 1.5 or 2.5 units are used as the abnormality cutoff, the prevalence of the marker will simply increase or decrease in step with the breadth of the inclusion rule. It is also possible for normal score fluctuations to make it appear as if the marker is present or absent. The influence of a patient's clinical state, symptoms, and medication, or simply the passage of time, may also serve to amplify or diminish a behavioral marker. What happens if a person is just below the cutoff during one evaluation and then slightly above it the next time? These are some of the vagaries of quantitative markers in general and behavioral ones in particular.

The imposition of a cutoff value on continuous data to achieve marker definition may seem unscientific, but it is not necessarily invalid if the patient and control groups are sufficiently different. Thus, neurofibrillary tangles in brain tissue are a pathological marker of Alzheimer's disease. Yet they occur in healthy elderly people as well as in dementia. Nonetheless, they appear in Alzheimer's disease at such elevated rates—rates never seen in healthy people—that the quantitative nature of the marker is not really a problem (Yamamoto & Hirano, 1985).

Marker prevalence in schizophrenia and healthy control samples is the most obvious way of evaluating a marker's validity. Unfortunately, investigators seldom report the actual number of patients who score above or below the critical two standard deviation cutoff in their studies. Hence it is hard to compile and summarize a marker's prevalence across a series of individual studies. Fortunately, the effect size methods introduced in chapter 1 provide an alternative, albeit less precise, way of estimating marker prevalence. An effect size of $d = 3.0$ corresponds to about 93% nonoverlap or separation of patient and healthy distributions. Allowing for some degree of error in diagnosis and task measurement, a potential marker that consistently yielded effect sizes in this neighborhood would possess impressive sensitivity to illness. However, Cohen's (1988) overlap percentages for effect sizes are based on the assumption that the sample distributions are equal and bell-shaped. This occurs seldom in practice, so the overlap percentage represents only a rough approximation of the actual distribution of measurements or scores. Such percentages must be tempered with consideration of actual marker prevalence figures whenever they are available.

With these considerations in mind, I will evaluate six well-researched potential markers—three cognitive-behavioral (digit span, Continuous Performance Test, visual backward masking) and three cognitive-physiological tasks (smooth pursuit eye movements, P300, P50 evoked potentials) in terms of their ability to identify patients with schizophrenia (see table 3.1).

Digit Span

It is well known that schizophrenia carries with it a decline in the ability to concentrate and possibly an increased vulnerability to distraction. Harvey and associates (Harvey, Earle-Boyer, & Levinson, et al., 1986; Harvey, Docherty, Serper, & Rasmussen, 1990) have provided strong evidence of a relation between patients' ability to recall a series of digits in the presence of distracting information and the severity of their thought disorder symptoms. However, the importance of the distraction component of the digit span task is unclear. Some studies of thought disorder in schizophrenia support the special contribution of distraction (e.g. Harvey & Pedley, 1989), but other studies suggest that digit span without distraction is still a powerful predictor of thought disorder (e.g. Harvey, Earle-Boyer, & Levinson, 1988). From a theoretical standpoint, it is conceivable that the effortful cognitive aspect of attention is the key ingredient of the task rather than the presence of competing information (i.e., distraction). In any case, digit span performance has been advanced as a possible disease marker for schizophrenia as a whole, quite apart from any tie that it may have to specific symptoms like thought disorder.

To assess the sensitivity of digit span to schizophrenic illness, my students and I searched the scientific literature since 1980 for studies that included schizophrenia patients and healthy control groups. Unfortunately, none of the studies reported actual prevalence figures or the number of patients who fell below two standard deviations of the control group average. The average effect size, in 29 studies that looked at a total of 1468 patients and healthy people, was d

Table 3.1 Effect Sizes for Candidate Markers of Schizophrena

Marker	Mean d	Confidence Interval	N
1. Digit span	.69	.48–.90	29
2. Continuous Performance Test	1.04	.90–1.18	29
3. Backward masking	1.27	.78–1.76	18
4. Eye tracking			
Root mean squared error	.75	.58–.92	16
Saccadic frequency	1.03	.56–1.50	14
5. P300 evoked potential waveform			
Reduced amplitude	.80	.64–.96	56
Increased latency	.70	.56–.84	49
6. P50 gating evoked potential	1.55	1.21–1.89	20

Note: The table shows effect sizes (Cohen's d) as absolute values, corrected for sample size and averaged over published studies. Confidence Interval is the 95% confidence interval for the mean d. N is the number of published studies in the meta-analysis. Published average marker prevalence rates in schizophrenia are 24.4% for the root mean squared eye tracking, 38.3% and 45% for P300 amplitude and latency, respectively, and 87.4% for the P50.

= .69 (table 3.1). This value is accurate within 21 decimal points 95% of the time. Thus many people with schizophrenia are deficient on the digit span task. However, using Cohen's (1988) normal curve estimates, this effect size also means that patient and control samples overlap by a factor of about 58%. Although this represents a respectable effect in many research contexts, it is not large enough to support digit span performance as a marker of schizophrenia. Only a minority of schizophrenia patients can be distinguished clearly from control values with an effect size of this magnitude. Moreover, there is considerable variability among individual study effects. For example, Salame, Danion, Peretti, and Cuervo's (1998) study yielded an effect size of $d = -2.16$, whereas Park and Holzman (1992) not only obtained a smaller effect of $d = .48$, their effect was in the "wrong" direction. In other words, the schizophrenia patients in their study actually did better than the control subjects in digit span performance. For the most part, however, the relatively tight confidence interval suggests that digit span abnormalities are reliable findings in schizophrenia research. Finally, three of the studies used a distraction version of the digit span task, and these studies produced a slightly larger average effect of $d = .81$. However, the number of studies is too small to allow for a statistical comparison. In any case, the difference between the distractibility effect sizes and the rest of the studies is small and well within the margin of error for the overall effect.

Thus schizophrenia patients as a group differ, on average, from healthy people as a group, but most patients and healthy people are indistinguishable on the digit span task. The relative insensitivity of digit span as a marker can be illustrated by considering Ruth, William, and James, the individual patients described in chapter 1. Application of Lezak's (1995, p. 359) rule of thumb that the average person can repeat six digits plus or minus one provides a way of determining whether the putative marker is present or absent in each of these patients. Two of the three patients had normal digit spans. Ruth, suffering from tactile and olfactory hallucinations, obtained a digit span of eight—slightly better than average. William, with grandiose delusions, obtained a normal span of six. It was James, convinced that his thoughts were controlled by a parasitic voice, who was impaired, with a span of only two. Indeed, he commented during the testing that the digit span task was very difficult. He said that his mind kept going blank when listening to the list of numbers or when he attempted the repetition. Strictly speaking, then, if digit span impairment was used as a marker to identify people with schizophrenia, Ruth and William would have been "missed" and only James would have been identified.

What could account for the modest prevalence of abnormal digit spans in schizophrenia? In his original description of the rationale for psychophysiological markers, Iacono (1985) briefly mentioned that all patients with a specific diagnosis could not be expected to possess the marker trait. The reasons cited include diagnostic invalidity and errors and illness heterogeneity. In other words, in the case of digit span, a number of the schizophrenia patients may have been misdiagnosed. Perhaps they had other psychiatric disorders. Conversely, in other cases, the diagnosis may have been accurate and the marker inaccurate. Measurement of the trait may have been faulty in some patients, leading to "false positives"—incorrect identifications—or leading to "misses": failures to identify a patient as impaired.

The problem with diagnostic error as an explanation for modest effect sizes and low prevalence rates is that there is no independent "gold standard" for diagnosis in schizophrenia research; no way of making the diagnosis other than through use of the *DSM-IV* (1994) or similar criteria (e.g., ICD-10; see WHO, 1992). Hence, there is also no way of finding out how accurate a patient's diagnosis is or of knowing the diagnostic error rate in a sample. Such error must exist, and diagnosticians can be trained to combat misdiagnosis by learning to make reliable, consistent judgments. But it is not possible to determine the accuracy of those judgments.

Accordingly, although both diagnostic error and marker measurement error can be invoked to explain low marker prevalence in schizophrenia samples, these are explanations that cannot be confirmed or even evaluated. In view of the fact that the candidate marker rather than the diagnosis is on trial in this research area, it is hard to escape the conclusion that an inaccurate marker is just that, inaccurate, and therefore not useful. Something else should be tried. This seems to be the case with digit span. However, what if schizophrenia is not a single disease?

The implication of Iacono's (1985) comment about heterogeneity is also worth considering. Suppose that the diagnosis is accurate—the patients really have schizophrenia, *and* the marker is accurate. What would this signify? Such an apparent contradiction is possible if there is more than one schizophrenialike disease. The marker is sensitive to one form of the illness but not to others. Hence numerous patients in an unselected "schizophrenia" sample will perform normally on the marker task. The diagnosis is too inclusive, like lumping Alzheimer's disease, cerebrovascular, and hydrocephalic disorders together under the diagnosis of "dementia." Perhaps schizophrenia is an overinclusive diagnosis too, binding unrelated disorders together into a single artificial illness.

Whether or not heterogeneity exists only at the level of symptoms or extends to the underlying causes of schizophrenic disease states is unknown, but in either case the difficulties of finding a single marker for a heterogeneous condition are apparent—at least in terms of digit span. On the other hand, there is no need to borrow trouble. Perhaps the modest effect size results are unique to the rather simple task of measuring the number of digits a person can repeat. Perhaps other attention-related and psychophysiological tasks index behaviors that occur in virtually all schizophrenia patients.

Continuous Performance Test

The popular Continuous Performance Test involves a task, or group of tasks, that requires a person to respond to a target that is embedded in a long stream of information. Most versions involve visual rather than auditory information. The original Continuous Performance task (Rosvold, Mirsky, Sarason, Bransome & Beck, 1956) involved a random sequence of letters with instructions to respond whenever an X appeared. In the easiest condition any occurrence of the letter X was a "hit." In the more difficult condition the instruction was to respond to X only when it followed the letter A.

A number of investigators have shown that these basic forms of the test are difficult for schizophrenia patients. Moreover, poor scores are not a simple function of general intellectual ability (see Cornblatt & Keilp, 1994). In addition to the requirement of sustained cognitive effort, the Continuous Performance Test measures the selective aspect of attention whereby information is scanned for a specific target. In this selective aspect the test is distinguished from the cognition involved in digit span.

Basic versions of the Continuous Performance test are hard for patients but relatively easy for subjects who are "at risk" for the development of schizophrenia. These are people, often children or adolescents, who have an increased liability for the illness because they are sons or daughters of a schizophrenia patient. The insensitivity of the basic test to preschizophrenia subjects is a drawback for attempts to establish the Continuous Performance Test as a trait or vulnerability marker. After all, the test defect should be there before the illness strikes if the defect is a true marker. However, this insensitivity has spurred the development of second and third forms of the test, all with an eye toward increasing the level of difficulty. Nuechterlein (1983), for example, developed a "degraded stimulus" version. In this form the test-taker is required to respond whenever the number zero appears within a sequence of single digits. However, the numbers are "degraded" by blurring, making them harder to see. Finally, a third version was developed by Cornblatt and Erlenmeyer-Kimling (1985) and referred to as an "identical pairs" test. The task rule was made complex so that a person taking the test must respond whenever the second item in a sequence is identical to its predecessor. For example, in the sequence "AB*B*DECF*F*ABC" both of the italicized letters would be considered "hits." No target is specified in advance, and the subject has to remember each item long enough to compare it to its successor. This flexible target rule has been applied to four-digit numbers and to nonsense shapes as well as to simple numbers and letters.

How accurate is the Continuous Performance Test in identifying patients with a diagnosis of schizophrenia? Before trying to answer such a question, it is important to note that several test scores as well as several test versions are available. These scores include the number of correct responses, or "hits," but also more sophisticated indices that reflect the patient's ability to discriminate "signals" from "noise." Thus there are scores that index a tendency to respond too readily and inclusively, or too cautiously and exclusively, to the task. For example, the "*d*-prime" statistic tempers the hit rate with the rate of incorrect responses, or "false alarms." Another statistic, termed beta, indexes a liberal (over-inclusive) versus conservative (underinclusive) response style. All of this is in addition to the different versions of the test described in the previous paragraph. Hence it is likely that test version and test score both play a role in the ability of the Continuous Performance Test to discriminate patients and healthy control subjects.

In the search for controlled comparisons, my students and I found 29 relevant studies representing 1892 patients and healthy control research participants, and we calculated effect sizes and related statistics for each of these studies. Unfortunately, the different versions of the test and the different scores pose a problem of interpretation. Any two researchers may or may not use the same version (e.g., identical pairs versus blurred target, etc.). Even when they do, different scores (e.g., hits versus beta) may be reported. This inconsistency makes it hard to judge accurately how important the different test versions really are in terms of sensitivity to schizophrenic illness.

Nevertheless, I examined the 29 studies in terms of different test versions and analyzed the same test score whenever possible. Four studies used the identical pairs version, yielding an average effect of $d = 1.2$, and five studies used the degraded stimulus version and yielded an average effect of $d = .84$. The rest of the studies used different versions or reported different scores. It is difficult to draw firm conclusions about the possible importance and differential sensitivity of versions of the Continuous Performance Test on the basis of relatively few studies. Nonetheless, the identical pairs version appears to be more sensitive to the illness than the degraded stimulus version. It is also possible that the patients in the different studies varied in terms of illness severity, medication, or general cognitive ability. Hence patient characteristics as well as the test version may figure in effect sizes. However, we found little evidence for relations between patient variables and effect sizes in our earlier study of this literature (Heinrichs & Zakzanis, 1998). It is probable that most of the variability between studies is due to the particular form of the Continuous Performance test employed by the researchers.

The average overall effect for the Continuous Performance Test came to $d = 1.04$. Despite the influence of different test versions, the margin of error for this average is only 14 decimal points 95% of the time. On the whole, schizophrenia patients are impaired relative to healthy people on the task, and impairment is a reliable finding. Actual prevalence statistics based on a two standard deviation cutoff were not reported in the studies. Hence, using Cohen's (1988) idealized distributions for an estimate of discrimination, about 43% of the patients and healthy control participants are indistinguishable in their test performance, or, conversely, perhaps 57% of the patients and controls are completely distinguished. This is a much stronger effect than the one obtained for the digit span tasks, yet it still falls well short of the $d = 3.0$ effect size required for 93% discrimination of patients and controls. Hence it fails to provide a reasonable degree of confidence in the marker's ability to identify the illness. All in all, a fairly consistent majority of schizophrenia subjects are impaired on the Continuous Performance Test, but the proportion is still too small to support the claim of this attention task to be a marker for a single illness.

Backward Visual Masking

Backward masking is a task that bears some similarities to the distractibility condition of the digit span task in that both reflect the disruptive influence of interference on memory performance. In the case of backward masking, however, the memory aspect does not involve recall of a number series. It involves the ability to recognize a very briefly exposed letter (figure 3.1). In the baseline condition, a letter is presented for a few fractions, thousandths, of a second. The critical measure in the baseline phase is the exposure time required to recognize the briefly flashed letter. However, this is not the phenomenon of greatest interest. Next comes the backward-masking condition itself, wherein the target letter is followed by a masking stimulus, such as an array of Xs. The mask degrades the fading target letter in the viewer's sensory memory. The question is: How long an interval between target and mask does a person need in order to preserve the letter memory from the degrading effects of the mask? Saccuzzo and Schubert (1981) showed that schizophrenia patients need more time than

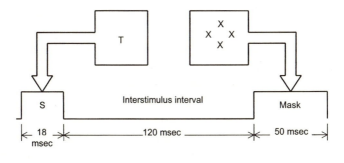

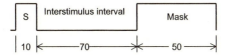

Figure 3.1. The visual backward-masking experiment: the durations of a stimulus (S), an interstimulus interval, and a visual mask in abnormal (upper) and normal (lower) performance. Abnormality is defined by the length of exposure time (18 versus 10 milliseconds) required to recognize a stimulus like the letter *T* and also by the length of interval (120 versus 70 milliseconds) needed to preserve the letter's image from the mask of *X*s. The second aspect of performance is the backward-masking effect. Many patients with schizophrenia perform abnormally on both aspects of the task. (Adapted from Willerman & Cohen, 1990, p. 310.)

healthy people do to preserve the letter from the degrading effects of the mask. These findings were interpreted as evidence that information processing is both slower and more vulnerable to distortion and inaccuracy (i.e., backward masking) in schizophrenia patients than in healthy people.

My students and I found 18 studies published between 1980 and 1999 that compared schizophrenia patients with healthy control participants on the visual backward-masking task. These studies were based on a total of 858 people. The compiled data reveal an abnormally enhanced vulnerability to masking in schizophrenia and an average effect size of $d = 1.27$. The moderately large confidence interval of 49 decimal points on either side of this average is due to some discrepant studies (e.g., Voruganti, Heslegrave, & Awad, 1997) that produced very large effects (e.g., $d = 4.42$). Most of the effect sizes are much smaller, including one as small as $d = .21$ (Slaghuis & Bakker, 1995). In the absence of actual prevalence statistics, the average effect implies that perhaps 35% of the patients and controls overlap in their performance during the backward-masking condition. This effect is considerably stronger than the one obtained with digit span and or with the Continuous Performance Test. Hence it is likely that more than half of patients with schizophrenia show an abnormal backward masking performance. However, individual studies vary rather widely in the strength of their findings, and backward-masking deficits are less stable than the other cognitive marker effects. The result of this variability is that the margin of error for the backward-masking effect encompasses the average effects for digit span and Continuous Performance. Hence any superiority of backward-masking may be more apparent than real. Arguably, Continuous Performance produces a more powerful average effect than digit span, but that is about all that can be said.

Therefore, the three research literatures considered thus far demonstrate that schizophrenia patients are disadvantaged as a group on attention-based information-processing tasks. However, none of these tasks consistently identify abnormalities in much more than half of the patient population. None can be considered a true marker of a single schizophrenic disease state. Backward visual masking demonstrates a fairly powerful effect, but the Continuous Performance results are much more reliable and still quite strong. Up to this point, I have considered only purely cognitive and behavioral tasks as potential markers. None of these tasks are anchored directly to physiology—they implicate physiological systems only vaguely and indirectly. It might be that tasks that link cognition with physiology more closely could be more accurate indicators of schizophrenic illness.

The Eyes Have It

Attention influences the ability of the eyes to follow, track, or "pursue" a moving stimulus like a point of light (Holzman, Proctor, & Hughes, 1973). If such a point moves continuously, our eyes will duplicate its pattern of movement. This pursuit of a moving stimulus can be measured objectively by placing electrodes beside each eye to detect the minute signals that accompany changing ocular position. The signals are amplified to yield a record of tracking movements and tracking errors or deviance like those illustrated in figure 3.2. Accordingly, such a record reflects the degree of resemblance between the stimulus pattern, usually a sinusoidal wave, and the corresponding eye movements of the viewer.

Research on eye movement abnormalities has its own technical and rather arcane language. Fast eye movements, or "saccades," reposition the eye in conformity with the stimulus. Hence, "catchup" saccades occur when the eyes lag behind the target, during pursuit tracking. Anticipatory saccades position the eyes ahead of the target, and backup saccades adjust for overshooting the anticipated stimulus path. Unlike catchup and backup saccades, which compensate for inaccurate eye position, anticipatory saccades actually take the eyes off the target path and then "wait" for its next movement. Patients with schizophrenia tend to have more deviations from the stimulus path than healthy people do and hence more errors like anticipatory saccades and "square wave jerks" (Levy, Holzman, Matthyse, & Mendell, 1993).

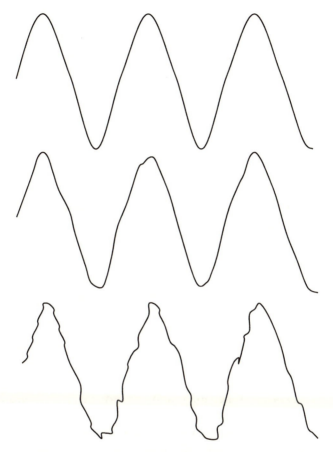

Figure 3.2. Normal and abnormal eye tracking of a sinusoidal wave. The top pattern is the target, the middle pattern is a record of normal tracking, and the lowest pattern is the kind of abnormal record produced by some patients with schizophrenia. (From Levy et al., 1993, p. 462.)

One of the attractive features of any physiological index of attention is that it may bear directly on the disturbed brain biology underlying schizophrenia. However, the neural structures and circuits that underpin eye tracking are extensive and multifocal, ranging from the brainstem through subcortical structures like the thalamus to the frontal eye fields in the cerebral cortex (Clementz & Sweeney, 1990). Disturbances in any part of this neural system may disrupt normal eye tracking. Moreover, the location of schizophrenic pathology is not known, so the neurological implications of deviant eye tracking in the illness are correspondingly vague and uncertain. Nonetheless, it seems possible that eye tracking could be closer than exclusively cognitive measures of attention and information processing to the biological basis of schizophrenia. If so, this candidate marker should generate much higher rates of accurate patient identification than the foregoing cognitive measures have managed to achieve.

The empirical literature on eye movement abnormalities in schizophrenia is huge when compared with the number of studies on cognitive tasks like digit span and backward masking. In their review, now 7 years old, Levy et al. (1993) wrote that the basic finding of a defect in schizophrenic eye tracking has been replicated more than 80 times in different countries, and they cite studies that go back as far as the early years of this century (i.e., Diefendorf & Dodge, 1908). However, not all studies used control groups, and many relied on qualitative ratings and impressions of abnormality rather than on quantitative indices of tracking performance.

The technical complexity of eye movement deviation and measurement has generated many scores designed to reflect the number or size of compensatory and intrusive saccades. Arguments have been advanced about the relative merits of each score as an index of tracking performance. In contrast, some researchers simply rate whether the eye movement record is normal or abnormal on the basis of a global impression (e.g., Weinberger & Wyatt, 1982). The problem with qualitative global ratings is that the specific nature of the observed abnormality remains unknown. Does it reside in the number of anticipatory saccades, the number of square wave jerks, or some other aspect of recorded performance? Moreover, qualitative rating methods may be peculiar to specific researchers and the scoring rules are hard to make explicit. There is even some evidence that impressionistic ratings lead to spuriously high estimates of eye movement abnormality in some schizophrenia patients (Iacono, Moreau, Beiser, Fleming, & Lin, 1992; Clementz, Grove, Iacono, & Sweeney, 1992). To correct this problem, a global quantitative index, root mean squared error, was developed (Iacono & Lykken, 1979) and advocated as the best way to calibrate the extent to which eye movements approximate a stimulus pattern. This too leaves the specific abnormality unclear, but a quantitative index has the virtues of objectivity and utility so that any investigator can calculate the error score. Finally, some researchers advocate the use of very specific measurements—the number of anticipatory saccades in a tracking record, for example, or "gain," the ratio of eye velocity to the velocity of the moving target.

My graduate students Carey Sturgeon, Konstantine Zakzanis, and Stephanie McDermid and I searched the literature between 1980 and 1999 for studies using quantitative indices of eye tracking and found 14–16 studies reporting results for both schizophrenia patients and healthy people (table 3.1). Consider first the global quantitative score, root mean squared error, introduced by Iacono and Lykken (1979). The average effect size for 16 studies based on 1332 patients and control participants was $d = .75$, which shows that indeed schizophrenia patients on average perform poorly on eye-tracking tasks. But this effect corresponds to a hypothetical group overlap of about 55%. An effect of this size is well short of a convincing discrimination and may in fact be an in-flated estimate. For example, several studies actually reported marker preva-lence results. Iacono et al. (1992) defined prevalence as a mean squared error score two standard deviations from the control group average. With this defi-nition, only 20% of their schizophrenia patients had abnormal tracking. The average abnormality prevalence for the four studies that reported data in this way was 40%. Hence no more than a large minority of patients show the pu-tative "marker" trait. Three of these studies also reported abnormality rates in their healthy control participants. These averaged to a rate of 8.2%. Accord-ingly, although the root mean squared error index of eye tracking suggests a low prevalence of tracking abnormality in healthy people and a much higher rate in schizophrenia patients, the majority of both populations have normal tracking.

Modest effect sizes always raise the twin possibilities that the phenomenon under study either is of minor importance in relation to schizophrenia or is es-sential only for a subgroup of patients. Unfortunately, it is usually hard to decide between these divergent possibilities. The 95% confidence interval or error margin in the accuracy of the average tracking effect is small, at 17 decimal points (table 3.1). Hence the eye-tracking abnormality seems stable and reliable across different studies. However, Clementz et al. (1992) and Iacono et al. (1992) reported a bimodal distribution of eye-tracking error scores in their patient sample. Bimodal distributions, where the score frequency seems to have two peaks instead of one, are often regarded as evidence for a mixed sample and more than one population of research subjects (see Levy et al., 1993). The ex-istence of subpopulations of schizophrenia patients with etiologically different forms of illness is the most likely explanation for the discovery of bimodal pa-tient samples in the eye-tracking results.

Another quantitative global indicator, saccadic frequency, reflects the number of times the eyes are repositioned relative to the stimulus track. This index does not distinguish between catchup and anticipatory saccades and groups them all together. We found 14 studies with normal control groups and useful statistics. The average effect size was $d = 1.03$, with a fairly large confidence interval or margin of error of 47 decimal points (table 3.1). This means that 95% of the time, the true average effect could be anywhere between $d = .56$ and $d = 1.50$. With so much variability among studies, the average effect is somewhat mis-leading. The range of individual effect sizes runs from $d = 3.85$ (Mather & Putchat, 1982) to $d = 0.07$ (Clementz, McDowell, & Zisook, 1994). Hence, sac-cadic frequency separated perhaps 97% of patients and healthy people in one study and failed to separate them at all in another study. Furthermore, the con-fidence interval is so broad that one researcher may obtain a relatively large ef-fect with perhaps only 30% overlap, while another may find an effect with a pa-tient control overlap as high as 64%. Altogether this suggests that saccadic frequency is a less stable indicator of schizophrenia–control group differences than the root mean error score.

Other and more specific indices of eye tracking have been reported in the literature on schizophrenia. Sturgeon (1998) calculated average effect sizes for anticipatory saccades ($d = .29$), catchup saccades ($d = .44$), and square wave jerks ($d = .12$), as well as for pursuit "gain" ($d = .94$). These other indices are all weaker than saccadic frequency, and only gain is superior to root mean squared error in terms of sensitivity to schizophrenia.

Instead of proving more accurate and reliable as an identifier and hence marker of schizophrenia, eye-movement deviations are, if anything, less accurate and less consistent than cognitive tasks. Even the "best" eye-tracking index from the standpoint of average validity, saccadic frequency, is undermined by its large error margin. If more reliable scores like root mean squared error are used, perhaps only a quarter of schizophrenia patients are truly distinguishable from normal subjects in their eye tracking. This poor discrimination contrasts with some published prevalence rates—based largely on qualitative ratings of eye-tracking abnormality—that are much higher (e.g., 51-85%, Holzman et al., 1988). Despite the popularity and frequently cited "validity" of eye tracking as the preeminent candidate for marker status, it is apparent that anchoring experimental tasks more closely to physiology does not necessarily make them more sensitive than cognitive tasks to the presence of schizophrenia.

Ironically, the eye-movement results provide the strongest evidence yet of illness heterogeneity. This evidence includes the distribution characteristics of root mean squared error results and the great range in effect sizes obtained with saccadic frequency. Indeed, recent studies suggest that eye-tracking researchers are gradually abandoning assumptions about schizophrenia as a single disease state. For example, Ross, Buchanan, Medoff, Lahti, and Thaker (1998) divided their schizophrenia sample into groups of patients with or without eye-tracking disorder. They found that schizophrenia patients with the disorder have more sensory and motor abnormalities than those with normal tracking. Hence eye tracking may be a marker for a specific variant of schizophrenia rather than for a unitary schizophrenic disease state.

On the other hand, perhaps eye movements are too indirect a measure of brain function to succeed as highly sensitive indicators of the disease process in schizophrenia. To explore this possibility, consider a group of tasks that link brain activity and information processing more directly.

Evoked Brain Potentials

One of the earliest ways of measuring brain activity involved the electroencephalograph. The technique records or amplifies ongoing electrical activity of the brain through application of electrodes to the scalp. This electrical activity is responsive to sensory stimuli like sounds or lights. Momentary changes in brain electrical activity caused by a sensory stimulus are termed evoked responses or potentials. These changes may be only fractions of a second in duration, and they are easily "lost" in the presence of unrelated but coexisting brain activity. However, technical advances have allowed researchers to obtain a "pure" evoked electrical reaction by eliciting many responses to repeated sensory events. The repetition of events allows the enormous cerebral "noise" of the conventional electroencephalograph to be removed by a computer, leaving behind the average evoked response.

An evoked voltage or potential that is measured as a person sits and listens to a series of sounds can be made psychologically interesting and significant. This is accomplished through manipulation of the stimulus or event that elicits the potential in the first place. Manipulations include embedding infrequent tones in a sequence of frequent tones. This induces informational novelty—surprise—into the task. Another approach is to present two sounds in close succession to create conditioning, or rapid habituation, whereby the response to the second sound is weaker than to the first. Both of these manipulations are associated with distinct kinds of evoked potential waveforms.

The P300 Component of the Evoked Potential

One of the most frequently studied evoked potentials in schizophrenia research is the P300 waveform that occurs in response to infrequent but task-relevant sensory events. In practice the paradigm that produces the waveform involves having a person listen to a series of tones that have the same low pitch. Once in a while, according to a predetermined ratio, a sound with a much higher pitch is heard. The research subject is asked to listen and count the number of high-pitched tones as they occur. While the subject engages in this task, electrophysiological recording is carried out. Following the infrequent high-pitched tones, a characteristic voltage swing like the one presented in the upper part of figure 3.3 is produced. A positive component of the voltage swing occurs from 300 to 1,000 milliseconds after the infrequent tone is heard. This component may vary from person to person in terms of its amplitude or size and in terms of its latency or time of occurrence. The P300 is altered in schizophrenia, so that people with the illness have a smaller, later waveform than the one seen in healthy people. It follows that alteration of the P300 potential has been advanced as a possible trait marker for the illness (Blackwood, St. Clair, Muir, & Duffy, 1991; Ford, 1999).

The precise psychological meaning of the P300 has been the subject of considerable debate (Siddle, Packer, Donchin, & Fabiani, 1991). In addition to attention, concepts such as subjective probability of events, perceptions of task relevance and stimulus meaning, and "equivocation" have been used to describe

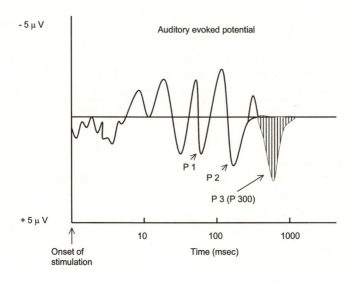

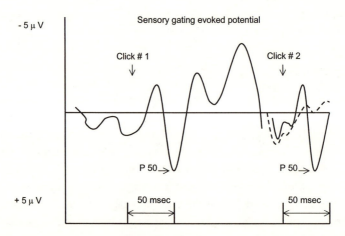

Figure 3.3. Two evoked potential paradigms used in psychophysiological research on schizophrenia. The top graph shows an averaged brain potential that occurs in response to a series of sounds. The graph includes the P300 component that seems to occur in response to a novel or infrequent sound. The length of time or latency before the P300 occurs and the sizes of the voltage swing or wave amplitude are often abnormal in schizophrenia patients. (Adapted from Hillyard & Kutas, 1983.) The lower graph shows averaged evoked potentials in response to two successive sound clicks. The positive component (P50) that occurs about 50 milliseconds after the click is smaller following the second click in most healthy people (dotted line). However, in a substantial number of schizophrenia patients, the second P50 is almost as big as the first (solid line), implying a failure of the brain to "gate" the stimulus. (Adapted from Adler et al., 1998, p. 190.)

the mental activity that is linked with the P300. Similarly, there is controversy about locating the origin of the P300 in a specific brain region or system. Because the waveform is measured in the brain through the scalp and skull with several electrode sites, exact localization is difficult to achieve. Some investigators argue for a focus in the central and parietal areas of the brain. Others suggest a neural P300 generator in the hippocampus of the medial temporal lobe, and still others hold out for the existence of many P300 generators that are located in a distributed fashion in several brain sites (Smith et al., 1990; Polich & Kok, 1995; Polich & Squire, 1993). Thus the evoked potential is a more direct measure than eye tracking of brain activity. But even evoked potentials are still fairly vague in terms of their neuroanatomical origins.

To index the ability of P300 amplitude and latency to satisfy the primary criterion for a marker, accurate diagnostic identification, we searched the literature and found 56 studies comparing a total of 3,213 schizophrenia patients and healthy people on amplitude. We found 50 studies that examined latency in 3,028 patients and controls. Evidently this is a very popular research field.

The P300 amplitude results confirm that schizophrenia patients, on average, tend to have smaller waveforms than healthy people do. However, with an average effect of $d = .80$, the degree of theoretical overlap between patients and controls remains in the neighborhood of 53%, clearly insufficient for a true marker. And the actual prevalence of the marker may be much lower. A handful of studies reported rates for abnormal P300 amplitudes in schizophrenia, and the average prevalence is only about 38%. This average masks some divergent individual prevalence findings that range from 5% (Obiols et al., 1986) to 75% (Jyoti Rao, Anathnarayanan, Gangadhar, & Janakiramaiah, 1995). The individual effects vary dramatically from a high of $d = 1.85$ (Eikmeier, Lodemann, Zerbin, & Gastpar, 1992) to a study by Rockstroh, Muller, Wagner, Cohen, and Elbert (1994) that reported an *increase* in P300 amplitude rather than a decrease for their schizophrenia sample. Nor was this the only study that found the reverse of the expected reduction in amplitude in the illness (see Shelley, Grochowski, Liberman, & Javitt, 1996). Unfortunately, the authors provide little insight into the reasons for their powerful and contradictory findings. Still, with so many studies in the pool, the discrepant findings do not grossly inflate the confidence interval, which is quite small, at 16 decimal places on either side of the average d.

The P300 latency meta-analysis complements the amplitude findings. The results show that on average schizophrenia patients have a delayed P300 waveform relative to healthy people, but the average effect ($d = 1.06$) yields only about a 58% group discrimination. Moreover, the average is spuriously inflated by the presence of one enormous and anomalous effect. A study by Frangou et al. (1997) reported latency data that yield an effect of $d = 15.22$. This is an implausibly large value and may be an error. With the questionable finding removed from the set of effects, the number of studies drops to 49 and the average drops to a much more modest $d = .70$, which is very close to the value for the amplitude effect. An effect size of this magnitude implies a distribution nonoverlap of about 43%. To underscore this poor discrimination, a subset of five studies reported the actual prevalence of latencies that were at least two standard deviations greater than the average control group value. Approximately 45% of the schizophrenia patients in these studies had abnormal P300 latencies.

In terms of error margin and stability of the average effect, the confidence interval indicates that, 95% of the time, the latency d will fall between $d = .56$ and $d = .84$. Thus the latency findings are fairly stable and similar in this respect to the amplitude results. Apart from the anomalous finding by Frangou et al. (1997) there are a few studies with quite large effects, notably St. Clair, Blackwood, and Muir (1989), who reported data consistent with a d of 2.27. However, there are many small or trivial effects, and one study even shows slightly shorter rather than longer P300 latencies in schizophrenia (Rockstroh et al., 1994). Thus the degree of overall discriminating power and reliability of the average effect size seems roughly equal in P300 amplitude and P300 latency research.

The P300 evoked potential is a psychologically intriguing aspect of electrophysiology because it appears to arise predictably in association with mental events. Furthermore, it is a direct, albeit poorly localized measure of brain activity. Nonetheless, its validity as a marker for a unitary schizophrenic illness is clearly inadequate. This much can be concluded: the P300 is not sufficiently sensitive to the presence of schizophrenia to constitute a trait marker for a single illness.

The P50 or "Gating" Evoked Potential

The gating paradigm is based on the idea that schizophrenia involves an impaired sensory filter (see also chapter 2). A person hears two "clicks," with the second occurring 500 milliseconds after the first. When electrophysiological instruments are applied, a waveform is detected in association with each click. In healthy people the evoked potential to the second click is smaller than to the first. This can be seen in the relative amplitude of the two responses in the lower part of figure 3.3. From a psychological perspective, the weaker response to the second click reflects a filtering, dampening, or "gating" of sounds in the environment. From a neurophysiological perspective, the origins of the gating effect are unknown. Adler et al. (1998) have speculated that the gating phenomenon reflects a kind of learning and therefore may originate in brain centers involved in learning, like the hippocampal formation of the temporal lobes. Many patients with schizophrenia show a pattern that differs from the normal evoked response: they fail to gate the stimulus. The amplitude of the potential evoked by the second click is almost as large as the amplitude associated with the first click. The brain reacts as strongly to a repeated event as it does to a new event. The positive component of the potential occurs about 50 milliseconds after the second click, hence the shorthand term "P50" to describe this phenomenon (Siegel, Waldo, Mizner, Adler, & Freedman, 1984).

In searching the literature we found 20 studies comparing P50 amplitude in 742 schizophrenia and control participants. With an average overall d of 1.55, P50 amplitudes are definitely larger, on average, in schizophrenia patients than in healthy people. This must reflect the failure of many patients to gate or reduce the processing of the second click they hear. With a normal curve approximation of about 72% nonoverlap between patients and controls, the d is a relatively impressive effect size. In addition, prevalence results based on a two standard deviation cutoff are available for patients in three studies and for controls in two studies. These results show that an average of about 87% of schizophrenia patients have abnormal P50 amplitudes, whereas only about 3.5% of healthy control subjects demonstrate the defect. Two studies (Waldo, Adler, & Freedman, 1988; Waldo et al., 1994) surpass $d = 3.0$ in terms of effect magnitude, which means that perhaps 95% of the patients and controls did not overlap in their P50 scores. However, the margin of error for the average of all 20 studies indicates that an effect between a d of 1.21 and one of 1.89 best describes the research results on the P50 in schizophrenia. This makes the margin of error substantially broader than what was found for the P300 potential. Overall, however, the P50 appears to be the most sensitive, if not the most stable, of all the putative attention-related markers of schizophrenia.

Perspectives on the Prevalence of Candidate Markers

Six cognitive and psychophysiological performance indicators have been considered here in relation to the primary criterion that any marker must satisfy—accurate case identification. The analysis of effect sizes suggests that only the P50 evoked potential can be considered a possible marker of a single illness. Although the average effect size for the P50 is well below values required for complete schizophrenia–normal control group discrimination, the handful of studies reporting prevalence data on their patients suggest that a substantial majority demonstrates the P50 defect. Hence, if very liberal allowance is made for diagnostic error, these results are sufficient to support the P50 evoked potential as a marker for a single schizophrenic disease state. Although several other criteria figure in the evaluation of potential markers, there are tentative grounds for believing that the P50 has passed the initial hurdle.

Ironically, the literature on illness markers also raises the possibility that schizophrenia is not a single disease state. One aspect of eye-tracking disorder, the root mean squared error score, may be a marker for a subtype or variant of schizophrenia. Any time a marker effect is too small to separate patients and healthy people but too large to be dismissed as trivial, the effect may index a subpopulation of patients. This situation applies to each of the putative marker candidates, with the possible exception of the P50 waveform abnormality. However, in the case of eye tracking, there is explicit evidence that the distributions underlying root mean squared error scores are too complex to reflect a single population of patients. Moreover, there are recent studies (e.g., Ross et al., 1998) that support the division of schizophrenia into at least two illnesses, on the basis of the presence or absence of eye-tracking abnormalities. It is possible that complex distributions also underpin digit span scores, Continuous Performance results, backward masking, and P300 potentials, not to mention other aspects of eye tracking like saccadic frequency. However, researchers have either not examined or not published the distribution characteristics of these variables. Still, at least two candidate markers provide competing visions of schizophrenia. Is this one disease (P50) or perhaps two or more diseases (root mean squared eye tracking)? Perhaps the issue can be resolved by considering the extent to which the attention-related and psychophysiological tasks satisfy the other criteria required of a disease marker.

Traits and States

To what extent do the attention-related and psychophysiological tasks constitute genuine traits? Temporal stability, independence from treatment, and symptom expression and remission relate to the concept of a trait as an enduring cross-situational consistency in behavior. If eye movements, evoked potentials, backward masking, and attention fluctuate greatly with time, or if they are altered by drug treatment, then their sensitivity to schizophrenia itself is compromised. From a statistical standpoint, a group of patients may "improve" on a marker task yet remain impaired relative to the performance of healthy people. Furthermore, on an individual patient level, the marker may enter the normal range of values. A patient shows the marker abnormality at first admission to hospital, but it disappears once medication is introduced. Alternatively, the abnormality shows up early in the illness, vanishes after a few years, then reappears. In such a situation using the marker to identify patients would be a hit-or-miss affair even if group differences relative to healthy people persist. Some marker tasks may be inherently unstable and unreliable over the course of illness, much as the measurement of a person's blood pressure fluctuates with a variety of situational and psychological factors that have little to do with the presence of physical disease.

The published literature provides an incomplete but still helpful evaluation of the candidate markers and their traitlike qualities. Digit span distractibility deficits persist even after the symptoms of schizophrenia improve (Frame & Oltmanns, 1982). However, performance on this test may be influenced by the kind of symptoms a patient experiences (Rund, 1989). The Continuous Performance Test is also vulnerable to a patient's clinical state (Nuechterlein, 1991; Knott et al., 1999) and there is evidence that medicated and unmedicated patients differ in their scores on some versions of the test (Earle-Boyer, Serper, Davidson, & Harvey, 1991). Several studies show that medication improves Continuous Performance scores, although the improvement is not sufficient to elevate scores into the normal range (Harvey et al., 1990; Serper, Bergman, & Harvey, 1990; Cornblatt & Keilp, 1994; Judd Finkelstein, Cannon, Gur, Gur, & Moberg, 1997). Older studies show that the visual backward masking effect is susceptible to medication (Braff & Saccuzzo, 1982) and diminishes when symptoms remit (Zaunbrecher, Himer, & Straube, 1990). But against this trend, Rund's (1993; Rund, Landro, & Orbeck, 1993) studies provide some countervailing evidence of stability for masking effects, and Green, Nuechterlein, Breitmeyer, and Mintz (1999) found a very large ($d = 3.53$) effect in unmedicated patients whose disease was in remission.

With respect to smooth pursuit eye movements, stability is acceptable over a two-year period, according to Iacono and Lykken (1981), and tracking performance does not appear to change with the length of illness (Amador et al., 1991; Mather & Putchat, 1982). Furthermore, there is solid evidence that eye movements are not affected by antipsychotic medication (Holzman, Solomon, Levin, & Waternaux, 1984; Levy et al., 1993; Siever et al., 1986). In the evoked potential literature some studies suggest that medication and clinical state are largely unrelated to the P300 (Pritchard, 1986; Blackwood et al., 1987). However, recent studies contradict this view (Coburn et al., 1998; Ford et al., 1999). Unfortunately, there are few longitudinal studies of P300 stability, so little is known about how the evoked potential responds to changing clinical features and states in schizophrenia patients (Friedman & Squires-Wheeler, 1994; Rao, Ananthnarayanan, Gangadhar, & Janakiramaiah, 1995).

The P50 or "gating" defect is the most promising single disease marker candidate from the standpoint of its prevalence in schizophrenia patients. Therefore it is disappointing to find studies by Boutros, Overall, and Zouridakis (1991) and Kathmann and Engel (1990) showing that the defect varies over time and even from trial to trial within a testing session (Patterson et al., 2000). Other studies have found that smoking can influence the P50 (Adler, Hoffer, Wiser, & Freedman, 1993; Adler et al., 1998). Moreover, Sturgeon (1998) found evidence across 14 published studies that P50 findings diminish with the proportion of study patients receiving antipsychotic medication. This conclusion is augmented by recent studies showing that the P50 gating abnormality is related to depression, anxiety, and feelings of low energy (Yee, Nuechterlein, & Dawson, 1998; Yee, Nuechterlein, Morris, & White, 1998). Therefore, it is very unlikely that the P50 abnormality constitutes a highly stable illness trait.

In summary, a vulnerability marker is most valuable when it remains stable and does not wax and wane with time, with how a patient is feeling, or with the drugs the patient is receiving. Although the trait properties of putative markers have received insufficient study, there is considerable support for smooth pursuit eye movements in this respect and some limited evidence in favor of digit span distractibility, while the situation for the P300 potential is mixed. There is minimal support for the Continuous Performance Test, backward masking, or the P50 gating waveform. What this means is that a patient's performance on most marker tasks may either "normalize" at some point or change into impaired ranges, depending on random score fluctuations or on a variety of clinical influences. Group performance differences between schizophrenia patients and healthy people may persist. But the instability of many marker tasks introduces uncertainty into the hypothesized equation that links these tasks with the presence or absence of disease vulnerability.

Convergence of Putative Markers

Do different psychophysiological and attention-related tasks identify the same patients as abnormal? For example, is deviant eye tracking found in the same schizophrenia patient who has a reduced P300 amplitude and an impaired score on the Continuous Performance Test? Convergent findings would imply that different markers are identifying a single disease. Divergent findings imply that different markers are identifying different schizophrenia-related disorders. High concordance among psychophysiological tasks in the presence of poor agreement with the DSM-IV (1994) diagnosis might even call the validity of the DSM-IV (1994)–based diagnosis into question. If the marker tasks collectively disagree with the diagnostic system, there may be something wrong with the system.

There is very little evidence on these important questions. Blackwood et al. (1991, 1994) found no association between deviant eye tracking and the P300 component of the evoked potential, and Grove, Lebow, Clementz, Medus, and Iacono (1991) found no association between eye tracking and the Continuous Performance Test. This kind of research is the logical next step for marker studies, but early results are not encouraging.

The reasons for the neglect of the crucial topic of marker convergence are not obvious. There is no shortage of research on the individual marker tasks themselves. More than 50 controlled studies have been carried out on the basic P300 phenomenon since 1980. However, the use of multiple marker tasks in individual studies remains rare. Some tasks like eye tracking and the evoked potential paradigms require sophisticated instrumentation, and this may make the use of batteries of marker tests expensive. But technical requirements in the area of psychophysiology are considerably lower than in areas like brain imaging and post-mortem neuropathology. Expense seems to be an inadequate reason for neglect. Even when more than one putative marker is employed in the same study, correlation between marker tasks is frequently not reported (e.g., Blackwood, Young, et al. 1991). Such omissions are puzzling, given the importance assigned to the search for valid markers and objective indicators of schizophrenic illness.

Specificity

If the sensitivity of cognitive psychophysiology to schizophrenia is only modest, if convergent validity is uncertain, and if temporal stability is unequal across tasks, perhaps supportive evidence for the putative markers lies elsewhere. For example, one of the secondary criteria for a good illness marker is its specificity. This involves the extent to which the candidate marker manifests itself selectively in schizophrenia and not in other psychiatric or neurological disorders. Perhaps these attention-dependent tasks are performed poorly by patients with any kind of disabling mental condition, from mental retardation to dementia. On the other hand, evidence that marker task performance is impaired only in schizophrenia would suggest an association between the tasks and the illness even in the presence of poor sensitivity.

Research is available on the specificity of some of the tasks considered in this chapter. Continuous Performance Test deficits occur more frequently in schizophrenia patients than in alcoholics (Mussgay & Hertwig, 1990). There is evidence in some studies that mood-disordered patients—patients with depression or mania—perform differently on the task from schizophrenia patients (Cornblatt, Lenzenweger, & Erlenmeyer-Kimling, 1989; Walker, 1981). However, this differential sensitivity is not found consistently (see Rund, Orbeck, & Landro, 1992; Walker & Green, 1982), and the number of illnesses studied in relation to schizophrenia is small. Similarly, visual backward masking differentiates mood-disordered from schizophrenia patients in some studies (Braff & Saccuzzo, 1985; Elkins, Cromwell, & Asarnow, 1992) but not in others (Green & Walker, 1986b; Rund, 1993).

With respect to eye movement abnormalities, there is also evidence for and against specificity to schizophrenia. The discrimination of mood disorders with psychotic features from schizophrenia is always a difficult challenge. In addition to mania and depression, these disorders include bipolar illness, where the person swings between mania and depression. In a review of the eye-tracking literature, Levy et al. (1993) argued that some findings, especially those pertaining to comparisons between schizophrenia and mania, suggest that eye movement abnormalities occur in both conditions, while other findings support specificity. One interpretation is that nonschizophrenic psychotic patients show eye-tracking deviations only during acute illness episodes or as a consequence of medications like lithium. In contrast, the argument continues, schizophrenia patients manifest deviant tracking as a stable trait. Nevertheless, several studies have found deviant tracking in alcoholics (Kobatake, Yoshii, Shinohara, Nomura, & Takagi, 1983) and in a variety of other psychiatric disorders (Van den Bosch, Rozendaal, & Mol, 1987). This evidence is difficult to assess because of technical variations in how different laboratories measure and evaluate eye movements.

The research on evoked potentials, and especially the P300, is less equivocal —this evoked potential waveform component is not found only in schizophrenia. Reduced amplitudes or increased latencies are seen in the elderly and in dementia (St. Clair, Blackwood, & Christie, 1985), Down's syndrome (Muir et al., 1988), alcoholism (Begleiter, Porjesz, Bihari, & Kissin, 1984), and bipolar psychosis (Salisbury, Shenton, & McCarley, 1999). The P50 gating abnormality is more common in schizophrenia than in other psychiatric conditions, but patients with any serious psychiatric condition may show some degree of reduced gating (Baker et al., 1987; Yee, Nuechterlein, & Dawson, 1998). Psychotic patients with mania are indistinguishable from schizophrenia patients in terms of their P50 gating evoked potentials (Waldo et al., 1986).

In view of these findings, the specificity of the six putative marker tasks has not been demonstrated. Eye tracking seems to have the most specific relationship to schizophrenia. There is no compelling evidence to support the specificity of the P300 evoked potential, while all the tasks have difficulty discriminating schizophrenia from manic or bipolar mood disorder patients. Accordingly, specificity research provides little compensation for the equivocal sensitivity and stability findings; indeed the validity of the tasks as markers is called further into question.

The possible reasons for weak specificity are the same as those for weak sensitivity and low marker prevalence in the illness. The diagnosis may be at fault; some "schizophrenia" patients may actually have, say, bipolar illness with psychosis. This then leads to poor discrimination between groups of inaccurately diagnosed patients. Conversely, diagnosis may be accurate but the marker task may be incidental or peripheral to the disease process or may only "mark" a subpopulation of patients, perhaps those with a distinct pathological variant of schizophrenia. There is no easy way out of this scientific conundrum except to discover a valid marker that could serve as a true gold standard for the diagnosis of schizophrenia. And it seems that all of the candidates considered here fall well short of such an ideal.

In conclusion, specificity research generally underscores the questionable status of the attention-related and psychophysiological tasks as disease markers. Even if an abnormal task performance occurs only in schizophrenia and not in any comparison illness, low prevalence or instability of the marker in schizophrenia creates problems of interpretation. Thus eye-tracking dysfunction may be relatively specific to schizophrenia; it seldom occurs in other illnesses. But large numbers of schizophrenia patients have normal tracking. Inevitably, the absence of powerful and convincing findings on the sensitivity front constrains research on specificity. Perversely, the best marker from the standpoint of sensitivity, the P50 gating effect, with an average d of 1.55, has inadequate support for specificity. All in all, the current state of trait marker research on schizophrenia is that none of the tasks show unequivocal specificity to the illness.

Marking Genes

Despite the inadequacy and ambiguity of marker research, the story of illness markers for schizophrenia does not end with the issues of sensitivity and specificity. The possibility has also been explored that putative marker traits are inherited along with the illness, thereby qualifying them as genetic trait markers. In theory, a person who shows the marker trait will eventually show schizophrenia as well, having inherited both the illness gene and the trait. It follows that the marker trait must show signs of being genetically transmitted from parents to offspring. The marker should be apparent in the relatives of patients with schizophrenia, especially those relatives who have a close genetic relationship to the patient and those who develop the illness themselves. In other words, parents and children of a person with schizophrenia must show telltale signs of carrying both the marker and the genetic vulnerability to the illness (see Iacono, 1985).

The methodology needed to study putative markers in terms of genetic criteria seems obvious at first glance: test people known to have a first-degree relative—parent, child, sibling—with schizophrenia, and then "follow" these people to see if they show the marker and develop the illness. Concurrently, examine the healthy relatives of ill patients to see if they lack the marker trait as well as the illness. Yet because the genetic liability for illness in first-degree relatives is so low (10–12%), the vast majority of patients will not have schizophrenic relatives. So it is hard to find enough cases to study. In addition, the onset of schizophrenia is most frequent early in the third decade of life for men and somewhat later for women. Thus, even with a candidate marker and young "at risk" subjects in hand, the researcher will have to wait many years to see who shows the marker and who actually becomes ill. Nonetheless, despite these obstacles and drawbacks, work has proceeded to gather evidence that several of the attention-related and psychophysiological tasks are not only illness traits but genetic markers as well.

Each of the six putative marker tasks has received some support in terms of its heritability and increased prevalence in subjects at risk for developing schizophrenia. Smooth pursuit eye-tracking researchers have marshaled considerable evidence that first-degree relatives of schizophrenia patients show elevated rates of eye-tracking deviance (Levy et al., 1993). There is also evidence that Continuous Performance Test scores are under genetic influence (Cornblatt et al., 1989; Grove et al., 1991; Judd Finkelstein et al., 1997). There is less abundant support for digit span distractibility (Harvey, Winters, Weintraub, & Neale, 1981), but the P300 (Blackwood et al., 1991) and the P50 evoked potentials (Braff, 1993; Clementz, Geyer, & Braff, 1998) seem to be familial. Siegel et al. (1984) reported that about half of the first-degree relatives of schizophrenia patients had abnormal P50 waveforms. This could mean that the P50 has a straightforward kind of dominant gene transmission. However, linkages to specific chromosomal locations have been relatively unsuccessful, and the genetic basis for the P50 is probably complex (see Adler et al., 1998). Backward masking has been studied in personality types "at risk" for schizophrenia, like schizotypal personality, but the masking task has received little study in biological relatives of patients with the illness itself (Saccuzzo & Schubert, 1981; Balogh & Merritt, 1987).

The interpretation of this support for a genetic, or at least familial, basis for the putative markers must be informed with two qualifying principles. First, wide ranges of behaviors, from reading ability to intelligence to psychopathology, show genetic influence, if not genetic control (Plomin et al., 1994). Accordingly, it is not surprising that the cognitive and psychophysiological performance of schizophrenia patients resembles the performance of their first-degree relatives more closely than the performance of the general population. This resemblance is not a unique property of the psychophysiological tasks proposed as markers and does not necessarily tie the marker to the illness. Second, schizophrenia patients are likely to be disadvantaged relative to healthy people on a variety of behavioral tasks by virtue of their mental illness and its negative effect on general cognitive efficiency (Chapman & Chapman, 1973; Heinrichs & Zakzanis, 1998; Miller, Chapman, Chapman, & Collins, 1995). So any comparison between a patient and a healthy person, relative or not, is likely to reveal a disadvantaged patient.

These principles are important to keep in mind because the evidence showing that markers run in the families of schizophrenia patients and segregate with ill relatives seems to be convincing support for a genetic marker. However, this is only conditional and very tentative support. Much more specific questions have to be asked and answered. For example, are any of the putative markers useful in predicting which relative of a schizophrenic individual will also become ill? The short answer to this question is no. None of the markers are found invariably in a majority of patients with the illness, and none of the markers can accurately predict who will develop it (see chapter 7).

In the case of eye-tracking disorder, the "latent trait" hypothesis has been advanced to account for the fact that some people who are at genetic risk for schizophrenia do not have deviant eye tracking and still go on to develop the illness (Matthysse, Holzman, & Lange, 1986; Holzman & Matthysse, 1990). At the same time, some at-risk individuals have poor eye tracking but never become ill, and some have healthy relatives who also show only the trait and no schizophrenic illness. According to latent trait theory, a person may inherit a genetic liability that expresses itself as eye-tracking deviance, or as schizophrenia, or both.

The marker concept has also been broadened to include sensitivity to a spectrum of vulnerabilities and characteristics in addition to schizophrenia itself (Iacono, 1998). The eye-tracking tasks described in this chapter may work as markers of a more general "endophenotype" if they do not work as markers of a schizophrenic disease state. This endophenotype may include personality characteristics and cognitive traits that are loosely linked to schizophrenia. Yet the very complexity of such a notion shows how far the marker concept has strayed from the basic idea of identifying cases with a specific disorder. The association between putative markers like eye tracking and schizophrenic illness is indeed loose and uncertain, and demonstrating that there is some degree of heritability in this connection does not resolve the uncertainty.

Conclusions

The study of potential illness markers for schizophrenia has arisen in part because of dissatisfaction with the vagaries of symptoms and personal history as the basis for identifying cases of the illness. The quest for markers has also arisen because of the hope that their successful discovery will pave the way for breakthroughs in understanding like those achieved with other diseases. Researchers and clinicians alike seek objective signposts to flag the nascent illness, signposts that allow its wandering course and hidden origins to be charted, if not explained.

In some ways, the evaluation of marker candidates can be thought of as a race composed of hurdles. The first hurdle is prevalence or sensitivity. If schizophrenia is a single disease state, how well does the putative marker identify people with this disease? The next hurdle is the requirement for stability and independence from clinical state influences like medication or symptoms. Then come specificity and the question of whether a marker candidate occurs selectively in schizophrenia or unselectively in a variety of psychiatric and medical conditions. Finally, the hurdle of heritability looms before candidate markers that seek the greatest prize—success as a genetic marker, the sign that follows the illness through families and into chromosomes.

This chapter has focused most on the first hurdle, the prevalence or sensitivity of candidate markers. This topic is seldom addressed directly in traditional literature reviews (e.g., Iacono, 1985; Levy et al., 1993, 1994; Szymanski et al., 1991), yet it is arguably the most important criterion for an illness marker, and its omission in favor of a concern with other problems like heritability or stability is puzzling.

There are numerous prospective candidates for markers of schizophrenia, and I have considered only six from a meta-analytic standpoint. Of these six marker candidates, all but the P50 evoked potential abnormality fare equivocally or even badly at the first hurdle. The P50 abnormality, which seems to reflect an inability to filter, dampen, or habituate to sensory experience, has the largest average effect size of the candidate markers and therefore probably has the highest prevalence, in schizophrenia of all candidate markers. It is difficult to be precise about prevalence, because effect sizes and associated overlap statistics are only idealized approximations and sample prevalence rates are rarely reported. It would help if all researchers indicated prevalence in their patient samples based on the two standard deviation cutoff as a matter of course, but they do not. The P50 abnormality may occur in up to 87% of schizophrenia patients, if the available studies are accurate and represent the field as a whole (see table 3.1). From this standpoint it is the best of the putative markers, and if it does not sail over the first hurdle, at least it is still in the running.

Unfortunately, the available evidence also suggests that the P50 falters at the second and third hurdles, making its performance at the final obstacle of genetic criteria largely irrelevant. The P50 abnormality waxes and wanes with the patient's emotional state and improves with antipsychotic medication. It may occur widely in illnesses other than schizophrenia. Therefore, the P50 is at best a generic psychopathology episode marker. The gating defect may flag any serious mental illness and come and go with the rise and fall of symptoms and acute distress that most psychiatric patients must endure. Indeed, the disorder in question may turn out to be a mood disturbance rather than schizophrenia. Moreover, the P50 abnormality could disappear the next time a patient is tested. It is unlikely that many clinicians or researchers will consider the P50 to be a helpful tool in diagnostic decision-making.

None of the other tasks do as well as the P50 in terms of the primary obstacle of showing high prevalence in schizophrenia patients. However, there is intriguing evidence that a reliable index of eye tracking, root mean squared error, identifies a subset of patients within the schizophrenia population, a subset who may have a different kind of illness. In addition, this aspect of eyetracking outperforms the other candidates at the stability and specificity hurdles, although its genetic aspects are complex and hard to interpret. In recent years researchers have been turning to eye-tracking measures as a way of parsing schizophrenia into component disorders.

Several of the other marker candidates may also harbor complex distributions that reflect the existence of multiple schizophrenic illnesses. These candidates include the Continuous Performance Test, which has the advantages of easy administration and relative simplicity when compared with tasks like eye-movement tracking and evoked potentials. Unfortunately, this attention measure exists in many versions, and some appear to be influenced by a patient's clinical state and treatment.

The visual backward-masking effect does well at the first hurdle, with a strong average effect size. This task bears some psychological resemblance to the P50 abnormality in that both seem to involve the perceptual consequences of stimulus order, of sequential mental events and their interactions. Perhaps the two tasks are related in some way. However, the trait status of backward masking has to be resolved, and there is little research evidence supporting its specificity to schizophrenia or its genetic basis.

Ironically, the most frequently studied marker candidate, the P300 evoked potential, fares poorly in many respects. The P300 is at best a generic marker for mental illness, and even then its prevalence in schizophrenia is too low to make it really useful from a diagnostic standpoint.

Simply put, there are no convincing attention-related or psychophysiological markers for schizophrenia. On closer examination, the very concept of a behavioral or psychological marker, rooted in both biology and behavior, is suspect. Behavioral markers may not exist for any illness. There is a very heavy assumption at work here: that attention-related behavior is in some way analogous to physical traits like eye color and blood type or analogous to microbiology and chromosomal abnormalities. This assumption has received little discussion or justification and may be completely misguided and indefensible. Behavior is indeed mediated by biology and influenced by genetic factors. The evidence in favor of such influence is overwhelming. However, the relationship between genes, biology, behavior, and illnesses like schizophrenia is not absolute or sufficiently direct to make finding a behavioral illness marker a feasible project. If the candidate markers "mark" anything, it is a fragmented illness or perhaps several illnesses—or perhaps they mark a wide spectrum of vulnerabilities that may or may not lead to psychopathology. These possibilities remain largely unexamined and unexplored, but they seem to indicate where marker research is headed in the future (see Cadenhead, Light, Geyer, & Braff, 2000; Iacono, 1998).

Finally, even the markers with a physiological component, like eye tracking and evoked brain potentials, only hint at the neural intricacies that underlie madness. The failure of marker research makes the need to look directly at the schizophrenic brain apparent. After all, marker research never promised an explanation for madness, just signposts to describe its outlines and a way of detecting its presence with certainty. To find explanations for schizophrenia it is necessary to leave the hurdles of marker research behind and to pursue the illness into the brain.

4

···············

EXECUTIVE
INCOMPETENCE

Why does the brain generate spurious experience? Why does it create the plagues of voices, the unfounded suspicion and impossible beliefs, and then the gray desolation of the schizophrenic mind? The brain, the organ of the mind, acquires knowledge of the world and experience and then reshapes and twists this knowledge into the strange forms and elaborate counterfeit of psychosis. What peculiar fault of neurology allows this to take place?

At the turn of the century, researchers and clinicians wondered about the answers to these questions. They could turn to two schools of thought for guidance. On the one hand, there was an evolving medical science that had already made breakthroughs in locating some behavioral disturbances, including the aphasias—language impairments within the brain. In other words, they could seek the neurogenesis of schizophrenia: the disordered brain that must underlie disordered thought and feeling. Or, in a very different vein, they could look to the new field of psychoanalysis and seek the genesis of the illness in the unconscious secrets of family life and the intimate failures of parents.

Consider the first option. The research techniques available to the neuroscientists of the early twentieth century were limited largely to clinical observation of patient behavior and to post-mortem inspection of the human brain. Nevertheless, these techniques had borne fruit in the case of expressive aphasia, the loss of speech despite preserved comprehension, that was seen frequently in stroke survivors. Broca (1861) had localized expressive aphasia to a lesion of the third frontal convolution of the left cerebral hemisphere (figure 4.1). Similarly,

Wernicke (1874) localized sensory aphasia, wherein speech was fluent but non-sensical while comprehension was impaired, to lesions involving the superior temporal convolution and the area around the Sylvian fissure (see chapter 5). Localization of other disabilities of mental life followed. Defective arithmetic calculation (Lewandowsky & Stadelmann, 1908) and impaired block construction and spatial skills (Kleist, 1923; Poppelreuter, 1917) were linked with damage to specific brain regions. It seemed as if the major categories of behavior and behavioral disorder could be mapped onto the brain. Unfortunately, however, schizophrenia did not join the list of localized disturbances. The inspection of post-mortem brain tissue yielded no lesions that could be ascribed convincingly to the illness instead of to the cause of death. This resulted in many years of pessimism and neglect in the search for brain abnormalities that might underpin schizophrenia (see Shorter, 1997, pp. 69–112).

At the same time that researchers were looking unsuccessfully for the neuropathology of schizophrenia, psychoanalysts theorized about possible psychological causes of the illness. These theories emphasized the formative role of parenting (Fromm-Reichmann, 1948), childhood experience (Alanen, Hagglund, Harkonen & Kunnenen, 1968), and destructive family dynamics (Bateson, Jackson, Haley, & Weakland, 1956; Laing & Esterson, 1964) in psychopathology. Such ideas held sway for several decades. Psychoanalysts even tried psychotherapy with schizophrenia patients to help resolve the infantile traumas and early rejection experiences that were believed to cause the disease. Although its power in Europe was never pervasive, by the 1960s the psychoanalytic approach dominated North American psychiatry (Shorter, 1997, pp. 145–189).

Then, with gathering momentum, a revitalized biological psychiatry emerged in the 1970s and 1980s (see Andreasen, 1985). Lack of scientific support, new drug therapies (see Chapter 6), and a changing intellectual climate forced psychogenic approaches to recede in favor of a return to the neurogenic view of serious mental illness. With the advent of powerful new instruments for observing the brain and with the harvest of decades of basic research in brain biology in hand, madness became, once more, a puzzle for the neuroscientist to solve.

The Search for the Schizophrenic Lesion

If schizophrenia is a brain disorder, where in the brain does the pathology lie, and what is its nature? Neurological damage may be a consequence of vascular insufficiency, whereby blood supply to neurons is reduced, causing the death of brain tissue, as in stroke. It may arise in the form of neoplasia, where tumors displace or infiltrate the neural architecture of the brain. In common dementias

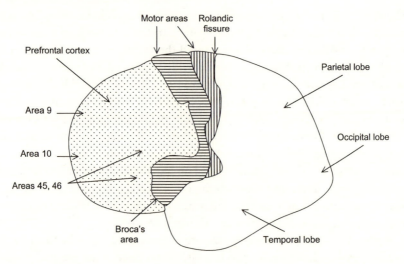

Figure 4.1. The frontal lobe of the human brain. The figure shows a lateral view of the left cerebral hemisphere. The primary and secondary motor regions are indicated, along with Broca's expressive speech center and several Brodmann areas of the prefrontal cortex. The functions of the prefrontal region are primarily psychological, poorly understood, and of special interest in relation to schizophrenia.

like Alzheimer's disease, nerve cells degenerate, lose connections to other nerve cells, and die. Still other pathological agents break down the supportive cellular structure or insulating sheath around nerve cells, as in the demyelinating diseases like multiple sclerosis. Infectious processes and inflammation have their own destructive role to play in neurological disease. And brain disorder may occur in the course of neural development, even before birth, so that normal neuroanatomical systems fail to form or function.

Brain damage not only has many causes, it can be coarse or subtle, static or progressive in nature, and it may occur at many levels of observation, from the manifest to the molecular. Neuropathology is often selective and prejudicial, striking preferentially at certain structures or systems and leaving others untouched. Thus the herpes virus that causes encephalitis has a predilection for inflaming the medial temporal lobe as it creeps along the trigeminal nerve (Walton, 1985, p. 280). Small hemorrhages associated with the thiamine deficiency in alcoholic Korsakoff's syndrome occur primarily in the medial thalamus and mammillary bodies near the base of the brain (Walton, 1985, p. 654). Neurological disease can be surprisingly discriminating in what it strikes and what it spares.

The early brain researchers quickly ruled out coarse, obvious brain damage, like strokes and tumors, degeneration, hydrocephalus, and similar pathologies, as a likely cause of schizophrenia. It was known that the pathology of madness must be subtler, of a different order, and must exist at the cellular or neuro-chemical level. And special techniques would be needed to find this subtle pathology. But where to look?

One of the first brain regions postulated as a site for schizophrenia was the frontal or, more accurately, the prefrontal region of the brain. It comprises about a third of the human cerebrum and is intricately and extensively connected with other cerebral structures and regions (see figure 4.1). Moreover, the frontal lobes appear to be especially well developed and prominent in humans, as opposed to lower animals (Heilman & Valenstein, 1993, p. 14). Therefore, this brain region must be involved in capacities that are inherently human in nature: higher intellectual skills and reasoning, language, self-awareness, planning, imagination and—madness? Surely the same brain region is also involved in schizophrenia, the most human of mental illnesses.

The psychiatric pioneers believed that capacities ascribed to the frontal brain were affected in schizophrenia (e.g., Kraepelin, 1919, p. 219). A series of case studies of people with frontal brain damage showed that personality change, impaired self-awareness, disorganization, loss of emotional inhibition, and inappropriate social behavior were common consequences of damage to this brain area (Ackerly & Benton, 1948; Brickner, 1934, 1936; Harlow, 1848, 1868; Hebb & Penfield, 1940). Likewise, schizophrenia patients often spoke incoherently, engaged in distorted reasoning, lacked planning ability, and seemed bereft of insight into their condition. Bleuler (1950) observed that the illness involved a kind of disintegration of the personality and alteration of normal emotional life. At least on the surface there were provocative similarities between schizophrenia and frontal brain disease.

More recently, as well, researchers have drawn further parallels between the behavior of schizophrenia patients and the behavior of neurological patients with prefrontal lesions (e.g., Benson & Stuss, 1990; Randolph, Goldberg, & Weinberger, 1993; Weinberger, 1988). Although few researchers are willing to argue that schizophrenia is exclusively a frontal brain disorder, the frontal hypothesis represents and remains one of the earliest and most consistent attempts to relate the illness to a specific brain system. But before evidence bearing on this attempt can be appreciated (table 4.1), more basic information about the structure and function of the human frontal lobes must be considered.

Neuroanatomical Landscape of the Frontal Brain

One remarkable and rather obvious feature of the frontal lobes is their relative size and the proportion of cerebral volume they occupy (figure 4.1). The Rolandic and Sylvian fissures border the frontal lobes in the cortex. The corpus callosum, the large band of nerve fibers that connects the two cerebral hemispheres, forms another boundary deep within the brain. Neuroanatomists have subdivided the frontal lobes in a number of ways. The sides, or lateral convex cortical surface, are termed the dorsolateral cortex, the floor or base of the lobe that rests in the cranial orbit is termed the orbital-basal cortex, and the region between the left and right frontal lobes is termed the mesial area.

Immediately in front of the Rolandic or central fissure is the motor strip, a long convolution of gray matter, a gyrus that extends from the dorsolateral into the mesial area. This is a famous region in neurology. In the 1870s Gustav Fritsch and Eduard Hitzig discovered that the prefrontal gyrus mediates the control of movement and does so in a highly specific or somatotopic fashion (see Fancher, 1996, pp. 90–91). Parts of the body, the hands, limbs and face, project onto discrete areas of the motor strip. Accordingly, damage to this area in the form of a disease like stroke produces paralysis of the body parts that are represented at the site of stroke. The brain is no longer able to direct movement because the "command and control" center for movement has been damaged.

The supplementary motor cortex and the premotor area are large regions in front of the precentral gyrus or motor strip. As the names imply, these areas also have motor functions. However, instead of simple movements, the secondary motor regions seem to mediate complex movements that comprise a series of related steps. Damage here may not prevent a person from, say, opening and closing their hand, but it may prevent them from using a computer keyboard or even buttoning a coat. Broca's area, identified with speech production, lies just below and in front of the premotor cortex.

Stretching out in front of both the motor and premotor areas is an even larger expanse of cortex, termed the prefrontal cortex. This is the area that clinicians and researchers often conflate with the more inclusive term "frontal lobes." One small area, the frontal eye fields, is involved in mediating the smooth pursuit eye movements described as a putative marker of schizophrenia in chapter 3. However, most of the functions ascribed to the prefrontal cortex are psychological, relating to attention, mental flexibility and planning, high-level or "executive" control functions, and the regulation of motivation and emotion.

At the microscopic level the cortex differentiates itself into layers of nerve cells or neurons. The traditional division for the prefrontal cortex includes six layers, whereas other brain regions may comprise fewer layers. As a general rule, the upper four cortical cell layers are recipients of neural messages from other brain regions. In contrast, the deeper layers send axons and information out to the rest of the brain. The neurons distribute themselves in varying densities across the different layers and across the different cortical subregions. Thus in the primary motor area of the frontal lobes there are many more neurons in layer V than in layer IV. However, frontal areas outside the primary motor region have greater densities of neurons in the upper neocortical layers (I–III).

The neurons themselves are also described and classified in various ways. Pyramidal cells, which are very roughly described by their shape, occur in layers II, III, and V. They project to other brain regions. Stellate neurons, also termed interneurons, are roughly star-shaped. They receive input from regions below the cortex and provide interconnections within layers and between incoming and outgoing neurotransmission. They are especially common in the middle cortical layers.

Further, increasingly complex subdivisions of the frontal system can be made on the basis of neuronal structure and function. This is the field of architectonics, and associated maps, like those of Brodmann (1909), provide further articulation of the frontal brain landscape. Thus the dorsolateral prefrontal cortex is fractionated into areas 9, 10, 45, and 46, based on features of cellular architecture (see figure 4.1). And this is not to mention the intricacies introduced by neurochemical properties of individual neurons and neuronal systems (see chapter 6). It stands to reason that observation and measurement of brain tissue at this microscopic level requires sophisticated technologies that are most easily applied to the human brain after death, when it can be preserved, dissected, and analyzed in detail. It also stands to reason that neurological abnormalities at this level may be hard to detect with instruments that lack the requisite degree of sensitivity and resolving power.

Another major feature of the frontal brain region is the degree of interconnection within and between frontal areas and the rest of the cerebrum. The prefrontal cortex is connected directly to the premotor cortex, which in turn connects to the motor strip. In addition, there are extensive links between the frontal area and the temporal, parietal, and occipital lobes. These links have been studied more thoroughly in monkeys than in humans (see Pandya & Yetarian, 1996). However, the available evidence indicates that most areas of visual (occipital), auditory (temporal), and somatosensory (parietal) cortex project to the frontal lobes. In reciprocal fashion, the frontal areas project to each of the postcentral lobes, especially to the temporal lobe.

Some of the most interesting and psychologically important brain structures are found below the cortical surface. Here, too, the frontal brain has numerous reciprocal connections. There are projections to frontal areas from the hypothalamus, amygdala, and hippocampus. The ties from the amygdala and hippocampus to the orbital-medial frontal region are particularly strong. The amygdala is a neural structure implicated in emotional behavior, and the hippocampus is critical for memory formation (see chapter 4). Another vital subcortical structure that projects to frontal areas is the thalamus. The thalamus is a complex structure comprised of nuclei that contribute to memory and sensory processing. It also has a relay function whereby the prefrontal cortex is linked via the thalamus to diverse other brain systems and to the peripheral nervous system.

The frontal region receives fibers from many other brain regions, but the frontal lobes also send their own projections outward, and these projections probably exercise an influence on numerous neural systems. Thus the medial-orbital frontal cortex sends projections directly to the amygdala and indirectly to the hippocampus. There are projections to many other subcortical structures, including the septum, the thalamus, and the striatum. The striatum, for example, comprises parts of the basal ganglia, an important group of nuclei that mediate some aspects of movement and motor skill (see chapter 7). Frontal regions also project to the claustrum, to the subthalamic and red nuclei, and to the central gray area.

The most common interpretation of the high degree of reciprocity and linkage between frontal and nonfrontal brain regions is that frontal neural activity both mediates and is mediated by the rest of the brain (Luria, 1978; Kolb & Whishaw, 1996, pp. 307–310). The frontal brain seems to be equipped anatomically to integrate and coordinate what the rest of the brain does. This kind of formulation has led most investigators to assign a superordinate or executive control function to the prefrontal regions of the brain. That sounds fine in theory, but what do these brain regions really contribute to mind and behavior, and how much do we know about this contribution?

The Frontal Brain and Its Mind

An early and attractive idea was that the frontal brain governs the highest mental processes, from intellectual synthesis and abstraction to ethical behavior and judgment. This idea persisted in simple form until Hebb (Hebb & Penfield, 1940, 1945) provided dramatic evidence that conventional measures of intelligence, like the IQ test, were unaffected by surgical removal of large amounts of frontal brain tissue. How could this be? Clearly, frontal brain activity was more complex and also less obvious than initial speculations suggested. Whatever the frontal brain did, it was hard to grasp objectively and could not be captured with the visual puzzles and verbal problems posed by standard intelligence tests.

As a result, during the first half of this century, views of the frontal brain region ranged widely between overstatement and dismissal. On the one hand, it was the seat of the highest intellectual processes and the springboard for human advance over other animals. On the other hand, the frontal brain had no demonstrable involvement with measured intelligence (see Damasio & Anderson, 1993, pp. 416–419). At the same time, it was apparent that the frontal brain was not exclusively cognitive in nature. Like schizophrenia, frontal brain disorders involved emotional and social problems. In fact, the earliest descriptions of the effects of frontal damage were basically case histories that documented personality change and altered interpersonal behavior (e.g., Harlow, 1848, 1868). Indeed, it often appeared as if frontal damage revealed itself more directly in loss of emotional inhibitions and in altered social behavior than in loss of intellectual ability. However, the apparent independence of intellectual function from the frontal brain diminished as neuropsychologists developed tasks that provide glimpses of what the frontal brain really does, even if these glimpses seem remarkably diverse and hard to integrate.

Neuropsychological Studies of the Frontal Lobes

Perhaps the best-known behavioral effect of frontal brain lesions is the expressive aphasia or speech disturbance that Broca (1861) associated with lesions of the third frontal convolution of the left hemisphere. However, other language-related deficits have also been observed, and some of these deficits occur following lesions to the prefrontal cortex in front of Broca's area (see figure 4.1). One of the most common deficits is an inability to generate words rapidly and fluently. According to studies with healthy people, the average person can come up with a total of 30-35 words that begin with letters like *F*, *A*, and *S* in three one-minute trials (see Lezak, 1995, pp. 544–546). Milner (1964) and Benton (1968) initiated studies showing that patients who had sustained surgical removal of frontal brain tissue generated very few words. This "dysfluency" occurred even when the speech area itself was spared any damage and the patients were not aphasic. In addition, Jones-Gotman and Milner (1977) developed a nonverbal analogue of word fluency in the form of a design fluency task. Instead of producing words, subjects were asked to produce geometric shapes as quickly as possible. Patients with frontal damage, especially if it involved the right frontal lobe, performed at below average levels on this nonverbal task. Hence the fluency defect occurred with both language and nonverbal kinds of information, and both cerebral hemispheres appeared to be involved.

Provocative parallels have been noted between word and design generation skills and some aspects of schizophrenia. The difficulty frontal patients have with fluency tasks may reflect a loss of behavioral spontaneity and initiative (Kolb & Whishaw, 1996, pp. 315-316). The same loss has been observed in schizophrenia patients, many of whom seem inexpressive, sluggish, and slow in responding to the environment, while others seem "avolitional," or lacking in will and drive (Andreasen, 1989; Bleuler, 1950; Kraepelin, 1919). Liddle (1994, pp. 43–44) termed this cluster of behaviors the "psychomotor poverty" syndrome. Schizophrenia patients with psychomotor poverty show decreases in blood flow to the left prefrontal region in brain-scanning studies—the same region that influences fluency skills. Here, then, is a suggestive link between the behavior of schizophrenia patients and the behavioral functions of the prefrontal brain region.

Another behavior that is difficult for patients with prefrontal brain lesions involves making judgments about events or objects. For example, patients are often impaired on cognitive estimation tasks that require them to guess prices of common objects (Smith & Milner, 1984) or to answer questions about dimensions, weights, and physical properties (Axelrod & Millis, 1994). These estimation tasks are selected to avoid obvious answers. For example, a patient might be asked to estimate the average length of a man's spine. Frontal lesions seem to induce highly improbable or unrealistic estimations. Other kinds of judgment tasks include those that require the accurate perception of time and how events are embedded in the flow of time. Research participants are shown a series of pictures or words. Periodically, a pair of previously presented pictures or words is shown again and the participant is asked to indicate which word or picture was seen most recently or most frequently in the series. Patients with frontal brain damage have little difficulty remembering what they have seen, but they are poor judges of how often or how recently they have seen it (Milner, Corsi, & Leonard, 1991; Smith & Milner, 1988). Hence the ability to locate single and repeated events in their correct temporal order seems to be an aspect of executive cognition (see also Tulving et al., 1994; Tulving, Markowitsch, Craik, Habib, & Houle, 1996).

Frontal brain damage does not appear to cause memory impairment in the everyday sense. However, there are several tasks that involve learning, or changing behavior in response to feedback, and these are compromised by frontal damage. For example, Petrides and associates (1985, 1990; Petrides, Alivasatos, Meyer, & Evans, 1993; Canavan et al., 1989) have shown the importance of the prefrontal brain in conditional or associative learning. This involves learning to associate, say, a color with a spatial location, or a color with a hand position. Patients with prefrontal lesions are poor learners of such tasks in comparison with healthy people or in comparison with patients who have damage elsewhere in the brain.

More conceptual and abstract kinds of learning have also been studied. One of the most popular clinical tasks is the Wisconsin Card Sorting Test (Heaton, 1981; Heaton, Chelune, Talley, Kay, & Curtiss, 1993). Most versions involve presenting four "key" cards that depict different shapes, colors, and quantities. The person taking the test is provided with a succession of cards and asked to match each one to a key card. Cards may match on the basis of color, shape, or number, but only one matching principle is "correct" at a given time. The examiner controls the matching principle and gives feedback about the correctness of each attempted match without ever disclosing the actual principle. Then, after a succession of correct matches, the examiner changes to a new principle (e.g., shape instead of color) without telling the test-taker. The object of the test is to discover the new principle each time it changes and to respond with correct matches.

The Wisconsin Card Sorting Test is easy for healthy people with average intelligence. But Milner (1963) showed that patients with neurosurgical excisions of lateral prefrontal cortex achieved abnormally few successively correct matches, or "categories." They also tended to repeat or perseverate erroneous responses. However, more recent studies have cast doubt on the idea that the test has a specific sensitivity to the frontal brain. Many neurological patients without frontal damage also find the test hard, and some patients with frontal damage manage surprisingly good scores (Anderson, Damasio, Jones, & Tranel, 1991; Heaton et al., 1993).

Another task that requires conceptual learning and problem solving is the Tower of Hanoi and its derivatives, the Tower of Toronto and the Tower of London (see Lezak, 1995, pp. 657–658). Subjects are given a board with three pegs and asked to move from three to five disks of different sizes from one peg to another, with the requirement that the disks are kept in the same order. The third peg can be used to "park" disks during the transition (Morris et al., 1988; Saint-Cyr, Taylor, & Lang, 1988; Shallice, 1982). Several studies have shown that patients with frontal brain lesions are particularly slow or unsuccessful at this task (e.g., Goel & Graffman, 1995).

On the face of it, problem-solving tests like the Tower paradigm engage anticipation, planning, and decision-making about alternate courses of action. However, Goel and Graffman (1995) point out that the Tower puzzle is not a true planning task. The person taking the test is allowed to reverse or change individual moves and therefore does not really have to "think ahead" to any great extent. All incorrect moves can be reversed, making it more of a trial-and-error procedure than a planning task.

Problems with mental inhibition and initiation, the use of experience to guide behavior, crop up in some form in many of the tasks used to find the primary cognitive defect caused by frontal brain damage. Moreover, even some tasks that are termed tests of attention appear to require the ability to inhibit and initiate behavior in a smooth and flexible manner. The Stroop task (MacLeod, 1991; Stroop, 1935) is a case in point. When people are presented with a list of color words like "red," "blue," and "green" printed in inks that do not match the word meaning, they can read the words as quickly as if they were printed in black ink. However, when they are asked to name the color of the ink instead of reading the word, performance slows down. It takes most people much longer to name the ink colors of discrepant color words (e.g. the word "green" printed in red ink) than to simply name ink colors of printed shapes. The increased time required for color-naming discrepant words is called the Stroop effect.

There is evidence that patients with definite or probable frontal damage have exaggerated Stroop effects (Brown & Marsden, 1988; Perret, 1974). Similarly, Owen, Roberts, Polkey, Sahakian, & Robbins (1991) found that even with nonverbal material, patients with frontal lesions are slow to shift between different aspects (e.g., visual shapes versus visual patterns) of information when solving a problem. Thus mental flexibility and the ability to inhibit incorrect responses without losing sight of the "big picture" or overriding goal seem to be involved in this classic test of selective attention.

Most recently, the construct of "working memory" has been proposed as an aspect of frontal function (Baddeley & Hitch, 1994; Gathercole, 1994). The term is slightly misleading and does not actually refer to the activity of a generic memory system in an everyday sense. Working memory is the active maintenance of information in awareness to serve or guide behavioral goals and purposes. The concept is similar to the idea of a computer's random access memory (RAM), a storage capacity that keeps information "on-line" to serve processing requirements. However, this on-line capacity is more than just a brief store of information. Working memory comes into play whenever information must be manipulated or analyzed in some way, kept in awareness, and used to accomplish a goal or task. For example, a straightforward digit span test where a person has to repeat a long string of numbers is really just a test of immediate memory. However, if the person has to repeat the number string with the number order reversed, working memory is required (see Lezak, 1995, p. 367). The number string has to be kept available, or "in mind," and it has to be manipulated concurrently to accomplish the task requirement. The same ability has been implicated in skills as diverse as mental arithmetic, sentence processing, and vocabulary learning (Gathercole, 1994). In some ways, working memory refers to nothing less than the conscious control of behavior. Hence it must play a role in abilities like planning and problem solving that require a person to hold and manipulate information in consciousness. In other words, working memory must play a role in most of the cognitive tasks that have been studied in relation to the frontal brain.

None of the various tests of executive cognition can be regarded as a definitive neuropsychological test of frontal brain activity. No such test exists. Many cognitive tests show some sensitivity to frontal damage, but inconsistencies and equivocal findings dog the field (e.g., Anderson et al., 1991). Indeed, clinicians and the relatives of neurological patients with frontal damage know that even specialized cognitive tests may not capture a patient's essential disability. Instead, the disability is seen in daily life: a sudden apathy and carelessness, a loss of social awareness, a declining capacity for empathy. The effects of frontal brain damage may involve emotion and personality as much as they involve cognitive skills and functions.

For example, I recall a man from my own clinical experience, a man who had a left frontal stroke in middle age. Although he was impaired on some cognitive tests, his intelligence was in the superior range and his recovery was regarded as complete. Shortly after discharge he wrote one of his rehabilitation therapists a passionate and sexually explicit love letter, suggesting that the two of them run away together to another country. Not surprisingly, the patient's wife and family were upset and shocked when he, without any hesitation, disclosed the contents of the letter to them after the therapist complained. This impulsive, uninhibited behavior was a complete change for someone who had been straitlaced, considerate, and emotionally controlled before his stroke. His own reaction to the whole event was one of mild amusement, and he appeared bewildered by the strength of the emotional responses of his family and the therapist. It was as if he could not understand why they might be upset.

In another case the dissociation between standard cognitive measures and social behavior was even more striking. A school vice-principal was referred to me for neuropsychological assessment after a car accident. A brain scan revealed frontal lobe contusions but no other focal brain damage. I was unable to detect *any* cognitive deficits when I tested him with an 8-hour battery of measures, including the Wisconsin Card Sorting Test, fluency tests, problem-solving and intelligence measures, and other tasks. His general intelligence, for example, was superior. Nonetheless, he experienced serious problems at work and had been passed over for promotion and almost fired because of his inappropriate social behavior. These social problems included making sexual comments in class to his students, which they subsequently reported to their parents. In addition, at parents' association and school board meetings he cracked jokes and told people not to take life so seriously. Like the first case, this man was surprised that his behavior elicited negative reactions, and he showed no ability to consider the impact of his behavior on other people. Asked to indicate if, in his own view, he experienced any interpersonal difficulties, his response was invariably no.

This kind of social awareness deficit is remarkably similar to the "theory of mind" deficits that Frith (1994) has described in relation to schizophrenia. (These deficits were outlined in chapter 2.) The person with no theory of mind is unable to imagine another person's mental life or perspective. They are unable to put themselves in another person's shoes. As a result such people develop faulty inferences about the intentions of other people, leading to delusions, and perhaps leading to the defective social awareness of both the schizophrenia and the frontal lobe patient.

Such clinical cases illustrate two related points concerning psychological functions of the frontal brain. First, these functions are not always tapped by putative executive-frontal cognitive tests and instead tend to emerge in the realistic context of everyday life and in response to the demands of work and family. Second, the effects of frontal damage cannot be regarded exclusively in cognitive terms. Emotional life, self-awareness, personality, social attitudes, and interpersonal skills often appear to be more altered than cognitive abilities by frontal damage (Damasio & Anderson, 1993, pp. 419–427).

The tie between schizophrenia and the frontal brain would be strengthened if research showed that neurological patients with frontal lesions experience delusions as well as social problems and impaired self-awareness. Here the evidence is very scant but nonetheless intriguing. In rare cases, awareness-related deficits after frontal brain injury take a severe and profound form as disturbances of consciousness. Benson and Stuss (1990) gathered together several of these cases wherein patients appear to suffer from delusional beliefs about their surroundings. One type of delusional belief is termed reduplicative paramnesia. A person with this disorder believes that he is no longer in the hospital or at home but in some previously experienced environment. For example, one man was convinced that his hospital was located on a distant army base where he had served many years before. He knew the correct name of his current hospital but relocated it to a different time and place. Brain scans showed frontal brain damage in the form of hematomas and contusions.

From my own clinical experience on a neuropsychiatry ward, I recall a man who had served on a ship in the navy as a pipe fitter and mechanic. He was convinced that he was not in the hospital but back on board ship and in charge of repairing all overhead piping and ductwork. He became a major behavioral problem on the floor because he could often be found perched precariously on an assemblage of chairs, removing ceiling tiles and tampering with water pipes and other mechanical apparatus. He not only placed himself in danger from a fall but managed to dismantle extensive sections of the ward's sprinkler and water supply systems. When confronted he protested that the last thing he wanted to do on his day off was more maintenance work, but "orders are orders" and he was in the navy, so the "repairs" had to be done. Computerized tomography brain scans revealed a very large area of excised right frontal brain tissue due to neurosurgery and an earlier large cerebral hemorrhage. However, he also had nonfrontal and diffuse brain damage, especially affecting the right cerebral hemisphere. He was severely impaired on a variety of cognitive tests, and his intelligence was compatible with dementia rather than with a selective disturbance of consciousness. This broadly based impairment is not peculiar to this case. Reduplicative paramnesia has been associated with several brain regions and not just with the frontal lobes (Feinberg & Shapiro, 1989).

There are other disturbances of consciousness seen in patients with frontal lesions, but a specific connection between lesion site and these bizarre forms of behavior is hard to demonstrate conclusively. Many patients have lesions in nonfrontal as well as frontal areas, and many lesions are very large. In addition, the link with psychotic behavior and symptoms is not as strong as may appear at first glance. For example, reduplication syndromes are qualitatively different from the most common psychotic delusions. In reduplication, the duplicated pasts or environments actually existed at some point. In contrast, delusions like the belief in self-divinity, special powers, or conspiracies and plots are creations, fabrications—and highly implausible ones at that—of the schizophrenia patient. As mentioned, patients with disturbances of consciousness often have large, extensive lesions. Hence it could be argued that the extent or severity of brain damage is more important than the involvement of frontal regions per se in producing these disturbances. Finally, reduplication and related syndromes are very rare. They are seldom reported in literature reviews of frontal behavioral effects and usually consist of occasional single case reports. They do not provide a very firm basis for associating schizophrenia, or its constituent positive symptoms, with the typical behavioral effects of frontal brain dysfunction.

Summary and Assessment of Frontal Brain Function

The frontal regions of the brain mediate a variety of behaviors that range from simple movements to complex movement sequences and speech patterns. These motor-related behaviors are associated with the cortical areas that comprise or border the precentral gyrus. Knowledge concerning more anterior areas, the prefrontal region proper, and reciprocal connections with subcortical and posterior regions is inadequate. A number of executive deficits, involving mental rigidity and poor problem solving, reduced word fluency, and impaired working memory have been discovered. These deficits occur in frontal patients despite their preserved general ability on standard intelligence tests. Hence executive impairment cannot be attributed readily to the effects of global cognitive impairment. Many patients with frontal damage also show defective social and emotional functioning. Yet there is no invariant picture of psychological deficit following frontal brain disease. The frontal lobes are a large and anatomically complex region. Different patients show different kinds of deficits, and many patients with frontal damage perform normally on putative executive control tasks. Therefore, is it possible to characterize or unify all of the psychological processes involved in these tasks and to provide a coherent account of the frontal brain's role in mind and behavior?

In contrast with theoretical ideas that draw primarily on cognitive psychology, Goldman-Rakic (1996; Levy & Goldman-Rakic, 2000) draws heavily on neuroanatomical considerations and on research with nonhuman primates in her approach to executive function. She argues that the dorsolateral prefrontal cortex has a generic working memory function that is used to support a number of cognitive processes. However, she breaks the frontal brain down into divisions, each of which has its own working memory capabilities and its own connections with the rest of the brain. In her view only this kind of anatomically differentiated model can account for the diversity and inconsistency of deficits seen in cases of frontal brain damage and in laboratory animals. Thus primate research suggests that area 9 in the prefrontal cortex (see figure 4.1) is a working memory–processing region that is specialized for visual-spatial information. Lesions in this region prevent animals from revising and remembering the locations of hidden objects. The animal cannot maintain a working memory representation of where things are in space or use these locations to guide behavior. The same region of prefrontal cortex also has connections with motor systems and with portions of the parietal lobe that are specialized for spatial perception. Frontal area 9 acts like a dedicated circuit that controls the sensory, cognitive, and motor aspects of responding to situations that involve changes in spatial location. Goldman-Rakic maintains that the prefrontal area is comprised of numerous working-memory processors and local circuits, each specialized for different kinds of knowledge and behavioral tasks.

This kind of model explains why neurological patients with frontal lesions are not invariably impaired on tasks like card sorting or word fluency and why patients with nonfrontal lesions sometimes have executive deficits. Special-purpose processors are localized in specific regions of the frontal brain, and they have specific connections with the rest of the brain. If the region that supports the processing required by a task like card sorting is spared in frontal brain, damage, then the patient will be able to perform the task. At the same time, damage elsewhere, outside the frontal lobes, may create problems if the sensory-perceptual analysis that card sorting requires is no longer available to the frontal executive.

Theories of frontal function provide a framework that is helpful in understanding the consequences of damage to this brain system. But it is hard to choose between different models of what the frontal brain does. The relevant knowledge base is still undeveloped and insecure. A compendium of cognitive tests and clinical observations has emerged that provides an incomplete and often unreliable but still provocative picture of the frontal lobes as a kind of engine of mind and behavior. And many allusions and parallels to schizophrenia drift through the rich mix of conjecture and data that characterize the frontal brain puzzle. Perhaps the neurobiology of the frontal brain is fundamentally altered in schizophrenia. Perhaps the frontal brain acts not only as the engine of mind and behavior in normal life but, when compromised, as the engine of madness as well.

Schizophrenia and the Frontal Mind

To what extent do the various cognitive and behavioral defects that have been studied in relation to the frontal brain create a picture that resembles schizophrenia? It is clear that frontal damage does not produce positive symptoms like hallucinations and delusions, or anything like them, except in rare cases of reduplicative paramnesia. And in these rare cases brain disease is usually massive and often extends outside the frontal region. The most documented effects of damage to the more posterior parts of the frontal lobes, including Broca's area, are seldom observed in schizophrenia. For example, in severe expressive aphasia, the patient is unable to produce articulated speech of any kind, something that occurs rarely in schizophrenia (Straube & Oades, 1992, pp. 59–62). Moreover, there is little to suggest that schizophrenia patients suffer a primary loss of movement control like what is seen in neurological patients with precentral gyrus or premotor damage. The most frequently reported motor problems in schizophrenia are side effects of antipsychotic medication, not direct effects of the illness itself. Nor is the picture of frontal emotion and personality change, with its unrestrained and impulsive social behavior, an obvious echo of what is seen in the course of schizophrenia.

The closest parallels between schizophrenia and the behavior of frontal patients are seen in negative symptoms like inattention, slowing, psychomotor poverty, reduced behavioral spontaneity, apathy, and loss of initiative. These symptoms seem to occur in both disorders. The neurological basis of positive symptoms may lie elsewhere, but perhaps the roots of negative symptoms are here, in the prefrontal brain and in its executive control of behavior. If there is a connection between schizophrenia and prefrontal brain dysfunction, the various executive tasks and abilities that are hard for patients with frontal brain disease should also pose problems for the person with schizophrenia.

Given the popularity of the frontal brain hypothesis in schizophrenia research, it is surprising that investigators have not been more comprehensive in their examination of patients' abilities with executive tasks. Konstantine Zakzanis and I (Heinrichs & Zakzanis, 1998) surveyed the literature between 1980 and 1997 and found that the most frequently used task was the Wisconsin Card Sorting Test (Heaton et al., 1993), with 43 studies. The oral version of the word fluency test (Lezak, 1995, pp. 545–546) came second, with 29 studies. We found two studies that used the Tower of Hanoi (Lezak, 1995, pp. 657–658) and six that used the Stroop test (Lezak, 1995, pp. 373–376). The great emphasis on the Wisconsin Card Sorting Test is troubling because its validity as a behavioral index of frontal brain activity has been questioned (Anderson et al., 1991). The word fluency test has received stronger support in terms of validity (e.g., Damasio & Anderson, 1993; Kolb & Whishaw, 1996, pp. 474–476; Warkentin, Risberg, Nilsson, & Karlson, 1991). Nonetheless, it seems that inclusion of the Wisconsin Card Sort has become almost obligatory in neuroscience-based clinical studies of schizophrenia.

There are several indices of card-sorting performance, but the number of successfully sorted categories—strings of 10 consecutive correct responses— and the total number of correct, incorrect, and perseverative responses and errors are the most frequently reported scores. We calculated effect sizes for each Wisconsin Card Sorting Test score and combined them into an overall effect ($d = .88$) to maximize the number of contributing studies. Milner's (1964) original study showed that patients with frontal lesions are prone to impairment in both categories and perseveration, so separate effects were calculated for these scores. The average effect for categories was $d = 1.05$. This average d is accurate within 20 decimal points 95% of the time. The average effect for perseveration was somewhat smaller at $d = .87$, but the margin of error was also smaller (.14). Thus there is certainly a reliable tendency for many schizophrenia patients to perform poorly on the Wisconsin Card Sorting Test. However, effect sizes of these magnitudes correspond to nonoverlap percentages of about 50% using Cohen's (1988) idealized normal curves. Therefore, a large proportion of patients, about half, also perform the test normally.

To gain a perspective on the strength and meaning of the average effect sizes in this situation, consider how they compare with card-sorting results obtained from neurological patients with documented frontal lesions. As expected, data reported in the manual of Heaton et al. (1993) show that frontal patients do poorly relative to healthy research participants. With the categories score as the basis for comparison, an effect size of $d = 1.04$ is obtained for frontal patients— virtually the same as the average effect obtained for schizophrenia patients. An associated overlap percentage of about 43% indicates that the test will yield many normal scores in both patient populations, despite the substantial effect. So it appears that the Wisconsin Card Sorting Test is about as sensitive to the integrity of the frontal brain as to the presence of schizophrenic illness.

The second most popular "frontal system" test is the oral-phonemic form of the word fluency task, sometimes referred to as the Controlled Oral Word Association Test (see Lezak, 1995, pp. 545–546). The task requires a person to generate as many words as possible beginning with a specified letter. Proper nouns are excluded, and there is a one-minute time limit for each of three letters. A total of 27 studies reporting usable schizophrenia–control comparisons for letter fluency was published between 1980 and 1997. The average phonemic fluency effect for these studies is $d = 1.09$, which corresponds to a nonoverlap of about 60%. This is larger than the result for the Wisconsin Card Sort perseveration score and about the same size as the category score. The margins of error are also quite similar for the two tests. The effect suggests that indeed, on average, schizophrenia patients are impaired in word generation when compared with healthy people. Nonetheless, once again, there must also be substantial numbers of patients with normal fluency rates.

For a neurological comparison I went to a study of patients with tumors of the frontal lobes by Butler, Roisman, Hill, and Tuma (1993). I also looked at results from a more etiologically mixed group of patients with bilateral frontal disease reported by Stuss et al. (1994). In the first study, the patients were significantly less proficient than healthy people in generating words. The effect size was $d = .81$, a moderately large finding. In the second study the effect size was $d = 1.27$. These results are fairly similar to the range of ds obtained for schizophrenia. Hence it appears that word fluency is roughly as sensitive to space-occupying frontal brain lesions as to schizophrenia. But as in the situation with the Wisconsin Card Sorting Test, there are also sizeable numbers of patients who cannot be distinguished from healthy subjects on the basis of their performance.

There were only six studies reporting Stroop results in our original meta-analysis, so I looked for more and found three new studies published in 1999. The average for all nine studies is $d = .97$, with a confidence interval ranging from $d = .66$ to $d = 1.28$. This average effect is extremely close to the size of the word fluency and Wisconsin Card Sorting categories score effect. All Stroop studies except the one by Mohamed, Paulsen, O'Leary, Arndt, and Andreasen (1999) found moderate or large effects. When schizophrenia patients are asked to report the ink colors of printed words and they see a word like "blue" that is printed, paradoxically, in red ink, they find it hard to ignore or inhibit the "pull" of the word meaning. Although even healthy people show some susceptibility to the word meaning over the visual sensation, schizophrenia patients, on average, clearly have exaggerated Stroop effects. An effect size of $d = .97$ corresponds to a nonoverlap percentage between control and patient populations of about 54%. Conversely, slightly less than half of schizophrenia patients may have normal Stroop performance.

Finally, there are very few studies reporting data on schizophrenia–control comparisons with the Tower problem-solving task. Goldberg, Saint-Cyr, and Weinberger (1990) used four trials of increasing difficulty, and the corresponding effect sizes ranged from $d = .5$ to $d = 1.3$. A more recent study by Morice and Delahunty (1996) reported a remarkably large effect size of $d = 2.58$ with the London version of the Tower problem. But this contrasts with the modest effects ($d = .25$) obtained by Rushe et al. (1999) and ($d = .46$) by Bustini et al. (1999). Therefore, it is not surprising to find a fairly large ($d = 1.05$) but unstable (confidence interval: $d = .16 - d = 1.94$) average effect for the Tower studies.

As a reference point, Goel and Graffman (1995) obtained an effect size of $d = .72$ when they used the Tower of Hanoi version with frontally damaged neurological patients and healthy control participants. Their neurological sample comprised primarily penetrating head injury patients with multifocal lesions that included the prefrontal region. Yet schizophrenia and focal frontal brain damage may impair this kind of problem solving in different ways and for different reasons. Rushe et al. (1999) found that neurological patients with frontal lesions have a special difficulty in dealing with conflicts between the goals of different moves, whereas schizophrenia patients have a more generalized difficulty across all aspects of the test. Unfortunately, studies using this task in the schizophrenia population are so few and far between that it is hard to draw any conclusions. It is perhaps fair to say that the evidence accumulated thus far is about as powerful, but more variable, than the results obtained for other executive tasks.

So are many schizophrenia and frontal brain-damaged patients impaired on the same kinds of cognitive tasks? The short answer is yes. The evidence shows that schizophrenia patients have executive cognitive deficits that are similar in magnitude to those found in neurological patients with focal lesions of the pre-frontal region. The problem is that these magnitudes are modest, and even frontal lobe–damaged patients are not always impaired on executive tasks. In both neurological and schizophrenia–control comparisons, the effect sizes are not large enough to separate completely the patient and control groups.

In view of theses results, it is understandable why texts on clinical neuropsychology always place heavy qualifications on the use of tests like the Wisconsin Card Sorting Test to localize brain lesions (i.e., Lezak, 1995, pp. 623–625). Clinicians and researchers know that a substantial proportion of any given patient group will perform normally on the task or perform abnormally but fail to show the expected neurological damage. It is hard to say to what extent such limited validity simply reflects the current rudimentary knowledge about psychological functions of the frontal brain region. However, it is also important to remember that the full range of executive tasks has not been applied to schizophrenia. The most popular task, the Wisconsin Card Sorting Test, also has the most questionable validity as a predictor of frontal pathology, and the focal neurological validity of the Stroop test rests on very few studies. The next most popular frontal system test is the word fluency task, which has a fairly large average effect size and is also fairly reliable. Indeed, from the standpoint of validity, reliability, and ease of administration, oral word fluency is probably the best of the widely used frontal-system tests.

The Problem of General and Specific Deficits

There is an additional issue that requires attention whenever cognitive abilities are evaluated in schizophrenia: not only are effect sizes often modest but also the demonstration of a specific task deficit is not as straightforward as it may seem. Any putative executive task deficit may be a product of a much more general cognitive impairment that is likely to affect most aspects of cognition and performance. A traditional strategy to combat this possibility is to show that the patient group has the same general intelligence as the control group but differs on the specific task of interest. This strategy proves feasible when studying neurological patients with focal lesions because intelligence is usually spared in such conditions. However, the same strategy is hard to implement in the case of schizophrenia. As a group, schizophrenia patients have lower IQs than the general population, corresponding to an effect size of about 1.0 standard deviation units of difference (Heinrichs & Zakzanis, 1998). To match schizophrenia patients to control participants, a researcher has to find patients with unusually high IQs or healthy people with unusually low IQs. In either case, the samples are unrepresentative of the patient or healthy populations.

Accordingly, a researcher who wishes to show that schizophrenia patients have a specific problem with executive ability has to show that any observed

Table 4.1 Intellectual and frontal-executive cognitive test results for three patients

Patient	Symptom	IQ	Wisconsin	Fluency	Stroop
1. Ruth	Feeling and smelling a leech	108	6	50	+4.5
2. William	Divine connections, powers	105	6	31	−2.0
3. James	Penetration by a parasite	84	0	25	−8.0

Note: IQ = Full-scale intelligence quotient from Wechsler Adult Intelligence Scale-Revised; Wisconsin = number of categories achieved on the Wisconsin Card Sorting Test (0 = severe impairment; 6 = normal); fluency = number of words produced in three one-minute trials; Stroop = interference effect score, with negative scores indicating greater interference.

deficit is independent of general intellectual ability. And this will always be hard to accomplish. For example, we (Heinrichs & Zakzanis, 1998) found 33 studies that reported both card-sorting and IQ results and correlated each study's card-sorting effect size with the average IQ of the schizophrenia sample. A substantial correlation of $r = -.54$ was found between IQ and the Wisconsin Card Sorting Test effect size. No such relationship with IQ was found for word fluency. However, relatively few studies reported both fluency and IQ test results.

Thus at least one of the executive task effects can be predicted partly on the basis of the patients' average intelligence, and larger executive effects and group separation can be associated with lower patient intelligence. Indeed, a few individual studies confirm that IQ correlates directly with card sorting in schizophrenia patients (Heinrichs, 1990; Van der Does & Van den Bosch, 1992). Thus researchers may be measuring a broad ability factor when they think they are measuring executive ability selectively, at least some of the time. Such a mistake is most likely with respect to the Wisconsin Card Sorting Test—the most popular of the frontal system tasks. It is not known to what extent the same problem exists with regard to the Stroop effect and the Tower tasks because of the small number of available studies.

What does this all mean for individual patients with schizophrenia? The patient profiles introduced in chapter 1 are helpful as an illustration of these issues of test validity and the contamination of selective and general ability influences. Test scores along with the patients' symptoms are shown in table 4.1. Ruth and William both have normal Wisconsin Card Sorting Test results and average intelligence quotients. These quotients are actually above average for the schizophrenia population. James, the man with delusions of alien control and parasitic penetration, has a low−average IQ and a very impaired Wisconsin Card Sort. Similarly, the word fluency and Stroop interference effects are within normal limits for Ruth and William, the patients with average intelligence. James, with a lower level of intelligence, also has a moderately abnormal Stroop effect. Ruth and William's results show that it is possible to have schizophrenia and powerful positive symptoms and to perform normally on tests of executive cognition.

Table 4.2 Summary of Evidence of Frontal-Executive Deficits in Schizophrenia

Index	Mean *d*	Confidence Interval	N
Wisconsin Card Sorting Test	.88	.76–1.00	43
Word fluency	1.09	.92–1.26	27
Stroop effect	.97	.66–1.28	9
Tower problem-solving	1.05	.16–1.94	4
Intelligence (IQ)	1.10	.86–1.34	35
Frontal brain volume (magnetic resonance)	.33	.23–.43	39
Left frontal volume (magnetic resonance)	.42	.20–.64	23
Positron emission (resting state)	.68	.47–.89	27
Positron emission (cognitively active state)	.80	.53–1.07	17
Left frontal positron emission (resting state)	.48	.16–.80	22

Note: The table shows effect sizes (Cohen's *d*) in absolute values, corrected for sample size and averaged over studies in a research domain. All *d*s are based on differences between schizophrenia patients and healthy participants. N is number of contributing studies; Confidence Interval is 95% confidence interval for the mean *d*. The true population mean effect is likely to fall in the indicated range, while confidence intervals that include zero reflect highly unstable findings. Two word fluency studies were deleted as outliers from the Heinrichs and Zakzanis (1998) literature base.

Although some schizophrenia patients have executive impairments, they may also have a broad intellectual dysfunction that manifests itself in many different kinds of cognitive tests and abilities.

Accordingly, drawing conclusions about the cognitive deficits presented as average effect sizes in table 4.2 is fraught with uncertainty. The uncertainty stems from our rudimentary understanding of what the prefrontal brain contributes to behavior. The number of valid and reliable tasks is small, and only some of these tasks have been applied to schizophrenia patients. These applications show that the illness does associate with poor performance on some executive tasks. But this performance is not always distinguishable from poor performance on tests of general intellectual ability. Moreover, many schizophrenia patients (and many neurological patients with frontal damage) perform normally on executive tasks. This underscores the heterogeneity that is found in both patient populations. It also underscores the difficulty of making inferences about frontal brain integrity in any illness on the basis of psychological data. In the end, the question of whether the frontal brain contributes to schizophrenic illness cannot be resolved with behavioral methods alone. Fortunately, the same question can be addressed with biological methods that offer a much more direct picture of frontal brain structure and physiology. Consider what these methods have to say about the neurological basis of schizophrenia.

Pictures of the Brain

Neuropsychological tests are one rather inexact means of searching for evidence of brain dysfunction; recent developments in brain scanning and imaging provide a more accurate way of studying brain biology. First, there are imaging techniques that yield a visual or quantitative display of neuroanatomical structure —a picture of the living brain. These techniques include computerized axial tomography and nuclear magnetic resonance imaging. Magnetic resonance in particular is able to provide very clear, detailed images of many brain structures that were previously only observable after death under conditions of post-mortem examination. Since schizophrenia does not involve frank pathologies like infarctions, hemorrhages, or neoplasms, most structural imaging research on the illness is based on volumetric comparisons with healthy control groups. The assumption is that brain structures with abnormally small tissue volumes must have sustained some kind of pathology, including, for example, cell loss or abnormal neural development.

A second methodology comprises "functional" imaging techniques. These include positron emission and single photon emission tomography as well as xenon inhalation procedures. Functional imaging involves introducing a mildly radioactive tracer into the bloodstream and the application of a sensory apparatus, a kind of camera, to detect the tracer's perfusion in the brain's blood circulation. Depending on the tracer, this can furnish a display or readout of blood flow changes, glucose metabolism, or neurotransmitter receptor binding in different brain regions. Regions with high activity or affinity for a particular tracer can be "imaged" and discriminated from less active regions. Recent technology also includes an amalgamation of techniques whereby chemical products of physiological processes are displayed in the form of magnetic resonance spectroscopy brain images. Moreover, localized neural activity can be detected with "functional" magnetic resonance imaging. This most recent technology is in its infancy and has been used in relatively few studies (see Curtis et al., 1999). In contrast, the structural magnetic resonance imaging literature has exploded over the last decade (McCarley, Hsiao, Freedman, Pfefferbaum, & Donchin, 1996).

The revolution in brain imaging techniques offers the great advantage of studying the living brain in people with schizophrenia. Yet these techniques are limited in that their accuracy, and resolving power is not great enough to provide information about the cellular, microscopic level of detail in the brain. As a result, the new techniques are most helpful in detecting conventional neuropathologies, like space-occupying lesions. However, more subtle pathology —within small regions or in cell organization in different layers of the cortex —are hard to detect. Spatial resolution is especially limited in the case of functional imaging techniques. Furthermore, although it is possible to index cerebral blood flow or metabolism, these processes do not necessarily reflect cognitive or behavioral activity when they are measured with the research participant "at rest"—just sitting there in the scanning apparatus. Fortunately, this limitation can be surmounted in the "activation" study. Participants undergo functional scanning while engaged simultaneously in behaviors like word generation or problem solving. Such "cognitive challenge," or activation, studies allow patients to be scanned before and during an activation task, thus opening a window on the working brain as it engages in mental processing.

When very high degrees of neuroanatomical detail and resolution are required, post-mortem techniques provide a partial solution. Post-mortem analysis involves studying preserved brain specimens following a patient's death. This kind of approach began during the time of psychiatric pioneers like Kraepelin (1919) and Bleuler (1950). However, major advances in microscopy, tissue preservation, and neurochemical assay techniques have taken place. Hence the contemporary researcher can estimate the number of receptors for specific neurotransmitter substances in a schizophrenic brain. It is possible to examine the organization of nerve cells in different layers of the cerebral cortex and to identify telltale signs of pathology. The researcher can count different kinds of cells or cell aberrations in minute areas of the brain. Post-mortem tissue examination offers a level of inspection and observation not available to researchers who rely on brain scans to find the schizophrenic lesion. Unfortunately, the number of available specimens is often small. In addition, the manner of death—stroke is a good example—may itself affect neural tissue. Rapid tissue sample preservation with freezing is essential. Moreover, many brain specimens from schizophrenia patients were, during life, subjected to decades of powerful drug administration for the control of psychotic symptoms. Hence tissue preparation and medication exposure factors can introduce contaminating influences that may lead the post-mortem researcher astray.

Taken together, the new or improved methods of neuroscience are dazzling in their ability to display the previously hidden biology of the brain. These methods have generated enormous enthusiasm and optimism that the identification of neural causes of schizophrenia is just around the corner (Andreasen, 1985; Mesulam, 1990). The search for evidence that the frontal lobes of the brain, especially the prefrontal regions, are involved in schizophrenia has relied heavily on these techniques. If the psychological evidence linking madness to the frontal brain appears equivocal, perhaps the new imaging techniques, which measure the brain more directly, will provide the convincing proof that researchers have sought.

Prefrontal Neuroanatomy and Schizophrenia— Does Size Matter?

Raz and Raz (1990) reported an early meta-analysis that showed an average effect size for reduced frontal lobe brain volume in schizophrenia of $d = .66$. This suggests only very modest support for a specific frontal brain contribution to schizophrenia. However, the most recent articles cited by Raz and Raz were published in 1988, and most used computerized tomography scanning. In contrast, studies now employ the more accurate technology of magnetic resonance imaging and measure frontal volume in terms of a ratio of frontal to whole brain volume. In this way it is easier to detect a selective loss of frontal brain tissue. Hence my graduate students and I decided to look for more recent and specific evidence of reduced frontal brain volumes in schizophrenia. We found 39 studies, representing 2,794 patients and control participants, published between 1980 and 1999 that used the high-resolution magnetic resonance technique. The summary statistics in table 4.2 indicate an average effect size of $d = .33$. The associated confidence interval or margin of error suggests that the true average schizophrenia prefrontal brain volume effect is somewhere between $d = .23$ and $d = .43$. Accordingly, on average, schizophrenia patients do tend to have somewhat smaller prefrontal brain areas than healthy people do. However, it is a small difference, and with an estimated distribution overlap of about 75%, the vast majority of patients and healthy people are indistinguishable in terms of their frontal brain volumes.

It is worth pointing out that the older computerized tomography scans actually produced a larger average effect ($d = .62$; see Zakzanis & Heinrichs, 1999). In contrast, many of the prefrontal effects derived from magnetic resonance are close to zero. Hence older imaging technology probably produced spuriously high estimates of frontal volume reduction. It seems reasonable to conclude that only very small differences sometimes exist between schizophrenia patients and healthy people with respect to the size of the prefrontal brain region.

Yet this region is a very large expanse of cerebral cortex, and it has many subdivisions that reflect microscopic anatomical differences. Although magnetic resonance imaging provides remarkably accurate data and pictures of the brain, a focus on the entire prefrontal region may miss the critical subregion that is smaller or abnormal in schizophrenia. Hence it makes sense to examine volumes of smaller parts of the frontal lobe, parts that are of theoretical interest in relation to the illness. For example, some neuropsychologists have argued that the left frontal subregion has an executive role relative to the frontal system itself (e.g., Luria, 1973, pp. 79–99). The left frontal lobe is therefore a kind of executive within an executive. This idea stems from the evident importance of the left cerebral hemisphere in language functions and its "dominance" with respect to the control of movement. If the left hemisphere controls the rest of the brain, the left frontal region must control the whole cerebral system. To assess the importance of this subregion in schizophrenia, Davidson (1999) found 23 published studies that measured the left prefrontal region separately. However, the average effect for left frontal volume ($d = .42$) was only slightly larger than the value for the whole frontal region ($d = .33$). Both are extremely modest findings, and their margins of error overlap, so the slight difference may be meaningless (see table 4.2). Thus there is no convincing support for the idea that the left prefrontal region is more deficient than the whole frontal cortex in schizophrenia.

It is also noteworthy that magnetic resonance studies differ from each other in terms of a wide variety of technical features. These features may include the scanner's magnet strength, the scanning angle and plane of measurement, and, of great importance, the demarcation of the prefrontal region from the rest of the brain (see Bilder et al., 1994; Delisi et al., 1991; Wible et al., 1995). Such differences in method may introduce noise and inconsistency between studies. For example, Davidson (1999) found a strong relationship between increasing spatial resolution and decreasing effect sizes across magnetic resonance studies. It would also be preferable if all investigators used the same consensus-based method for determining the boundaries of the prefrontal brain region. Still, it is unlikely that technical variations between studies can, by themselves, account for the very small neuroanatomical differences between schizophrenia patients and healthy people (Zakzanis & Heinrichs, 1999).

Nonetheless, the argument for examining smaller cortical regions could be made again. For example, the left prefrontal region is also a differentiated expanse of cortex. A number of investigators have argued for the importance of subregions like area 9 in relation to working memory functions (Goldman-Rakic, 1996; Levy, & Goldman-Rakic, 2000; see figure 4.1). These small areas are "lost" when the volume of the whole left prefrontal cortex is measured. Other researchers have examined subcortical structures, like the thalamus, that have a strong association with the prefrontal area. Thus Andreasen et al. (1994) applied an improved system for measuring neuroanatomy with magnetic resonance scans to samples of schizophrenia and control research participants. This system yielded effect sizes for imaging segments across the entire brain. The largest effect sizes ($d = .75 - 1.0$) were in the right cerebral hemisphere and involved the lateral thalamus and possibly the fibers connecting the thalamus with the prefrontal region. Yet specific inferences about small regions of neuroanatomy are hard to justify because the scanning technology is at the limits of its sensitivity in such applications. Indeed, any attempt at fine-grained tissue analysis must grapple with the limited resolving power of even the best scanning machines. If examination of microscopic neuroanatomical detail is needed, post-mortem studies of brain tissue are the preferred option.

Post-Mortem Analysis of Prefrontal Neuroanatomy

Observation of human brain tissue under an electron or fluorescent microscope, with the assistance of selective neuron staining, or with histochemical techniques that highlight specific nerve cells and tracts, offers the most detailed and accurate way to find neuropathology. The degree of spatial resolution achieved with post-mortem analysis is far beyond what even the best magnetic resonance imaging has to offer. And in principle it should be possible to look closely at neuroanatomical subdivisions of the frontal cortex like those described by Brodmann (see figure 4.1). Area 9 is of special interest because it has been implicated specifically in relation to schizophrenia and the neuroanatomical substrate of working memory. Yet when I looked for recent studies of patient–control comparisons of prefrontal cortex, I found only three reports that provide area 9 measurements and two studies that provide data on the adjacent area 10. I also found three studies (Akbarian et al., 1993, 1995, 1996) reporting results relevant to neurodevelopmental ideas (I discuss these in Chapter 7).

Recall that the cerebral cortex is organized into six layers of cells. These cells differ in kind and include pyramidal cells and interneurons. Therefore, a good question to ask at this level of observation is whether area 9 of the schizophrenic brain is abnormal in terms of neuronal density—numbers of neurons per unit area or volume. Markedly reduced density might indicate neuronal degeneration in the illness. In fact, a study by Selemon, Rajkowska, and Goldman-Rakic (1995) did find evidence of abnormal cell density in area 9. However, the schizophrenia samples had *higher* densities than the control samples ($d = 1.09$). Moreover, the total number of neurons was normal. This raised the possibility, that abnormally tight "packing" of neurons in a thinner cortex caused the elevated density. To test this possibility, cortical thickness in area 9 was measured in the schizophrenia and control tissue samples. The associated effect size was moderately large ($d = .79$), meaning that about half of the schizophrenia samples probably had a cortical thickness in the normal range and half had thinner, more densely packed cortical layers in area 9. Then the same research group (Rajkowska, Selemon, & Goldman-Rakic, 1998) reported detailed data on both cell size and density in each cortical layer of the same region. The overall cell density was again elevated in schizophrenia tissue, but the effect was much smaller than in the first report ($d = .40$). Furthermore, Woo, Miller, and Lewis (1997), looking at the density of a subpopulation of neurons that form local circuits within area 9, found essentially no difference between patient and control tissue ($d = .06$). However, Rajkowska and associates were impressed with another aspect of their own research—the reduced size of nerve cells. Yet here, too, although schizophrenia samples tended to have smaller neurons than control samples, the average effect was modest ($d = .53$).

Area 10 is immediately below area 9 in the far frontal region of the cortex (figure 4.1). Two studies by Benes and associates (Benes, Davidson, & Bird, 1986; Benes, McSparren, Bird, SanGiovanni, & Vincent, 1991) reported data on cell densities in this region. Densities were reported from cortical layer V in both studies, but the results are inconsistent, with abnormally low densities reported in the first study ($d = -.52$) and moderately *increased* density in the second study ($d = .64$). Part of the inconsistency may derive from the fact that all kinds of neurons were counted in the older study, perhaps leading to loss of crucial distinctions among subpopulations of neurons. Thus in 1991 the research group reported a decrease in the number of small interneurons in layer II but an increase in pyramidal cell numbers in layer V. The relative increase in pyramidal cells was moderate, but the reduction in small interneurons in layer II was extremely large ($d = -3.01$), with very little schizophrenia–control group overlap. Unfortunately, this finding remains unreplicated at present.

The post-mortem findings on the prefrontal brain in schizophrenia are too few and varied to be aggregated into a meta-analysis in table 4.2, but this literature can be characterized as follows. There are interesting demonstrations of abnormalities in neuronal distribution, cell size, and laminar density in schizophrenic brain tissue. These demonstrations have not been replicated, so the evidence, with so few studies in hand, is weak and inconsistent. Moreover, even in the positive findings, only one study (Benes et al., 1991) produced the kind of effect size expected of a neuropathological marker. The definitive evidence for prefrontal brain involvement in schizophrenia does not lie in post-mortem studies, at least not yet.

The scarcity of post-mortem data deserves some additional comment from a different perspective. Consider the fact that we found only a handful of post-mortem studies that looked at the prefrontal cortex. In comparison, we found 39 magnetic resonance brain scanning studies reporting data on 2,794 patient and control participants. The great disparity in the two bodies of evidence is striking. It may be due in part to the difficulties involved in obtaining and preserving large numbers of specimen brains for research purposes. Kirch, Wagman, and Goldman-Rakic (1991) have described some of these difficulties. There are shortages of both control and schizophrenia patient tissue. A patient has to provide consent, during life, for eventual donation of brain tissue—a bizarre and unpleasant prospect for someone struggling with mental illness. For that matter, obtaining samples of normal brains for comparison involves asking a healthy person to consider the same prospect. Moreover, even when a brain is donated, there are many technical ambiguities that must be sorted out before useful research data are obtained. These ambiguities may include an uncertain retrospective diagnosis of schizophrenia and problems in tissue handling and preservation. The pathologist wants to be sure that the brain is useful for sophisticated analysis with light and electron microscopy. In view of the practical obstacles and shortage of specimens, it is not surprising that few recent studies exist. Nonetheless, this research approach has an important story to tell about the schizophrenic brain, and brain tissue banks deserve some of the resources and energy being expended on less accurate techniques like magnetic resonance brain imaging.

The Brain at Rest and in Action

Perhaps the abnormality of the frontal brain that underlies schizophrenia is an abnormality of the working brain. It may, therefore, be detected in physiological processes like blood supply and energy use. Perhaps this functional abnormality is not reflected in cell loss or in reduced tissue volumes in key brain areas. The answer to the schizophrenia brain puzzle may lie in the biological activity that the frontal system depends on. If so, positron emission tomography may provide the answer.

Positron emission tomography allows physiological events to be recorded in living people with schizophrenia. The two most common variations involve introducing tracer molecules either for glucose metabolism or for blood flow into the body. Since glucose is the only source of energy for the brain, a compound like fluorodeoxyglucose moves rapidly to the central nervous system and is taken up by the most active brain regions. The distribution in brain of this mildly radioactive tracer is detected with positron emission tomography cameras. In this way, regional energy metabolism or, with other tracers, regional blood flow can be assessed in living schizophrenia patients and healthy people (Sedvall, 1992). Reduced frontal brain function may take the form of "hypofrontality" or abnormally low blood flow or metabolism. In theory the frontal brain in schizophrenia is pathologically underactive and silent, unable to engage in the executive control of mind and behavior. If this is correct, hypofrontality should be extremely prevalent in people with the illness.

To explore the evidence in this area my graduate students and I located 27 studies that compared frontal metabolism or blood flow in samples of patients and healthy people under conditions of "rest." We did not include studies using the less accurate technique of single photon emission tomography. Research participants were not involved in any kind of directed activity at the time of the "resting" scan. They were awake and alert, perhaps looking at a picture or daydreaming, but they were not solving problems or expending large amounts of mental effort. Taken together the studies yield an average effect size of $d = .68$, which is accurate within a margin of about .21 (see table 4.2). In principle, the effect corresponds to about 60% overlap in frontal blood flow and metabolism values between normal and schizophrenia distributions. Thus only a minority of schizophrenia patients, albeit a substantial one, demonstrate reduced frontal brain physiological activity.

Apart from the modest size of the average effect, the positron emission findings on the frontal region show considerable inconsistency among studies. A number of researchers (e.g., Ariel et al., 1983; Clark, Kopala, Hurwitz, & Li, 1991) obtained effect sizes larger than $d = 1.0$, suggesting that at least half of schizophrenia patients are "hypofrontal." In contrast, many other researchers found no effect (e.g., Schroeder et al., 1994; Yuasa et al., 1995) or found small effects in the wrong direction. Thus Buchsbaum et al. (1984), Cleghorn et al. (1989), and Gur et al. (1995) all found that on average schizophrenia patients had *higher* than normal frontal brain activity. Hence some patients must show enhanced activity, others show the expected hypofunction, and still others have normal frontal physiology. But this patient heterogeneity may be more apparent than real. Davidson (1999) shows that effect sizes vary between studies partly as a function of positron emission image resolution. Echoing similar findings in the magnetic resonance literature, a more accurate image generally yields a smaller difference between a schizophrenic brain and a healthy one.

There is also nothing to suggest pronounced or selective hypofrontality in the left frontal lobe in schizophrenia. We originally found an average effect of $d = .50$ in 16 studies that reported functional imaging data separately for the left frontal region (Zakzanis & Heinrichs, 1999). Davidson (1999) updated the article base and found six more studies and an average d of .48. An effect like this implies that at most a third of schizophrenia patients show abnormal left frontal lobe physiology. Hence, if anything, there is less evidence of hypofrontality in the left frontal region than in the frontal lobes as a whole.

Finally, one study (Biver et al., 1995) reported detailed glucose metabolism rates in different subregions of the frontal cortex, including area 9 in the left hemisphere, the area that may support aspects of working memory. However, the associated effect of $d = -.54$ is not dramatically different from the values obtained for the left frontal lobe or for the whole frontal system.

Inconsistency in the results of positron emission studies may occur because the patient samples differ in some way. We examined some of these sample differences in an earlier meta-analysis of this literature (Zakzanis & Heinrichs, 1999). Effect sizes were largest in studies that used acutely ill patients. In a similar vein, recent work by Spence, Hirsch, Brooks, and Grasby (1998) suggests that hypofrontality may disappear as a patient recovers from the acute phase of psychosis. We also found a source of effect size inconsistency in the form of sample gender composition. Studies with a high proportion of male participants yield smaller effects. Finally, two of the studies that contribute to the average d in table 4.2 examined drug-free patient samples. These studies yielded "reverse" effect sizes, indicating that the patients had higher metabolic rates in the prefrontal area, on average, than the healthy people did. It may be that exposure to antipsychotic medication influences prefrontal metabolism in some patients and perhaps exaggerates the degree of abnormality in brain scan findings.

Weinberger and Berman (1996) suggest another way of looking at the variable and generally disappointing body of evidence on hypofrontality in schizophrenia. They argue that although technical and sampling differences between studies create some inconsistency in results, the basic problem is the nature of the "resting state" during which the brain is scanned for physiological activity. This state is inherently subjective and uncontrollable. Research participants who undergo scanning may engage in different kinds of mental activity as they pass their time in the scanner. Sometimes participants are given a picture to look at, or they are told to close their eyes. However, there is no way of knowing what they are thinking about or feeling. Many patient participants may be distracted by their symptoms; many healthy participants may daydream about a range of topics. The point is that this uncontrolled mental activity probably creates a great deal of physiological noise for the scanner. Moreover, the sensitivity of the scanner to subtle pathological signals may be inadequate. Subtle signals may simply be undetectable against a noisy background, lost in the physiological ebb and flow of the brain's "resting state."

One potential solution to the problem of uncontrolled mental activity during resting scans is to provide research participants with a structured task that engages the brain and directs mental and associated physiological activity during the scanning procedure. Hence "activation" conditions have been developed wherein participants are given mental work to do while the scan is conducted. Activation studies were initially much rarer than resting scans, and they have their own technical problems. For example, the kind of cognitive activation task that can be applied to positron emission scanning is limited by time constraints. The period of time during which the radioactive tracer is detectable in the brain is brief, so the activation tasks must be correspondingly short and in temporal step with the scanning procedure. Nonetheless, the activation technique is an exciting addition to the scanning literature, and its logic is compelling: make the brain engage in mental work, and the schizophrenic defect will reveal itself.

We originally located only 9 imaging studies that used activation or "cognitive challenge" paradigms (Zakzanis & Heinrichs, 1999). However, this is a burgeoning area of research, and a more recent search yielded another seven studies, for a total of 17. These studies produce a somewhat larger average effect at $d = .80$ than the resting studies (see table 4.2). An effect in this range means that close to half of schizophrenia patients are distinguishable from healthy people on the basis of frontal blood flow and metabolism values during activation scans. Put another way, perhaps half of the schizophrenia patient population demonstrates hypofrontality if activation paradigms are used in functional imaging studies.

An unexpected aspect of the results of activation studies concerns the range of tasks that seem to elicit impaired frontal function in schizophrenia patients. Not all of these are executive tasks. The largest effect ($d = -2.09$) was obtained by Volkow et al. (1986), who used a simple visual task where participants had to track a geometric figure as a way of activating the brain. However, even the resting baseline condition produced a large effect ($d = -1.65$), suggestive of lowered brain metabolism in the frontal regions of the patient sample. The well-known study by Weinberger, Berman, and Illowsky (1988), using the Wisconsin Card Sorting Test for activation, produced a much weaker effect of $d = -.89$. This is still above the average for resting studies. Yet it is noteworthy that only 4 of 16 patients in this study had blood flow values that were completely outside the control group range and only 2 of the 25 control subjects had values above the upper limits of the patient range. The point is that there is little to suggest that putative executive tasks like the Wisconsin Card Sorting Test are superior to simple perceptual tasks in terms of revealing frontal physiological abnormalities in schizophrenia patients (see also Buchsbaum et al., 1992). Instead, the use of *any* kind of activation task during scanning may yield slightly larger hypofrontality effects than results obtained with "resting" scans.

It is important to remember that the functional imaging literature is based on a technique that still provides a fairly crude picture of the working brain. Positron emission tomography is an amazing technical advance, but it still has limitations. The positron emission technique provides only a net estimation of alterations in activity in fairly gross brain regions, and its spatial resolution is much lower than the resolution of magnetic resonance imaging. All "in vivo" brain-imaging techniques are several magnitudes below what can be observed microscopically with post-mortem study. Given the weak, inconsistent, and theoretically ambiguous findings with respect to simple hypofrontality and schizophrenia, there is increasing interest in patterns of activation in different brain regions and in the extent to which these patterns are correlated into neural networks (e.g., Mallet, Mazoyer, & Martinot, 1998). This idea may be one of the springboards for future advances in the neuroscience of schizophrenia, and it shows how researchers are moving beyond simplistic notions like "hypofrontality" in searching the brain for madness.

The Frontal-Executive Brain and Its Contribution to Schizophrenia

The frontal regions of the human brain have been implicated in higher mental functions and thereby in mental illness since the turn of the century. Yet these regions continue to pose a challenge to neuroscience in terms of understanding their contribution to mind and behavior. The frontal brain seems to exercise an executive role in psychological life. It allocates working memory to the formation, maintenance, or elimination of plans and actions as the mind faces novel situations. When habit and routine no longer suffice, and flexibility, estimation, and initiative are required, the frontal system comes into play. Several cognitive tests of executive ability have been used to explore and document this executive role. However, they capture only part of frontal function, and many patients who sustain frontal brain damage perform standard tests normally. Moreover, it is hard to find an executive task that has an exclusive relationship with the frontal region. Indeed, the most frequently used psychological tests of executive ability probably reflect contributions from several distinct brain regions. Hence, progress has been made since the days when the highest human capacities were simply presumed to involve the frontal lobes. But understanding this brain region remains a major scientific problem in its own right.

To what extent, then, is schizophrenia a disorder of executive frontal brain function? The evidence reviewed and presented in summary form in table 4.2 provides no convincing support for the idea that frontal dysfunction is a necessary part of the illness. The biological literature seldom reports frontal abnormalities in more than about a third of schizophrenia patients, and often the proportion is much lower. Alternatively, the argument can be made that some corresponding minority of patients has an illness that affects the frontal brain, especially in acute, early stages. There are also theoretical possibilities that stress network models, where focal frontal dysfunction is not obligatory. But the empirical record on these possibilities is sparse at present. The general failure of frontal dysfunction as an explanation for a single schizophrenic disease state is inescapable.

It is really the cognitive tests that are most sensitive to the differences between people with and without schizophrenia. This is evident in the effect sizes obtained for the Wisconsin Card Sorting Test and the Stroop and word fluency tests. It seems that giving the brain of a person with schizophrenia mental work to do is the key to demonstrating a substantial difference between the schizophrenic and the normal brain. If the patient's brain is not "challenged" in this way, the evidence of frontal defect is quite weak.

Is it possible that technical limitations, rather than a faulty hypothesis, underpin the weakness of neurobiological findings on the frontal brain in schizophrenia? Perhaps the brain scanners are at fault. They still lack the degree of spatial resolution needed to detect the kind of microscopic neural abnormalities that must underlie the illness. It is possible to achieve much more powerful resolution with techniques used in post-mortem studies, but unfortunately these studies are too few and far between to draw conclusions. Post-mortem studies have supplied interesting ideas but not consistent, replicated evidence. Still, the near future may hold the answers. In this new millenium, the next generation of imaging developments, including functional magnetic resonance and magnetic resonance spectroscopy, may furnish the powerful evidence of frontal brain involvement in schizophrenia that is lacking. At present, techniques like magnetic resonance spectroscopy can index molecular and metabolic information about the brain, but their spatial resolution is still far below what can be achieved with structural magnetic resonance imaging (McCarley et al., 1996). Thus far, some spectroscopy studies have produced promising results (e.g., Stanley et al., 1995), while others have not (e.g., Buckley et al., 1994). Many aspects of neurobiology are under study, and the field awaits a succession of strong findings that converge on the same aspect of frontal neurobiology (see also Harrison, 1999).

But why are excuses being made for inadequate support for an idea? Faith that a technologically exquisite future will furnish what the past has denied underscores the weakness of the existing evidence. And scientific promissory notes are not really explanations; the predictions of incipient breakthroughs may prove misguided. Possibilities always abound, but in science, speculative explanations to account for weak findings are seldom satisfying. Perhaps the answer, or part of the answer, to schizophrenia simply lies elsewhere in the brain. Indeed, another brain region that has close connections to the frontal lobes—the temporal brain—also has a long history of being associated with mental illness, and that is the next place to look for answers and evidence.

5

•••••••••••••••••••••••••••••

THE BIOLOGY OF
MEANING

In some ways schizophrenia can be understood as a disorder of meaning. It is an illness that transforms the commonplace into the supernatural. A radio announcer's mundane chatter evolves into cryptic but strikingly personal references aimed at the listener. Newspaper headlines no longer disclose the private failings of politicians and film stars; they communicate the inner life, the biography, of the person with schizophrenia. To the delusional mind, the eyes of strangers in the street confirm conspiracies, challenge secrets, and dispute innocence. Dates in calendars now signal calamities or ratify mythologies. Coincidence is misinterpreted as causation; the irrelevant shouts with significance. What was once trivial is now monumental. The illness appears to construct meaning where there is none and to do so with such virtuosity that psychosis has been mistaken for creativity. Then, after the storm, a strange reversal often takes place: the madness recedes and leaves a profound vacancy of meaning in its wake. It leaves a mind of impoverished thought, diminished action, empty language, and sparse emotion, a mind devoid of imagination and interest. It is as though the very intensity of psychotic experience both generates and then extinguishes all meaning.

If there is a cerebral basis for schizophrenia, perhaps it lies in brain regions that store knowledge, assign meaning to experience, transform sounds into communication, sights into objects and people. Perhaps madness roots where the brain preserves these meanings in memory and gives them an emotional significance. Beginning with the work of Carl Wernicke (1874) on the deficit

119

of language comprehension, or aphasia, that bears his name, the temporal lobe of the left cerebral hemisphere has been implicated as part of the brain's semantic system. This implication was known to Kraepelin (1919) and to other psychiatric pioneers who suggested that along with the frontal brain, the temporal lobes were the place to look for the neurogenesis of schizophrenia. Indeed, the pioneers noted that schizophrenic symptoms like thought disorder were often most evident in a patient's nonsensical language. Moreover, there were suggestions and scraps of evidence that the temporal lobes were involved in emotional behavior (Brown & Schaefer, 1888). Here then was another brain region to explore in relation to schizophrenia, one that might prove to be responsible for the illness.

Yet, like the frontal lobes, the temporal brain region did not yield signs of an obvious disease process, at least not in response to the early and fairly crude observations of post-mortem brain tissue carried out at the turn of the century. Instead, over the ensuing decades, a number of behavioral and biological methods arose that were used to gather more subtle evidence on the temporal lobe hypothesis of schizophrenia. First, however, consider the nature of this brain system and how it contributes to normal mind and behavior.

The temporal lobes comprise the sides of the cerebral hemispheres below the Sylvian fissure and in front of a rather vague demarcation from the occipital lobe (see figure 5.1). The temporal cortex includes the neocortex, with six cellular layers, and "older" cortex, the archicortex and paleocortex, composed of three layers, found in the medial surfaces of the temporal lobes. The lateral aspect of the lobes can be divided roughly into superior, middle, and inferior temporal folds of gray matter, or gyrii, and associated creases, or sulcii, along with a small area called Heschl's gyrus at the lip of the Sylvian fissure. Behind Heschl's gyrus and hidden from view is the planum temporale. The temporal cortex is folded so extensively that there is cortical tissue, called the insula, deep within the Sylvian fissure. The cortex of the medial areas includes the fusiform and parahippocampal gyrii, the uncus (literally, "hook"), the hippocampus proper, and the amygdala.

From a functional standpoint, the temporal lobe consists of a primary sensory cortex that is involved in the perception of sound (Heschl's gyrus), an "association" cortex that has psychological importance, and a "limbic" cortex that has been implicated in memory and emotion. Like the frontal lobe, the temporal lobe is rich in connections within and without its own region of the brain, and these connections provide the architecture for the brain's semantic system. The left and right temporal lobes connect with each other and also with the rest of the neocortex and archicortex by way of the corpus callosum and anterior commissure. Neocortical-temporal connections include one system from the primary auditory area around Heschl's gyrus and from posterior visual areas

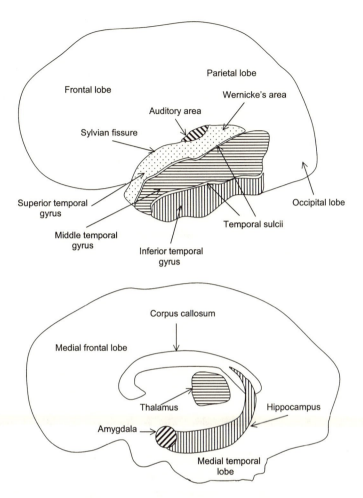

Figure 5.1. The temporal lobe of the human brain. The top drawing shows a lateral view of the left cerebral hemisphere and the three convolutions, or gyrii, of the temporal cortex. The temporal lobe is extensively folded, and the Sylvian fissure and adjacent frontal and parietal lobes hide portions of the auditory area, including Heschl's gyrus as well as the planum temporale. The superior temporal gyrus has been implicated in language perception and includes Wernicke's receptive speech area. However, the temporal cortex is not just a sound processor. It has other semantic and cognitive functions, including object perception and categorization and information selection. The lower drawing shows the medial temporal area, including the hippocampus, which is essential for memory formation, and the amygdala, which plays a role in emotional experience and learning, especially in relation to fear. The temporal lobe semantic system has strong connections with the frontal lobe and with the rest of the brain.

in the occipital lobe that link with the tip or pole of the temporal lobe. This tract brings sensory information, sights and sounds, to the temporal region. A second system brings information from the parietal, occipital, and superior temporal areas into cortical folds deep in the superior temporal sulcus. This information derives from sensations like touch and pressure, along with visual and auditory sensation, and forms an area of "polymodal" temporal cortex. A third tract relays auditory and visual information from the temporal cortex to the amygdala and hippocampus, and a fourth communicates with the prefrontal area of the brain (see Kolb & Whishaw, 1996, pp. 288–289).

It has been theorized that the first, or occipito-temporal, system mediates recognition of a stimulus event. In other words, it allows a person to identify a noise as a speech sound or a pattern of light as an object. The second, or "polymodal," system mediates categorization—what *kind* of object or sound has been identified, and what is its function or use? It is believed that this process, whereby sensory experience is organized into meaningful perceptions and then interrelated with broad classes of meaning, is a primary function of the temporal lobe region. The third system projects to medial structures involved in memory formation and emotion so that information processed into categories, perhaps with emotional associations, is preserved and available for future use. The fourth and final tract allows the frontal executive access to the identified, classified sensory information that is processed in the temporal region.

It is important to note that the left and right temporal lobes differ somewhat in their respective functions. The left side processes language-related information preferentially, while the right side processes nonverbal data like shapes and spatial patterns. To some extent anatomical differences between the temporal lobes mirror this functional asymmetry. Thus the planum temporale is substantially larger in the left than in the right temporal lobe in most people; this may be due to the greater degree of language representation in the left hemisphere. However, such specialization is not absolute, and there is considerable functional overlap between the two temporal lobes (see Kolb & Whishaw, 1996, p. 291).

Accordingly, functional neuroanatomy suggests that the temporal lobes are an essential part of the brain's semantic system: its basis for generating, analyzing, and storing meaning and knowledge. But what kinds of tasks do the temporal lobes actually execute, how are they effected by focal damage in this area, and to what extent do the effects of temporal lobe disorders resemble the behavior seen in schizophrenia? Is it justifiable to consider psychotic illness as a disturbance of the brain's semantic system?

The Temporal Lobe and Its Semantic Functions

Receptive Language

Neuropsychologists and other neuroscientists know a lot more about the psychological importance of the temporal lobes, especially the left, than they know about the frontal lobes and their "executive" role in mind and behavior. Since the trailblazing studies of Wernicke in the nineteenth century, the temporal lobes have been studied more intensively and more successfully than the frontal lobes. Wernicke (1874) discovered 10 patients who could speak fluently but spoke incoherently and were unable to understand language. Their incoherent speech was filled with mispronunciations, peculiar new words, and incorrect word substitutions. For example, a modern patient with Wernicke's aphasia, asked what had led him to the hospital, replied, "Boy, I'm sweating, I'm awful nervous, you know, once in a while I get caught up, I can't mention the tarripoi, a month ago, quite a little, I've done a lot well, I impose a lot, while on the other hand, you know what I mean, I have to run around, look it over, trebbin and all that sort of stuff" (quoted in Gardner, 1975, p. 68). The response has a grammatical structure that resembles normal speech, but is contaminated with errors that make no sense, words invented by the patient (e.g., "trebbin") and is full of empty stock phrases (e.g., "on the other hand . . . you know what I mean"). Here is a kind of speech that is different qualitatively from the expressive aphasia seen in frontal brain damage, which tends to be sparse and poorly articulated. But the cardinal feature of Wernicke's aphasia is an inability to *understand* speech rather than an inability to speak or articulate words correctly. This disturbance, also referred to as sensory or receptive aphasia, was localized to a portion of the posterior superior temporal gyrus (see figure 5.1).

The impairment of Wernicke's aphasia seems rooted in an inability to isolate and categorize speech sounds into established language patterns that carry meaning. Patients with sensory aphasia have adequate hearing and are able to recognize different sounds like a whistle or a telephone ring; but these sounds are nonverbal. As soon as language is involved, the impairment is evident. Aphasic patients not only lack the ability to understand spoken language ("word deafness"), they often cannot repeat back a word or sentence that is spoken by another person. Moreover, comprehension problems are not limited to the auditory modality. They also occur with visually presented language in the form of reading ("word blindness") and writing disabilities ("dysgraphia"; see Benson, 1993).

The brain's capacity to perceive meaning in sound patterns exists in forms that reflect the differential specialization of the right and left temporal lobes in right-handed people. Thus the left temporal lobe is better at processing sounds that are linguistic in nature, whereas the right temporal lobe has an advantage for nonlinguistic sounds like music or tonal passages. Kimura (1961, 1964, 1967) demonstrated these hemispheric advantages and differences with her dichotic listening paradigm. For example, if a person is given stereo headphones and presented with simultaneous but different digits in each ear, more digits will be recalled from the right ear presentation than from the left. This is due to the fact that neuroanatomy gives the right ear a more direct path to the language-specialized left hemisphere. It may even be that the other ear route undergoes suppression and inhibition in the course of language processing. The reverse advantage occurs when melodies, chords, environmental sounds, pitch differences, or emotional sounds are presented to each ear. Then it is the left ear, and presumably the right temporal lobe, that perceives these nonverbal sounds most accurately.

The asymmetries seen in dichotic listening–ear advantage studies have been demonstrated in normal healthy subjects, but they are relatively mild in magnitude. In contrast, dramatic deficits are apparent when clinical tests of receptive language are given to neurological patients with left hemisphere damage. For example, in the Token Test (De Renzi & Faglioni, 1978), a standard clinical task that involves commands of increasing grammatical complexity and comprises stimuli or "tokens" that vary in shape as well as in size and color, the patient has to carry out instructions that begin with simple statements like "touch the red circle" and progress to statements that require precise understanding of grammatical structure like "if there is a black circle, pick up the red square." Healthy people with undamaged brains have little difficulty on even the complex commands of the Token Test, but patients with left temporal lobe damage make many errors.

The traditional localization of sensory aphasia is on the posterior-superior portion of the first temporal gyrus (figure 5.1). However, more recent research suggests great individual variation in the location of receptive language areas (Ojemann, Cawthon, & Lettich, 1990). In other words, some people develop sensory aphasia from lesions in Wernicke's area, but others do not. A sensory aphasia can develop with lesions in adjacent parietal, middle, or inferior temporal areas of cortex. What this implies is that language comprehension may be localized to a specific area of the left temporal lobe in some people, but other people probably have comprehension represented elsewhere in the temporal lobe or even outside it in the parietal area. On the other hand, basic auditory sensation is localized consistently across people to Heschl's gyrus. Thus sensory functions like audition may have a relatively invariant location in the brain yet support associated cognitive functions that vary widely among people in terms of localization. All of which goes to show that psychological abilities resist simple, predictable mapping onto brain regions. Despite this qualification, however, the temporal lobe of the left hemisphere is the brain region most frequently associated with receptive language functions, and disorders effecting this region are expected to have an impact on language.

Selective Attention

The aphasic problems identified in Wernicke's discovery, the first and perhaps most dramatic indications of temporal lobe function, have been supplemented by other discoveries. One of these discoveries concerns the ability to focus attention on particular components of a message and to exclude other components. For example, at a social gathering many people may be speaking at the same time. A listener is unable to process simultaneously every conversation in the room. Two basic options are available to deal with the situation. First, one voice and speech message can be attended to while the others are ignored. Alternatively, attention can be switched rapidly from one speech to another in the hope that the gist of each statement reaches understanding. In either case, however, *selection* of information occurs. Analogous informational conflicts can be imagined in the visual modality. The high school student who attempts to do homework reading while watching television faces the same dilemma. Either one source of information is blocked out and not processed or attention must move back and forth between competing sources.

Psychologists have developed methods to examine this selective information-processing ability with techniques like dichotic listening and split visual-field stimulus presentation. The dichotic listening technique that Kimura (1961) used to study ear and cerebral hemisphere advantages for different kinds of information has many variations and can be adapted for use as a measure of selective attention. Thus message A is heard in one earphone, and message B is heard in the other earphone. The research subject is asked to attend to, or "shadow," one message and to ignore the other. In a sense, one message is the target and everything else is noise. Later, a report of the attended message is requested. The accuracy in reporting or recalling the target message constitutes the index of selective attention. When the dichotic listening–selective attention technique is applied to neurological patients with left or right temporal lobe damage, the expected right ear–left hemisphere advantage for verbal information is found. However, the overall number of words reported also drops markedly, especially with left-sided damage and regardless of which ear receives the target message. Accordingly, beyond its importance in language, the left temporal lobe plays a special role in our ability to attend to information from one source and to block information from another source. This psychologically vital brain system not only extracts meaning from sounds, it selects and ignores different or competing sounds in the environment. This finding is of special interest for psychiatry, because schizophrenia patients show a correlation between their dichotic listening performance and the severity of their thought-disorder symptoms (Wielgus & Harvey, 1988).

Visual Perception

The fact that the primary auditory area is within the temporal lobe system makes it natural to assume that the whole lobe is just a sound processor. However, the extensive intersensory connections that merge visual as well as auditory information in the temporal lobe point to a broader, or "multimodal," kind of role for the temporal lobes in mental life. This has been confirmed by numerous case studies of disorders like agnosia, wherein patients can see an object but are unable to recognize its meaning (Bauer, 1993, pp. 215–278). Studies with normal people also support the importance of the left temporal lobe in visual semantics.

For example, Sergent, Ohta, and MacDonald (1992) carried out positron emission brain imaging to index increases in metabolism during a perception task. Both the left and right temporal lobes showed increased activation when participants had to identify and discriminate photographs of different faces. In addition, when people were asked to categorize photographs of objects as either living or nonliving, a strong metabolic increase was seen in the left hemisphere and left temporal area. Such results highlight the role of the left temporal lobe in visual perception and categorical thinking. The temporal brain is a meaning generator, not just a language generator (see Kolb & Whishaw, 1996, p. 299).

Memory

Damage to the temporal lobes, especially their medial aspect, has been linked to impaired memory since Bekhterev's (1900) amnesia case study at the turn of the century. The anterior temporal cortex, the hippocampus, and the entorhinal cortex have all been implicated as important for the formation of memories (figure 5.1). Yet memory impairment or amnesia is not a unitary inability to recall the past but a syndrome of problems. First, amnesia has an anterograde component wherein new learning is impaired. In neurological patients, "new" usually means since the lesion or disease was acquired that is affecting brain tissue. Whenever the amount of information exceeds what a patient can hold in immediate awareness, a profound recall problem becomes evident. This is often of such severity that the patient never learns new surroundings and rapidly forgets new events. Anterograde amnesia patients are not aphasic; they can speak and understand conversations with little difficulty, and they are not intellectually impaired in general. However, a few moments after an event takes place, conscious memory of the event is gone.

In addition to anterograde amnesia for new events, patients with temporal lobe damage have a milder deficit remembering events that took place in the past, prior to their neurological damage. The famous patient "H.M," whose memory disorder was documented by Brenda Milner (Milner, Corkin, & Teuber, 1968; Corkin, 1984), had poor recall of events for the years immediately preceding his temporal lobe surgery. Yet his memory for very remote events and time periods, his youth and early history, was relatively preserved. Thus the characteristics of true organic amnesia are the complete opposite of the popular media stereotype wherein the amnesiac is unable to remember personal identity or early life experiences but has normal continuous memory for new events. In fact it is memory for new experience that fades in amnesia; people with the disorder do not forget who they are or where they come from.

In neuropsychological research a patient is understood as showing an amnesic syndrome if performance on tests of general intelligence, attention, and immediate memory are normal in the presence of impaired memory for new information and events. Hence amnesia has to be distinguishable from other cognitive deficits. Patients with dementias like Alzheimer's disease may also be diagnosed as memory-impaired, but they are not considered as showing a "pure" amnesic syndrome if evidence of broad intellectual deterioration is present.

There are many tests that can be used to measure the nature and severity of memory problems. This abundance reflects in part the intensive and extensive study that memory has received in biological and experimental psychology over the past century (Lezak, 1995, pp. 429–522). Most tests require the patient to recall or recognize a list of words or a paragraph and to retain information over a specified period of time. The best memory tests allow for an examination of the benefits of practice on learning and also assess the effects of various manipulations on memory performance. These manipulations include introducing new word lists that interfere with accurate recall of the original list. They also include test comparisons between recall that is prompted, or cued, and recall that is uncued, or "free." Finally, some testing paradigms measure recognition memory and not just recall. Recognition is distinct from recall in that recognition tests do not require the subject to produce the original items, just to identify them from a list of possibilities.

A widely used clinical task is the California Verbal Learning Test (Delis, Kramer, Kaplan, & Ober, 1987), which involves oral presentations of 16 words that are introduced as a list of shopping items. These words are organized into four semantic categories (e.g. spices, fruits). The list is initially presented five times, with free recall requested after each presentation. Subjects' responses are scored for the number of words correctly recalled and also for error types like repetitions (perseverations) and intrusions (off-list words). After the first five trials, a new list of 16 words is introduced to create interference with the original items. Following this, free and cued (e.g., "tell me all the words that were spices") recall trials are administered for the original list at short and "long" (20 minute) delay intervals. A recognition test rounds out the evaluation, wherein the original shopping items are read out, interspersed with related and unrelated new words. The patient has to indicate which words were from the original shopping list.

Patients with neurological damage that is confined exclusively to the medial temporal lobes are rare and hard to find. However, there are a number of diseases that preferentially affect the temporal lobes, and these diseases provide an indication of how temporal lobe damage can affect verbal memory. For example, Crosson, Sartork, Jenny, and Nabors (1993) reported California Verbal Learning Test results on two samples of patients with medial temporal lesions due to trauma or surgery. Although these patients did poorly on several aspects of the test, they were most markedly abnormal in their high rates of intrusion errors on the free and cued recall trials. They seemed unable to remember recent information selectively. Memory was not absent as much as it was contaminated by errors, false memories, or attempts at remembering that only approximated, inaccurately, the original information.

Accordingly, memory impairment associated with mesial temporal damage is fairly selective in that it strikes new learning but leaves old knowledge and intellectual skill largely intact. More specifically, current memory research designates the hippocampus in the medial temporal lobe as the structure that is crucial for new memory formation (Kolb & Whishaw, 1996, pp. 300–301; Bauer, Tobias, & Valenstein, 1993).

Emotion and Psychosis

The importance of the temporal lobes in mind and behavior is not limited to their contribution to cognitive function. The semantic brain influences emotional processes as well. In a sense, meaning is emotional and not just cognitive in nature. Recognizing a visual form as a person may be a cognitive process, but emotional experience adds context and significance to the act of recognition. The person we recognize evokes passion or interest, fear or apathy. This too is a kind of meaning.

Suggestions that the temporal lobes of the brain were important in human emotion came from early research on animal behavior. The Kluver-Bucy syndrome in monkeys (Brown & Schaefer, 1888; Kluver & Bucy, 1939) involves tameness, loss of fear, indiscriminate eating and sexual activity, intense reactions to any visual stimulus, and excessive "orality"—placing things in the mouth— along with cognitive defects in recognizing objects. Similar problems have been observed in a handful of humans when the amygdala and inferior temporal cortex are damaged through inflammatory disease or removed in the course of surgery (Kolb & Whishaw, 1996, pp. 418–420).

Clues to the importance of the temporal lobe in human emotion have also been accrued by studying patients with temporal lobe epilepsy. This condition arises from irritative lesions or other focal abnormalities in the temporal region that in turn cause local electrical disturbances in the form of seizures. In one study, the friends of patients with temporal lobe epilepsy were asked to rate the patients on a number of personality traits (Bear & Fedio, 1977). Many of the traits were cognitive in nature. For example, one was "circumstantiality," or a kind of speaking style that lacks a focal point and is full of irrelevant detail. Another trait ascribed to the epileptic patients was "philosophical interest"—a tendency to speculate about topics like the nature of existence, morality, and the origins of the universe. Emotional traits were also observed: the epileptic patients were seen as irritable, temperamental, elated, and hostile (see also Fedio & Martin, 1983; Kolb & Whishaw, 1996, pp. 453–455).

Of course, such idiosyncracies of personality and emotion hardly amount to psychotic behavior of the kind seen in serious mental illnesses like schizophrenia. However, a few epileptic patients do develop a "schizophreniform" syndrome as part of their illness, and there seems to be a link with the medial temporal region in such patients. For example, Jibiki, Maeda, Kubota, and Yamaguchi (1993) described two patients with epilepsy who developed psychotic symptoms, including auditory hallucinations and delusions of persecution. Functional brain scanning that indexed blood flow patterns revealed abnormalities in the left temporal lobes of both patients. Moreover, when the patients were scanned during an actual psychotic experience, one showed an abnormality in the amygdala region of the temporal lobe. On the other hand, the second patient had a normal scanning study. In addition, such cases of apparent epileptic psychosis may simply represent a situation where both schizophrenia and seizures develop independently in the same person. In this respect it is worth noting that only a minority of seizure patients, perhaps 10%, develop a syndrome that resembles schizophrenia (Roberts, Done, Bruton, & Crow, 1990). Even those who do develop the syndrome show patterns of positive and negative symptoms that differ from what is seen in schizophrenia (Crowe & Kuttner, 1991).

There are also occasional reports of patients with space-occupying brain lesions and frank psychosis. Thus Ferracuti, Accornero, and Manfredi (1991) reported psychosis in four patients with arachnoid cysts—fluid-filled cavities—affecting their left temporal lobes. The patients experienced brief paranoid delusions and strong mood-related changes that alternated between depression and excitement. They also showed aggressiveness, disturbed sleeping and waking behavior, and changes in eating habits. This syndrome is intriguing, but it resembles mood disturbances like manic depression (bipolar disorder) as much as schizophrenia.

In many ways, however, the strongest evidence for a relationship between emotion, if not psychosis, and the medial temporal brain regions comes from animal rather than human studies. This work has been synthesized by Ledoux (1995, 1996), who argues that the amygdala (see figure 5.1) is an important component in mediating emotions like fear and the perception of danger. According to Ledoux, animal studies of fear conditioning, in which a previously neutral event like a harmless sound comes to be associated with a threatening or unpleasant stimulus like a shock, show that the amygdala receives "crude" sensory data by way of a "fast" neural route through the thalamus. This connection is essential for simple fear conditioning, which does not take place if the route is damaged. A second connection carries information processed in the cerebral cortex. This route is slower but provides more complex, detailed cognitive analysis. Together the two neural pathways form a system that supports the learning of fear. Experiments with animals also demonstrate that learning to associate fear with a stimulus or event involves a contextual aspect so that the situation is learned along with the stimulus pairing. In other words, the animal associates threat or danger with surrounding contextual cues (i.e., the cage) rather than with just the conditioned stimulus (i.e., the sound). The surroundings come to evoke fear on their own. This context learning aspect depends on connections between the amygdala and the hippocampus. Accordingly, fear learning does not take place in animals if the lateral amygdaloid nucleus is destroyed, or if the hippocampus is damaged, in the case of context learning. Furthermore, another part of the amygdala, the central nucleus, interacts with motor systems to control defensive behavior like "freezing" and also influences brain regions that control stress reactions. The amygdala in turn not only influences other structures and neural systems but is influenced and inhibited by the prefrontal executive cortex. An animal that has been conditioned to fear a previously innocuous event or stimulus takes longer to extinguish and lose the association over time if the prefrontal brain is damaged. It seems that fear memories themselves are permanent, but behavior associated with such memories, like avoidance, can be suppressed by the frontal brain system.

Amygdaloid lesions in humans are rare, which makes it hard to compare animal and human behavior. Nonetheless, Ledoux (1996) extrapolated the animal literature to humans to provide a picture of how the amygdala regulates the psychological experience of fear. He gives the example of a hiker in the woods suddenly spotting a "snake" coiled on the path. The initial perception of a curved object occurs very rapidly and yields a quick transmission from the visual part of the thalamus to the amygdala. This sets up a rapid fear response in the hiker, who experiences a sense of danger and freezes or avoids the snake. However, this fear response is based on cursory and limited analysis of the perceived shape. Indeed, the perception *curved shape = snake* may be inaccurate. The object might be a curved branch, a rope left by another hiker, or a play of light from the sun shining through the trees. But such detailed analysis requires the second and cortically based link to the amygdala. Yet the price of accuracy and detail is time. Moreover, the hiker is better off mistakenly treating a branch as a poisonous snake than treating a snake as a branch. Not engaging in avoidance or freezing when it is called for can have dire consequences. Curiously, the next day, the hiker may feel uncomfortable just walking in the woods, with no snake in sight. The hippocampus has preserved the contextual memory and surroundings of the previous experience of fear and danger.

Support for the role of the amygdala in normal human emotional memory comes from positron emission tomography research by Cahill et al. (1996). Healthy research participants watched emotional and neutral film clips while being scanned for regional changes in brain metabolism. Three weeks later they were asked to remember as many of the film clips as possible. The number of emotional films recalled was related to the level of metabolic activity in the amygdala during the original viewing session. Hence, amygdala activation seems to be important for the formation of emotional memories in humans as well as in animals.

In further support of Ledoux's (1996) idea that the amygdala is a "hub in the wheel of fear," it is noteworthy that fear and anxiety are the most common emotional effects of temporal lobe seizures. During a seizure, an epileptic patient may become sexually aroused, laugh, and cry, but the most frequently seen behaviors suggest fear and anxiety (Heilman, Bowers, & Valenstein, 1993). Similarly, between seizures, fear and anxiety are the most common phenomena. Restriction of emotional expression, the "flat affect" commonly seen in schizophrenia, also occurs, but only in small numbers of epilepsy cases (Roberts et al., 1990).

Summary of Temporal Lobe Function

In view of the evidence, there is considerable justification for regarding the temporal lobes as a system that adds a variety of meanings to experience. The meanings may be cognitive, so that objects can be categorized or conceptualized or so that sound patterns can be recognized as language instead of as gibberish. At the same time, meaning may involve the emotional significance of a perception, the feeling or experience it evokes. The cognitive kind of meaning (e.g., what is this shape or sound?) appears to be mediated by the temporal neocortex, and the emotional kind of meaning (e.g., is this shape or sound to be feared?) is influenced by the amygdala. The ability to learn new associations on a cognitive basis seems to depend on the hippocampus. However, both the hippocampus and the amygdala contribute to emotional learning. True, the temporal lobe semantic system is not functionally or anatomically self-contained. It is closely related to executive and sensory and motor brain systems. Nonetheless, the temporal lobes contribute disproportionately to what theorists like Gazzaniga (1985) term the "interpretive module" of the brain: the categorizing, inferential network that interprets events and experience, assigns significance to events, and colors experience with feeling. Can the riddles of schizophrenia be solved by studying this psychologically powerful brain region?

Schizophrenia and the Semantic Brain

Damage to the temporal lobes in the form of conventional brain damage may occasionally produce a picture that mimics some of the symptoms seen in schizophrenia. However, this is indirect evidence, and it makes sense to ask whether temporal lobe function and structure are actually altered in the illness, and if so, in what way and to what degree. And if diminished function and structure exist, are they of sufficient magnitude to support a causal explanation for the neurogenesis of schizophrenia?

Receptive Language in Schizophrenia

Linguistic analyses of schizophrenic speech and comprehension were popular research subjects in the 1970s and 1980s (e.g., Morice, 1986; Rochester & Martin, 1979). This interest has waned over the last decade, at least in terms of trying to make the case for a schizophrenic aphasia. Relatively few studies still include language tests in their neuropsychological batteries. Nonetheless, Konstantine Zakzanis and I (Heinrichs & Zakzanis, 1998) searched the literature between 1980 and 1997 for studies reporting results with the Token Test—De Renzi and Faglioni's (1978) receptive language task—in patients and healthy control subjects. We located seven studies showing a fairly strong average tendency ($d = .98$) for schizophrenia patients to be impaired on the test. An effect size like this implies perhaps 45% score overlap between patient and control distributions. The effects are reliable in the sense that studies consistently yielded ds larger than 0. However, the range of values is considerable, from $d = .3$ to $d = 1.8$, which is mirrored in the fairly large margin of error (.36). Thus, on average, roughly half of schizophrenia patients probably have problems understanding basic language and speech structures. Therefore, Landre, Taylor, and Kearns (1992) may be correct in arguing that dysphasic schizophrenia represents a subgroup of the illness, especially in light of the range of effect sizes that exist in the literature.

Another question that emerges in relation to language function in schizophrenia is whether any deficit is of the same order as the impairment seen in neurological patients with aphasia. In other words, perhaps patients are disadvantaged when compared with healthy people. But the language difficulties of schizophrenia patients may pale in comparison with the deficits seen in true aphasia. As a perspective on this question, consider data drawn from Heinrichs and Awad's (1993) study. The schizophrenia patients in this sample had been ill for 17.1 years on average, which means that they were a relatively "chronic" sample. Using De Renzi and Faglioni's (1978) scores and severity categories for aphasia patients as a reference, only about 13% of the schizophrenia sample could be considered mildly to severely language-impaired. In contrast, 93% of the aphasic patients fell into this category. Such a large discrepancy suggests much greater impairment in true aphasia than in schizophrenia. To be fair, some schizophrenia patient samples may show much higher prevalence of severe impairment on the Token Test than our sample did. In the end, a dysphasic subpopulation of schizophrenia patients may be the most plausible explanation for the findings on language impairment in the illness.

Yet perhaps the temporal lobe dysfunction of the schizophrenia patient manifests itself most consistently elsewhere and not in receptive language tests and comprehension problems (Levin, Yurgelun-Todd, & Craft, 1989). Perhaps temporal lobe functions in schizophrenia are compromised more consistently and more severely on other tasks, such as those that require selective attention, verbal and object categorization, memory processes, and emotion.

Selective Attention, Memory and Schizophrenia

Recall that the dichotic listening task can be used as a measure of selective attention. Words or sound patterns are presented simultaneously to both ears, and the research participant must ignore one message and attend selectively to the other message for a period of time. The person is asked to report or repeat the target message, and this report is scored for accuracy and errors. Stephanie McDermid and I searched the literature between 1980 and 1999 and found 11 studies that compared 514 schizophrenia patients and healthy people on dichotic listening–selective attention tasks. These studies yield an average effect size of $d = 1.16$. Hence schizophrenia patients tend to do poorly when required to attend and ignore auditory information selectively. This effect size corresponds to less than 40% overlap of schizophrenia and control distributions. However, the range of individual effect sizes, from $d = .59$ to $d = 2.23$, is considerable. Moreover, older studies seem to yield much larger effect sizes than recent studies. All of the effects greater than $d = 1.0$ come from the early to mid 1980s, whereas recent work consistently shows much more modest findings. Nonetheless, perhaps 60% of schizophrenia patients are defective in selective attention, and this is consistent with impaired temporal lobe function.

The most frequently studied cognitive ability in relation to the temporal lobes and schizophrenia is undoubtedly memory. Psychiatric pioneers like Kraepelin and Bleuler were less prescient than usual in this respect. They maintained that the illness had little effect on memory. Indeed, interest in studying memory in schizophrenia with neuropsychological tests has a relatively short history in comparison with the longstanding interest in language and attention. Nonetheless, research on memory in the illness has burgeoned over the last decade. This growth parallels the availability of a wide variety of clinical memory tests and the fact that memory is probably the most studied ability in both cognitive psychology and neuropsychology. Indeed there is a proliferation of different tests and measures, all supposedly tapping different aspects of learning and memory. For example, the California Verbal Learning Test alone yields 28 different scores and indices.

Ironically, the abundance of memory tests and measures is a disadvantage from the perspective of research synthesis. Different investigators often use different tests or report different scores from the same test. Thus Randolph et al. (1994) reported total recall scores summed across the first five trials of the California Verbal Learning Test. In contrast, Paulsen et al. (1995), using the same test, reported a very specific aspect of memory, intrusion error rates on free and cued recall trials, along with the more general recall score. Both kinds of score reporting are valuable. Selective scores are of theoretical interest because they may involve processes that are especially prone to disruption in the case of medial temporal lobe dysfunction. Summary or aggregate scores are broader performance indicators that cast a wider net and may be sensitive to a larger variety of pathologies.

To organize the literature for the purposes of meta-analysis we (Heinrichs & Zakzanis, 1998) distinguished global from selective verbal memory and both of these from nonverbal memory. Global verbal memory comprises summed recall scores over trials and other similar general learning indices. Selective verbal memory comprises specific scores like intrusion rate, forgetting, recall, and recognition rates over a specified retention interval. Nonverbal memory tests in common use have not been fractionated into as many subcomponents as the verbal tests. Hence it was possible to include all measures that involved recall or recognition of visual shapes and patterns into one category.

In our search of the literature between 1980 and 1997 we found 31 studies that reported 33 global verbal memory scores. The average effect size for impaired global verbal memory in schizophrenia was $d = 1.41$. This corresponds to a hypothetical overlap of about 30% between schizophrenia and control group distributions. The confidence interval shows that the average global verbal memory effect has a margin of error of about 21 decimal points 95% of the time. Hence, this is a large and fairly reliable finding—one of the largest average effect sizes found thus far in the schizophrenia literature. Moreover, a recent meta-analysis by Aleman, Hijman, de Haan, and Kahn (1999), which used a somewhat broader definition of verbal memory and included 60 studies, had an average effect size of $d = 1.21$, which is within the margin of error of our own finding.

The selective verbal memory results are of greater theoretical interest because they probably index aspects of memory that are more specifically tied to the left temporal lobe as opposed to the brain as a whole. However, we only found seven studies, reporting nine "selective" scores that could be converted into effect sizes. These studies yielded an average effect size for impaired memory of $d = .90$, which corresponds to about 50% score overlap between schizophrenia and control distributions. This is smaller than the effect obtained for global verbal memory, but the margin of error is larger (.46).

One way of looking at the two verbal memory effect sizes is to argue that although verbal memory deficit is quite prevalent in schizophrenia, there is no evidence that patients are impaired disproportionately on those selective aspects of verbal memory that are implicated in medial-temporal dysfunction. Schizophrenia patients are most likely to show impairment on general aspects of memory that probably depend on large areas of the left cerebral hemisphere.

The nonverbal memory results reported in our meta-analysis of 14 studies (Heinrichs & Zakzanis, 1998) reveal an effect size ($d = .74$) that is substantially smaller than the ds obtained with verbal memory measures. Moreover, there is a much greater degree of variability and dispersion present in the nonverbal results, with effect sizes ranging between $d = 0$ and $d = 2.2$. An individual result like $d = 2.2$ is a powerful finding and corresponds to less than 16% overlap between schizophrenia and control group distributions. However, such findings are rare in the published literature. Nonverbal memory deficit is a rather unreliable finding that raises questions about both the nature of schizophrenia and the nature of the testing involved. For example, heterogeneous results may reflect the existence of a heterogeneous patient population, with variable proportions of memory-impaired and intact patients. It may also reflect different testing methods and differential contributions of the two cerebral hemispheres to nonverbal retention and recall. Recognizing previously presented photographs of faces may involve somewhat different processes and brain regions than drawing a previously presented geometric shape from memory. If this is true, then some nonverbal memory functions may be more impaired than others in schizophrenic illness.

Accordingly, schizophrenia–control comparisons on memory tests yield large effect sizes for verbal material, especially for more general aspects of learning and memory. The effect sizes are large, but are they large enough to indicate that verbal memory deficits are a feature of schizophrenia in general? Not really. A substantial minority of patients with normal memory functions must still exist.

Case Studies

A perspective on the magnitude and consistency of memory impairment in schizophrenia can be gained by considering Ruth, William, and James. Test results obtained on the three patients are presented in table 5.1. The table shows that Ruth, who experienced tactile sensations of a leech or creature around her neck, has normal scores on almost all of the temporal lobe tests. Her receptive language (Token Test) and verbal (CVLT) memory scores are average and her nonverbal recall is only slightly below average. William, who experienced delu-

Table 5.1 Intellectual and temporal-semantic cognitive test results in three patients

	Patients and Test Scores		
	Ruth	William	James
Symptoms			
Hallucinations	Strange smell	None reported	Voice
Delusions	Impending death	Divinity, power	Alien control
Negative	Withdrawal	None reported	Withdrawal
IQ (WAIS-R)	108 (90–110)	105 (90–110)	84 (90–110)
Token Test	35 (29–36)	35 (29–36)	27 (29–36)
California Verbal Learning Test (CVLT)			
Total words, trials 1–5	52 (51–66)	37 (46–61)	29 (49–63)
20 minute retention (%)	100 (90–100)	100 (90–100)	71 (90–100)
Intrusion errors	3 (0–5)	0 (0–6)	2 (0–6)
Complex Figure Recall/36	18 (21–24)	11 (21–24)	22 (21–24)

Note: WAIS-R = Wechlser Adult Intelligence Scale—Revised (Wechsler,1981). Values in brackets are score ranges for normal performance. The Complex Figure (Osterrieth, 1944) Recall Test is described in chapter 2 and by Lezak (1995), pp. 475–479.

sions of divinity, has no problems with language comprehension but learned a smaller number of words than average on the CVLT and also did poorly in recalling a complex geometric figure on the test of nonverbal memory. On the other hand, his other memory results are unremarkable. He remembered an average number of words after about 20 minutes' delay, had a normal rate of forgetting, and was not prone to making intrusion errors. Nonetheless, there is some evidence of impaired memory. Finally, James, who was convinced that a parasite had penetrated his brain, did poorly on all of the language-related, comprehension, and memory tests. Yet he performed within average limits in the area of nonverbal recall. James is clearly the most impaired of the three patients, but he also has a lower general intelligence than the other two patients.

The individual patient data, like the effect size analyses, indicate that deficits on psychological functions associated with the temporal lobes are not an invariant feature of schizophrenia. Ruth's results demonstrate that it is quite possible for someone with the illness to be almost completely normal on tests of receptive language and verbal and nonverbal memory. Moreover, the only major problem that William had was on the nonverbal memory task. Finally, James's test results again raise the issue of generalized deficits and the extent to which many patients do poorly on almost any kind of cognitive test.

How can the memory problems of the schizophrenia patient be characterized, and to what extent do they reflect pathological events in the temporal lobes? Memory problems are prevalent in the illness, but not all patients have them, and there is concurrent evidence of lowered general cognitive ability. In addition, many aspects of verbal memory are compromised by schizophrenia and not just those aspects, like intrusion errors, that are most tied to the temporal system. Therefore, the memory difficulties of the schizophrenia patient probably reflect a broad brain dysfunction that extends beyond the temporal lobes.

Emotion

Do patients with schizophrenia show emotional behavior that resembles the behavior of neurological patients with temporal lobe abnormalities? The question is almost impossible to answer. Schizophrenia patients and healthy people are seldom compared on measures of emotional functioning that reflect putative temporal lobe abnormalities. In fact, there is little consensus regarding what emotional effects are intrinsic to focal temporal lobe damage. The most common effects are believed to involve fear and anxiety. Perhaps schizophrenia patients suffer from intense and pervasive anxiety. But perhaps not. Although emotional disturbance has always been considered part of schizophrenia, its most frequently described features include "flat affect," an expressionless face, along with apathy and withdrawal. Such features imply a lack of feeling, or at least its outward supression, rather than a heightened experience of emotion (see Andreasen & Flaum, 1991). Still, the hypothesized role of the medial temporal region in emotion, especially the idea that the amygdala controls threat appraisal and fear conditioning, is intriguing in light of schizophrenic symptoms like paranoia and suspiciousness. To some degree a delusion of persecution is like an excessive and unwarranted appraisal of danger. Is this the telltale sign of a malfunctioning amygdala? Unfortunately, the literature is too sparse to say that schizophrenic illness is linked in any clear way to the amygdala by way of emotional behavior. However, the use of disordered behavior to find the location of abnormal brain biology is not the only available tool. There are alternative ways of pursuing the neurological roots of schizophrenia deep into the semantic and emotional brain.

Neurobiology of the Temporal Lobe in Schizophrenia

Cognitive tasks provide the most direct way of measuring the temporal brain's meaning-generation and storage capabilities. However, cognitive tests are an uncertain guide to the discovery of focal brain abnormalities. Most cognitive functions are mediated by more than one neural structure or are represented diffusely throughout the brain. At the same time, many aspects of perception, language, thinking, and reasoning have not been examined extensively in terms of their possible cerebral basis. As was the case with the frontal-executive hypothesis, the best way to find brain abnormalities is to look for them directly with biologically revealing instruments like brain imaging or post-mortem microscopy and tissue analysis. Yet some of the realities and disadvantages of the biological approach laid bare in chapter 4 are worth keeping in mind. Nuclear magnetic resonance and positron emission tomography provide pictures of brain structure and physiology but at a level of resolution that may fail to detect the fine-grained neural changes associated with schizophrenia. This limitation of resolving power is even more evident with less sophisticated techniques like computerized axial tomography and single photon emission tomography scanning. In the case of the frontal brain hypothesis and as seen in chapter 4, the brain-imaging research produced very modest effect sizes, and none were able to consistently separate even a majority of schizophrenia patients from healthy people. In addition, the most powerful imaging evidence was obtained when patients were first engaged in cognitive test–related behavior and then scanned for blood flow or metabolic changes. Will the temporal lobes tell a similar tale?

There are grounds for expecting stronger biological evidence in the case of the temporal lobes and schizophrenia. The scientific literature has implicated specific temporal lobe structures in the illness, like the hippocampus and amygdala, rather than just large expanses of cortex in the frontal brain. Although old techniques like computerized axial tomography are incapable of distinguishing structures like the hippocampus from surrounding tissue, magnetic resonance imaging does have this capability. Moreover, the symptoms of schizophrenia are easier to understand as the result of an abnormal semantic system than as the result of an incompetent executive. Consider table 5.2, then, and the neurobiological support for the temporal-semantic brain hypothesis.

Left Temporal Lobe Structure in Schizophrenia

Consider first the entire left temporal lobe, its relative size or volume in schizophrenia and healthy people, and the possibility that the lobe is abnormally reduced in the illness. Magnetic resonance studies have increased in frequency in recent years, so I was able to concentrate on this technique. I did not include computerized tomography (CT) studies in my search. My students and I found 25 studies published between 1980 and 1999 that measured the volume of the whole left temporal lobe in schizophrenia patients and in healthy people. The average effect size for reduced volume in schizophrenia ($d = .25$) reveals a very weak group tendency for the left temporal lobe to be smaller in the illness. This effect size corresponds to an average overlap of about 81% between patients and healthy people in terms of tissue volumes. There are no large individual effects (i.e., $d > 1.0$) in the set of studies; most of the ds are small, and the margin of error is small (.10). Overall, the evidence clearly shows that the vast majority of

Table 5.2 Left temporal lobe abnormalities in schizophrenia

Abnormality	Mean d	Confidence Interval	N
Language comprehension deficit (Token Test)	.98	.62–1.34	7
Selective attention deficit (dichotic listening)	1.16	.82–1.50	11
Global verbal memory deficit	1.41	1.20–1.62	31
Selective verbal memory deficit	.90	.44–1.36	7
Nonverbal memory deficit	.74	−.31–1.79	14
Magnetic resonance studies			
Reduced tissue volume (lobe)	.25	.15–.35	25
Reduced planum temporale area	.38	−.02–.78	7
Reduced planum temporale asymmetry	.30	−.07–.67	5
Reduced superior temporal gyrus	.59	.39–.79	12
Reduced hippocampal volume	.41	.25–.57	22
Reduced amygdala volume, area	.30	.02–.58	12
Post-mortem studies			
Reduced hippocampal volume, area	.92	.63–1.21	6
Reduced hippocampal pyramidal cells	.86	.38–1.34	4
Positron emission tomography studies			
Reduced metabolism at rest (lobe)	.13	−.29–.55	11
Reduced blood flow at rest (lobe)	.25	−.02–.52	10
Increased metabolism during activation (lobe)	.39	.17–.61	6
Reduced blood flow during activation (lobe)	.26	−.29–.81	5
Reduced hippocampal metabolism/blood flow	.25	−.23–.73	10
Reduced amygdaloid metabolism/blood flow	.55	.25–.85	6

Note: The table shows effect sizes (Cohen's d) as absolute values, corrected for sample size and averaged over studies in a research domain. Confidence interval is the 95% confidence interval for the mean d. The true average population effect probably lies in this range, and intervals that include zero indicate highly unstable effects. N = the number of published studies included in the meta-analysis.

patients with schizophrenia have left temporal lobe volumes that fall within normal limits.

Simply measuring the whole left temporal lobe is a relatively coarse index of possible brain abnormalities. The lobe is a complex system of cortical convolutions and subcortical structures, any or none of which may be abnormal in some way in schizophrenia. Accordingly, a number of specific regions within the temporal lobe have received attention. One of these is the planum temporale, located in the superior posterior area of the lobe. The planum temporale is of special interest because it is larger in the left than in the right temporal lobe in most right-handed people. This asymmetry in size is believed to reflect the asymmetry of language representation in the brain, wherein the left cerebral hemisphere is "dominant" for verbal functions. If schizophrenia is a disorder of the brain's semantic system, perhaps the disorder is manifest in language-related structures like the left planum temporale (see DeLisi et al., 1997).

To explore this possibility we located seven studies that used magnetic resonance imaging to measure the area of the planum temporale in schizophrenia patients and control subjects. The average effect size for reduced area in schizo-phrenia patients was $d = .38$, and four of the studies yielded effects that were close to zero. However, one recent study (Kwon et al., 1999) reported a large ef-fect ($d = 1.55$). Still, the results are so uneven that the margin of error for the average effect is large enough to include zero ($d = -.02 - d = .78$). Yet it could also be argued that the key schizophrenic abnormality lies not in a smaller left planum temporale relative to healthy people but in a reduced or absent asym-metry between the left and the right planum. This reduced asymmetry might reflect an abnormal functional organization of the brain in the illness. We were able to assess this possibility on a small scale by considering five studies that compared the degree of left–right asymmetry for the planum temporale in pa-tients and healthy people. The results show that although schizophrenia patients as a group tend to have slightly less asymmetry than healthy people, the aver-age effect size is very small ($d = .30$) and would be even smaller if the anom-alous finding ($d = -1.14$) of Kwon et al. (1999) was excluded.

The superior temporal gyrus is another cortical subregion in the temporal lobe that has received attention recently (see figure 5.1). This convolution of gray matter along the top of the temporal lobe, including Wernicke's area, has been implicated in disturbances of auditory sensation and perception (Kolb & Whishaw, 1996, pp. 446–453). These disturbances include defective language comprehension and selective attention. Davidson (1999), in her meta-analysis of this region, found 12 studies demonstrating that there was a tendency for schizo-phrenia to be associated with reduced volumes of the left superior temporal gyrus as indexed by magnetic resonance imaging. However, the effect is still modest ($d = .59$; confidence interval: $d = .39 - d = .79$), suggesting that about two-thirds of schizophrenia patients have tissue volumes in the normal range. This is stronger evidence than the support for whole lobe volume or planum temporale abnormalities, but still too weak to support the idea that most patients with the illness have reduced temporal lobe tissue volumes. It may be, therefore, that abnormal tissue reductions exist in the more medial and subcortical parts of the temporal lobe–semantic system, the parts that govern memory and emotion.

Verbal memory deficits are among the strongest findings in the whole liter-ature on schizophrenia. This leads to the complementary prediction that pa-tients should have abnormalities of memory-related brain structures like the hippocampus in the medial region of the left temporal lobe. To evaluate the outcome of this prediction, we again collected only magnetic resonance studies that reported volume comparisons in schizophrenia patients and healthy par-ticipants. These studies average to an effect size of $d = .41$ for a reduced hip-pocampus in the illness. However, this modest average value is somewhat mis-leading in that it hides the presence of both large and very small effect sizes. Thus Bogerts et al. (1993) measured the posterior portion of the hippocampus and reported values that correspond to an effect size of $d = -1.37$. In this study, a majority of schizophrenia patients had smaller hippocampal formations than the comparison subjects. In contrast, Marsh et al. (1997) found a slight tendency for schizophrenia patients to have *larger* hippocampal formations than the comparison subjects. Overall, two of the 22 studies discovered larger average hippocampal volumes in the patients than in healthy people, two studies yielded effects close to zero, two studies found strong effects in the expected direction, and the rest produced modest evidence for reduced hippocampal volumes in the illness. Some schizophrenia patients, a small minority, have abnormally reduced hippocampal formations in the left temporal lobe, but most patients are indistinguishable from normal values. There may also be a very small minority with abnormally large hippocampal formations.

The amygdala's central importance in at least one aspect of emotion—fear—has been supported strongly by research on animals (Ledoux, 1996). However, the amygdala is a very small structure and difficult to separate clearly from the adjacent hippocampus, even with the best scanning instruments. Nevertheless, to assess whether patients with schizophrenia have abnormal reductions, or increases, in the size of the amygdala, we searched the literature and discovered 12 studies that reported magnetic resonance scanning results. I only included studies that delineated the amygdala from hippocampus sufficiently for a separate measurement. The average effect size for a reduced amygdala in schizophrenia is $d = .30$. This is quite similar in magnitude to the hippocampal findings. The individual study effects range from fairly large values (e.g., $d = -1.14$; Egan et al., 1994) to modest values in the opposite direction (e.g., d = .42; Schneider et al., 1998). The average effect size corresponds to about 79% overlap between patient and healthy distributions in terms of amygdala volumes.

Hence, viewed collectively, the structural brain imaging research on the left temporal lobe has failed to yield strong support for abnormal tissue reductions in schizophrenia. In the case of planum temporale comparisons, the average effects are so unstable that there really is no evidence of any abnormality in this language-linked region of the cortex (see table 5.2). None of the other temporal regions examined are markedly abnormal either, even when stability is not an issue. However, the resolving power of magnetic resonance imaging is taxed to the limit when small structures like the amygdala are measured. It is hard to know whether the weak findings are a true picture of the schizophrenic brain or the result of a technology that cannot detect subtle pathology.

To emphasize these points, consider left temporal lobe magnetic resonance findings in Alzheimer's disease compiled by Zakzanis (1998). This form of dementia is known to involve extensive pathological changes in temporal cortex and hippocampus. The average d is 1.51 for volume comparisons of the whole left temporal lobe in Alzheimer dementia and healthy elderly people. The average comparison for hippocampal volumes yields $d = 1.11$. These values are much larger than the corresponding values obtained for schizophrenia. However, even in the case of Alzheimer's disease, the average d is not large enough to completely separate distributions of people with and without the disorder. Thus 30–40% of Alzheimer and healthy old people are still indistinguishable on the basis of magnetic resonance scans of their left temporal lobe volumes. It is not surprising that neurologists do not rely on brain scanning to make a diagnosis of Alzheimer's disease. The definitive diagnosis is made with a microscope by a neuropathologist after the patient's death.

If the pathological changes of dementia are hard to detect with brain-scanning techniques, then finding the pathology of schizophrenia is likely to prove even more difficult. The possibility of structural abnormalities in the semantic brain of the person with the illness persists. But if these abnormalities exist, researchers must look much more closely at the microscopic cellular landscape of this brain region. At present, only post-mortem brain tissue analysis allows for such a detailed look at the neurobiology of the semantic brain.

Post-Mortem Studies of the Left Temporal Lobe

The first question I asked of this literature was whether the greater measurement accuracy and precision available with post-mortem microscopy would yield estimates of left hippocampal volume and area that differed from the magnetic resonance findings. We found six studies that reported data on hippocampal area and volume in schizophrenia brain tissue samples. Unfortunately, only two of the studies focused on the left hippocampus, and the rest seem to have measured both the left and the right hippocampus together. Still, with an average effect of $d = .92$, the studies reveal the strongest evidence so far of reduced hippocampal volume in schizophrenia. An effect size of this magnitude means that in theory more than half the patient and control brain samples are distinguishable in terms of measured tissue volumes. Still, the studies are few in number, and there was appreciable variation in effect sizes, ranging from a low of $d = - .44$ (Heckers, Heinsen, Heinsen, & Beckmann, 1990) to a high of $d = -1.61$ (Bogerts, Meertz, & Schonfeldt-Bausch, 1985). Hence the rather sparse and somewhat dated post-mortem literature suggests that a variable but substantial proportion of preserved schizophrenia brain samples, perhaps half, have reduced hippocampal volumes.

Size alone is an uncertain indicator of dysfunction. Reduced area and volume in structures like the hippocampus imply rather than indicate pathology. More convincing evidence would be to find fewer hippocampal neurons in schizophrenia than in control brain samples. Such a result would imply neuronal death as a basis for the illness. In searching the literature, we found six studies reporting cell counts or densities in the hippocampus. Four of these focused on one cell type, the pyramidal neuron, and two measured all cell types. The average effect for reduced pyramidal cell counts and densities was $d = .86$. In contrast, the two studies that reported generic neuron counts produced trivial effects ($d = .06$, $d = .17$) suggesting no real differences between patient and control brain tissue. Three of the pyramidal cell assays yielded substantial effects greater than $d = 1$. Unfortunately, one study (Benes, Sorensen, & Bird, 1991) produced a result of only $d = -.01$—basically zero. Thus the most that can be said is that certain neurons, like the pyramidal type, are the most likely to show lowered densities in schizophrenia. But there is inconsistency here, with only a few studies reporting data.

We also located two studies that measured amygdala volumes post mortem. They yield contradictory results. Heckers et al. (1990) reported data that result in an effect of $d = .54$ in the "wrong" direction—the patients had slightly *larger* amygdalas on average than the controls. On the other hand, Bogerts et al. (1985) reported quite a large deficit finding of $d = -1.26$, showing that most post-mortem patient samples have reduced amygdala volumes. Nothing can be concluded from these two contradictory studies.

The post-mortem literature in schizophrenia is always intriguing because of the precise and detailed level of observation it affords the search for neurobiological abnormalities in the illness. It is also a frustrating literature. Studies are too few, and they are often inconsistent in their results. Nonetheless, the available evidence offers some support for the idea that schizophrenia involves reduced hippocampal volumes and possibly reduced numbers of pyramidal cells in particular. The most recent research is moving toward an examination of specific cell populations and a search for abnormalities that reflect anomalies of fetal growth and maturation. I consider these more recent directions in post-mortem research in chapter 7.

Overall, the question of whether temporal lobe structures are abnormal in schizophrenia depends partly on the research methods employed. The abundant brain-scanning findings with respect to the size of the temporal lobes and their component structures provide little support for the idea that schizophrenia patients have abnormally small or reduced tissue areas or volumes in this region. The post-mortem studies are more supportive of the tissue deficit hypothesis, but they are too few for firm conclusions. There is certainly no evidence to suggest that the illness involves the kind of pronounced atrophy found in degenerative temporal lobe pathologies like Alzheimer's disease. However, neurobiological abnormality may take the form of altered physiology, as well as altered tissue and cell numbers. If this is true for schizophrenia, the new functional brain-imaging techniques that reflect the working brain should furnish some answers.

Positron Emission Metabolism and Blood Flow Studies

Positron emission tomography provides images and data that reflect physiological processes like glucose metabolism and blood flow in regions of the brain that interest researchers. The highest resolution is obtained with tracers that index the brain's principal source of energy—glucose metabolism. However, blood flow tracers lend themselves more for use in cognitive activation tasks where data reflect the brain in mental action. In the activation paradigm, research participants are scanned during a baseline or "resting" phase and are then scanned again as they engage in mental activity of some kind. The original technology in this field measured blood flow by way of injected or inhaled xenon and its perfusion in the brain (Lassen, Ingvar, & Skinhoj, 1978). This technique can be used for both resting blood flow and activation studies. However, it has serious technical limitations and is being superseded by advances in positron emission methods that use a radioisotope based on oxygen to trace blood flow changes in the brain. Yet to some degree the cost of the brevity and flexibility of blood flow techniques is still their lower resolution—a relatively blurry image. Consider what these literatures have to say about the temporal lobes in schizophrenia.

In our search for studies of the left temporal lobe, my students and I looked, as usual, for research that included schizophrenia and healthy comparison groups and statistics that could be converted to effect sizes. We found 21 "resting" studies published between 1980 and 1999. Eleven of these studies measured glucose metabolism, and 10 indexed blood flow in the left temporal cortex. The overall average effect for reduced temporal lobe metabolism in schizophrenia was extremely weak, only $d = .13$. This suggests virtually 90% overlap between patients and healthy subjects in resting metabolism values. However, the average masks some large discrepancies between the findings of different studies. Several researchers found evidence of abnormally *increased* resting temporal lobe metabolism in the illness. For example, Post et al. (1987) reported glucose utilization rates in schizophrenia patients that were much higher than rates found for healthy people ($d = 1.13$). A few other investigators also found increased temporal glucose metabolism (Delisi et al., 1989; Gur et al., 1995) in schizophrenia. However, none of the other reports approach the relatively large effect of Post et al. (1987). In general, about half of the studies report reduced metabolism, and half report increases.

There is no obvious methodological reason for such inconsistency in results, despite the fact that technical differences exist between scanning methods used in different studies (McCarley et al., 1996). What could be responsible for the coexistence of abnormal increases and abnormal decreases in schizophrenic brain metabolism? The medication status of patients with illnesses like schizophrenia always raises questions about how drugs alter biological findings. Indeed, Post et al. (1987) studied medicated patients and found a large metabolic increase, whereas Wiesel et al. (1987) studied unmedicated patients and obtained evidence of a moderate decrease. Perhaps antipsychotic drugs enhance prevailing metabolic activity, and when the drugs are removed metabolism falls below normal levels. Yet Gur et al. (1995) studied drug-free patients experiencing their first psychotic episodes and also found evidence of mild increases in temporal lobe metabolism. Delisi et al. (1989) studied more chronic patients who were unmedicated at the time of the brain scan and found increased metabolism as well. It is difficult to escape the conclusion that extreme heterogeneity exists in temporal lobe metabolism in schizophrenia. Most patients resemble healthy people, but substantial minorities have abnormally increased or decreased resting metabolism.

The 10 blood flow studies yield a fairly similar picture of heterogeneous and often weak findings with respect to temporal lobe physiology. The average effect for reduced left temporal blood flow is $d = .25$, which means that roughly 80% of patients and healthy people have overlapping blood flow values. Several studies yield effect sizes close to zero (e.g., Nordahl et al., 1996), and two studies produced evidence of mild increases instead of deficits in temporal lobe blood flow in schizophrenia (Hook et al., 1995; Yuasa et al., 1995). Only one study produced a fairly large effect in support of reduced blood flow in the illness (Andreasen et al., 1997). The blood flow studies also echo the metabolism research, in that no obvious relation exists between discrepant findings and the presence or absence of antipsychotic medication in the patient participants. This implies that drug administration is not a major factor in producing the heterogeneity. There simply is no consistent picture of abnormal resting temporal lobe metabolism or blood flow in schizophrenia.

There are a smaller number of studies that report functional scanning data from medial temporal regions in schizophrenia patients. Functional brain scanning is at its technical limits when trying to isolate physiological changes in regions as small as the hippocampus and amygdala. For this reason, some investigators report data for generic "medial-temporal" or "limbic" regions rather than for specific structures. Nonetheless, we located 10 studies that reported blood flow and glucose metabolism data specifically from the hippocampal region. These were all studies done under "resting" conditions, and they yield a very small average effect of $d = .25$ in support of diminished activity in this region. However, once again, there is a great deal of variability, with evidence of both increases and decreases in physiological activity in schizophrenia relative to healthy people. For example, DeLisi et al. (1989) scanned patients who had been free of medication for 15 days and found evidence of increased hippocampal glucose use in the illness. In contrast, Wiesel et al. (1987) studied a small group of drug-free patients and found a modest decrease in glucose use. Tamminga's group (Tamminga, Burrows, Chase, Alphs, & Thaker, 1988; Tamminga et al., 1992) was alone in obtaining large effects ($d = -1.52$; $d = -1.32$) showing abnormal deficits in glucose use in schizophrenia.

In searching for studies that examined the amygdala we found five glucose metabolism and one blood flow study. These produced a somewhat more consistent picture than the hippocampal findings. All of these studies except one reveal a moderate deficit in physiological function of the amygdala in schizophrenia. The average d of .55 indicates that most patients do not differ substantially from control group values but a minority, perhaps a third, are distinguished from the control group by having less physiological activity in the region of the amygdala.

Part of the consistency problem that bedevils much of the research into resting temporal lobe physiology reflects an issue that relates to resting studies of the frontal brain. Researchers do not really know what subjects are doing as they sit in the scanning apparatus. Some may stare at the fixation point provided by the researcher, others may experience symptoms, and still others may engage in daydreams or mental reflection. This variability can wreak havoc with stable measurement and confound the possibility of assessing a true "resting" physiology in any brain region. Hence, the activation research strategy has arisen, whereby all subjects are given the same mental task or exercise to complete during the scanning procedure. Activation paradigms measure cerebral blood flow or glucose utilization patterns that occur in response to specific mental task requirements. The brain is thus scanned in the act of information processing rather than in a more passive baseline or resting state.

We found only one study that reported hippocampal or amygdaloid physiological changes during activation tasks (Ragland et al., 1998). However, 11 studies report positron emission findings under activation conditions for the whole temporal lobe. Most of these studies used fairly simple attention-related activation tasks that require detecting or tracking sounds or visual symbols. Two studies, Berman, Doran, Pickar, and Weinberger (1993) and Ragland et al. (1998) used the Wisconsin Card Sorting Test (see chapter 4). About half the studies measured metabolism and half the studies measured blood flow. The average effect for abnormal temporal lobe activation was only $d = .09$, but there is a remarkable degree of heterogeneity in these studies. Some of this heterogeneity derives from the two physiological indices. Thus activation studies of glucose metabolism yield evidence of an average mild ($d = .39$) *increase* in temporal lobe activity in schizophrenia. On the other hand, blood flow studies indicate the reverse, a mild ($d = .26$) *decrease* in temporal activation in the illness. Clearly, activation methods do not eliminate the problem of heterogeneous results seen in resting studies. In fact, these methods further complicate the picture by suggesting that metabolism and blood flow yield contradictory information about the brain's response to mental work.

Another possible source of inconsistent results is the activation task given to participants during the scan. Perhaps complex tasks like the Wisconsin Card Sorting Test (Heaton et al., 1993) effect the brain differently from simple tasks like the Continuous Performance Test (see chapters 3 and 4). Yet task differences are hard to disentangle from differences in physiological indicators. Both studies' using card sorting as an activation task also used blood flow as the physiological index. Berman et al. (1993) was the only study to yield a large effect (d = −1.13) in support of the idea that activation reveals diminished temporal lobe function in schizophrenia. Ragland et al. (1998) used the same activation task and obtained a much smaller effect for diminished activation. In contrast, all of the studies that used the Continuous Performance Test also used glucose metabolism as the physiological index. At the same time, most of the metabolism studies found increased physiological activity in schizophrenia, and most of the blood flow studies show a decrease. An exception to this trend is Hook et al. (1995), who used blood flow and a verbal memory task to activate the temporal region—surely a logical choice, given the importance of the region for memory functions—and found a moderate increase in patients' blood flow. It is simply not possible to sort out the relative contributions of activation task and physiological index to the confused findings in this literature.

With such high variability, lack of replication, and major technical differences in scanning methods, there is little that can be said about the temporal brain in schizophrenia when it is given mental work to do. Perhaps the most intriguing finding is that some studies suggest the existence of abnormally increased rather than deficient temporal brain activity in the illness. When patients are actively engaged in a mental task and scanned at the same time, some of them show temporal metabolism and blood perfusion rates that exceed what is found in healthy people. Is this the sign of an abnormally active brain, a brain that also produces psychosis, or is it the sign of a brain that has to work harder to achieve the same outcome as a healthy brain? Unfortunately, no sufficiently reliable or powerful finding has emerged to answer these questions.

One promising trend for the future is the increased feasibility of imaging small regions like the hippocampus and amygdala with activation tasks that tap the functions of these regions. For example, Heckers et al. (1998) reported that 7 out of 8 healthy participants but only 1 out of 13 schizophrenia patients activated the hippocampal region during a verbal recall task. Similarly, Schneider et al. (1998) report failure to activate the amygdala in schizophrenia patients during episodes of sad emotion even though the patients "feel" sad. Unfortunately, these literatures are too small and undeveloped for evaluation at present.

The Right Temporal Lobe

I have concentrated almost exclusively on the evidence for left temporal lobe abnormalities in schizophrenia. The right temporal lobe plays a role in nonverbal perception and semantics. Its importance lies in relation to music, voice quality, and environmental sounds and in understanding, discriminating, and remembering human faces and complex spatial patterns. Although the language and categorical functions of the left temporal system seem most implicated in schizophrenia, the semantics of space and nonverbal sound may also be involved.

Davidson (1999) examined neurobiological findings on the right temporal lobe in schizophrenia and generally found magnitudes of difference between patients and healthy people that approximate those found for the left temporal lobe. Thus right temporal lobe volume comparisons with magnetic resonance scanning yield an average effect of $d = .36$ (versus $d = .25$ for left temporal lobe). Right hippocampal comparisons yield an average d of .58 (versus $d = .41$ for left hippocampus). Positron emission studies of right-brain resting metabolism and blood flow show an average effect of $d = .05$ for the whole right temporal lobe (versus $d = .13$ for left) and an average d of .19 for the right hippocampus (versus $d = .25$ for the left). Hence there is no strong reason to believe that either lobe is preferentially involved in schizophrenia, and both bodies of evidence yield results of similar strength.

The Temporal-Semantic Brain and Its Contribution to Schizophrenia

Is there a region of the brain that is more suggestive and richer in clues about schizophrenia than the left temporal lobe and its semantic functions? Probably not. What is known about this brain region and its importance for generating and preserving intellectual and emotional meaning seems to cry out for a connection to the illness. Surely schizophrenia is a disturbance where meaning rages unchecked, where danger and threat invade perception only to collapse into a kind of mental vacuum, an empty mind, where meaning and passion have no place. Surely the neurological engine that drives madness is located in the semantic brain.

The neuroscience evidence summarized in table 5.2 does not live up to expectations. On the one hand, some psychological functions associated with the left temporal lobe, notably memory but also language comprehension and selective attention, are probably deficient in about three-quarters of schizophrenia patients. Although there is no replicated evidence of complete separation of patient and healthy samples, the findings of disturbed semantic processing in many patients are substantial in magnitude. On the other hand, there is no evidence that defective temporal lobe cognition is a *necessary* part of schizophrenia. There are substantial numbers of patients with the illness who perform normally on these tests. Moreover, as neurobiology is measured more directly by structural or physiological imaging, effect sizes and deficit rates seem to diminish rather than gather strength and become more heterogeneous rather than more consistent.

In the case of the volume of the left temporal lobe, together with its medial regions, the question of whether an inclusive schizophrenic deficit exists can be answered with a fairly unequivocal no. The overlap of healthy and ill people is so extensive that the hypothesis of temporal lobe abnormality underlying schizophrenia is simply implausible. Only in the post-mortem data indexing hippocampal volumes and cell densities is there the suggestion of substantial findings, and this suggestion is based on a very small number of older studies.

The situation hardly improves when the results of brain metabolism and blood flow studies are considered. Average resting physiological activity seems to be almost identical in patients and control subjects. The qualification on this conclusion is that heterogeneity exists whereby some studies actually show enhanced physiological activity and other patient samples show decrements in activity. The same overall evidential weakness and inconsistency applies to studies where subjects engage in cognitive tasks while undergoing the brain scan. The tendency for both increments and decrements to appear also occurs here and proves hard to disentangle from study differences in method and patient samples. The possibility of multiple disease states exists as a further complication in this confusing body of evidence.

The biology of meaning is not the biology of schizophrenia, at least not in terms of existing evidence. However suggestive the semantic brain hypothesis may be, the link between the illness and this vital cerebral region has not been demonstrated in a convincing way (see also Harrison, 1999). The evidence does not appear to provide the answers that the frontal-executive hypothesis failed to provide.

Where to look next? Perhaps the limitations of the scanning technology really are critical. This technology is the primary means of finding biological abnormalities in living people with schizophrenia. Yet the level of resolution of these techniques may be too coarse. The neurology of madness may lie in the temporal lobes or in the frontal lobes and remain undetected because the sensitivity of available instruments is inadequate. The neurogenesis of schizophrenia may exist at the cellular or molecular level. Therefore, it is time to consider a much finer level of observation: the world of neurotransmitters and receptors, where the dynamics of chemical action and neurotransmission may yet reveal the causes of schizophrenia.

6

• •

NEUROCHEMICAL
TEMPEST

For many decades following Kraepelin's (1896, 1919) seminal descriptions of schizophrenia there was no effective medical treatment for the illness. Unfortunate patients might be "treated" with "great and desperate" methods like prolonged barbiturate-induced sleep therapy, insulin coma, or psychosurgery (Valenstein, 1986). These were treatments to be feared. Insulin coma involved creating a hypoglycemic state, low blood sugar, through administration of high doses of insulin. This resulted in loss of consciousness and frequent convulsions. A few reports suggested that a series of such insulin shocks might reduce a patient's psychotic episodes. However, the technique was never carefully evaluated, and it posed risks in terms of heart attacks and strokes. Other schizophrenia patients underwent surgical operations in the form of frontal lobotomies or leukotomies, wherein nerve tracts in the frontal brain were cut. As a hospital psychologist I once met a survivor of this grim era, an elderly woman who had undergone psychosurgery decades before, in a dim past that she could barely remember. She was left with brain damage and cognitive deficits due to the surgery —and she retained her schizophrenia. Many thousands of patients were operated on with little demonstrable benefit and little concern with ethical requirements like informed consent to treatment.

Limited therapeutic options and prospects during the first half of the twentieth century meant that large numbers of schizophrenia patients were "warehoused" in huge psychiatric hospitals. Pilgrim State Hospital in New York, for example, once had a population of almost 14,000 patients. The wards were understaffed, and it was hard to tell what was worse, the unchecked illness or the custodial environment. Mary Holt, a physician at Pilgrim, was in charge of two buildings of severely ill or "regressed" female patients. She describes what psychiatry and serious mental illness were like in 1950:

> They were so wild that I just couldn't keep them decent. They'd soil themselves, tear their clothes off, smash the windows, and gouge plaster out of the walls. One of them would even rip radiators right off the wall. We'd sometimes have to surround them with mattresses in order to give them sedative injections, and these would help for a little while, but then they'd get addicted to the sedative and we'd have to take them off it. (quoted in Hunt, 1962, p. 26)

Sidney Cohen, chief psychiatrist at a Veteran's Administration hospital in Los Angeles remembered "the lobotomies—the broken glass—the subhuman screams in the night—the windows under which you would not walk lest excreta of some sort drop on you." And he remembered "the interminable locking and unlocking of doors" and the "beat-up patients and beat-up attendants" (Cohen, 1964, p. 95).

By the middle years of the 1950s, the United States and Canada alone had over half a million psychotic inpatients, many with schizophrenia, who were hospitalized on an indefinite basis. Accordingly, despite the efforts of the psychiatric pioneers in bringing medical science to bear on the problem of schizophrenia, a patient in 1850 may have been better off in terms of quality of life, if not the disease process itself, than a patient of 1950. Yet within a few years this overwhelmingly negative picture was to change as the treatment and then science of schizophrenia underwent a biological revolution.

It did not come from an obvious direction. It came from the observations and somewhat eccentric ideas of a young French naval surgeon named Henri Laborit (see Swazey, 1974). Laborit was not interested in schizophrenia; he was interested in the syndrome of circulatory shock that occurred during and after surgery. This syndrome included symptoms of depression and apathy along with marked physiological problems, ranging from shallow respiration to a bloodless, pale clinical appearance. Shock was progressive in some cases and could lead to death within hours. Surgeons knew that the immediate cause was abnormal blood circulation, whereby the heart was unable to supply the body with sufficient blood flow. This in turn deprived tissues of needed oxygen and nutrients. The challenge was to find a way of treating and reversing the syndrome. Laborit and his associates began experimenting with a variety of drugs in an attempt to combat the shock syndrome in surgical patients. One of the drugs was a new agent called promethazine, and Laborit noted that it had a number of intriguing properties. The primary reason for using this drug was its effect on the autonomic nervous system and its indirect effect on blood vessels. However, the "secondary" properties of the drug proved even more important: it made patients drowsy, reduced pain, and created a feeling of "euphoric quietude." In other words, promethazine had psychological effects. Surgical patients receiving the drug were conscious but without apparent pain or anxiety. The secondary or psychological effects must arise from promethazine's action in the central nervous system. Laborit reasoned, correctly as it turned out, that the drug must reach the brain as well as the autonomic system.

The psychological effects and psychiatric implications of the new treatment did not escape Laborit, but, ironically, they did seem to escape the army psychiatrist who was asked to observe how calm and relaxed postsurgery patients were if they received the drug. Nonetheless, Laborit's (1950) published observations on promethazine stimulated researchers at the laboratories of the firm of Rhône-Poulenc to modify the formula of promethazine in an effort to enhance its curious, brain-related effects. The result of these efforts was chlorpromazine, the first effective antipsychotic medication, and the rest is history, although it is a rather prolonged and circuitous history. It took another 10 years before the new drug's value in treating schizophrenia was fully recognized and established. The initial observations of promethazine and chlorpromazine in psychiatric patients reflected short-term effects of the drugs rather than their longer term antipsychotic effects. It took the clinical trials of Delay, Deniker, and Harl (1952) and Sigwald and Bouttier (1953) in Europe, Lehmann and Hanrahan (1954) in Canada, and finally the large collaborative National Institute of Mental Health (1964) study in the United States to demonstrate the full value of the new medication. Chlorpromazine reduced more than agitation, mania, and mood disturbances. It reduced the bizarre mental symptoms suffered by the person with schizophrenia.

A large and diverse clinical research literature now attests to the value of chlorpromazine and its derivatives and related compounds in reducing the frequency and severity of hallucinations, delusions, positive thought disorder, and even some of the negative symptoms of the illness. Patients who receive these medications require less time in hospital; they have fewer relapses and show enhanced life functioning when compared to untreated patients (Julien, 1995, pp. 269–300; Kane, 1989; Meltzer, 1993). To be sure, a minority of patients responds poorly to antipsychotic drugs, and even responsive patients may have to deal with unpleasant and occasionally disabling side effects of the medication. The drugs based on chlorpromazine are an aid to illness management and not a cure. Many patients suffer a return of their symptoms if medication is discontinued. Moreover, the advent of antipsychotic drugs had a problematic consequence. Chronic hospital patients were often given the new medication and then discharged into the community, yet they were without the occupational and daily living skills or social supports needed to ensure successful functioning outside of the hospital. Patients were "liberated" from institutions only to be cast adrift in city streets with nowhere to go, nothing to do, and no one to meet. Poverty and stigma replaced confinement and dependency—poor alternatives for the person with schizophrenia (see Torrey, 1995).

The arrival of the first therapeutic drug treatments for psychotic symptoms also provided impetus for the science of schizophrenia, which had been languishing since the early and largely unsuccessful attempts to discover a biological basis for the disease. If the new drugs were effective in reducing symptoms, it must be because they influenced brain chemistry in some way. It seemed that schizophrenia consisted of an aberration in neurotransmission—the chemical transactions that comprise communication between nerve cells at the molecular level. Instead of a structural defect or lesion, or a death of neurons, an abnormal alteration of neurochemistry might be the cause of madness.

Dopamine: Modulator of Mind and Movement

The early 1960s implicated a group of brain chemicals in the therapeutic effects of antipsychotic drug action. In particular, dopamine, a member of the catecholamine family of neurotransmitters, appeared to play a role in therapeutic drug effects. Dopamine is one of approximately 10 substances that are regarded as "classical" neurotransmitters because they share certain characteristics, which include being present in nerve cell terminals and being released when a neuron fires. In addition, to qualify as a neurotransmitter, a substance must be subject to an inactivation process whereby it is removed from the synaptic cleft between nerve cells. Furthermore, there must be evidence that chemicals placed in the synapse that inactivate the putative neurotransmitter also prevent neuronal firing. In practice, each of these characteristics cannot always be demonstrated for a given transmitter substance. However, there is general consensus that the catecholamine chemical group of substances including norepinephrine and dopamine are neurotransmitters.

If schizophrenia represents an aberration in dopamine transmission, a kind of neurochemical storm, this aberration could be present in any of the following five processes. First, a neurotransmitter is produced from existing or precursor chemicals. Second, once synthesized, it is stored in the presynaptic neuron. In dopaminergic neurons, the neurotransmitter is transported down the axon and into the terminal for storage. Third, the neurotransmitter is released into the synaptic cleft. Fourth, once it has reached the postsynaptic membrane of the next nerve cell, the neurotransmitter interacts with receptors and has an effect on the postsynaptic nerve itself. In the case of dopamine, these receptors fall into two major classes based on their biochemical properties: the D1-like and the D2-like receptor families. Further subtypes exist within each class (e.g., D1,

D5, in the D1-like group; D2, D3, D4 in the D2-like group). Receptors bind the transmitter substance and activate or inhibit the postsynaptic neuron. Dopamine is generally considered to be inhibitory in nature, reducing and constraining the activity of nerve cells that it targets. Fifth, the postsynaptic effect is ended by inactivation of the transmitter. Inactivation occurs when enzymes break down the transmitter or it is taken back up into the presynaptic neuron. Enzymes that eventually yield homovanillic acid as a by-product or metabolite degrade and destroy dopamine. However, enzymatic degradation is relatively slow, and dopamine can be removed more rapidly through uptake, wherein neurotransmitter is returned across the presynaptic neural membrane and stored in vesicles for later use. A critical component in the inactivation and recycling of dopamine is the dopamine transporter, a chemical mechanism that "pumps" neurotransmitter back into the nerve terminal (see Cooper, Bloom, & Roth, 1996, pp. 293–351; Johanson, 1992; Vallone, Picetti, & Borrelli, 2000; Weiner & Molinoff, 1994). These processes are presented diagrammatically in figure 6.1.

Dopamine-Related Drug Effects

A drug may effect any of the stages of neurotransmission, from synthesis to uptake, and thereby influence psychological brain function by increasing, decreasing, or destabilizing neurotransmission. A drug like reserpine inhibits the storage of neurotransmitter in the presynaptic vesicles. Amphetamine, or "speed," causes release of newly synthesized dopamine from nerve terminals. In contrast, cocaine binds to the dopamine transporter and prevents uptake. This in turn increases the amount of dopamine remaining in the synaptic cleft that is available for binding with postsynaptic sites. Drugs may also stimulate (agonists) or block (antagonists) dopamine receptors. Indeed, it is here, at the postsynaptic dopamine receptors, that antipsychotic drugs like chlorpromazine are believed to exercise their effects by acting as dopamine receptor antagonists. These drugs displace dopamine on the receptor site, so the net effect of their administration is to decrease dopamine-related activity. The brain in turn may compensate for prolonged receptor blockade by making more receptors on the postsynaptic neuron and by increasing the sensitivity of receptors to dopamine (see Cooper et al., 1996, pp. 313–330; Dykstra, 1992).

Dopamine-Containing Brain Systems

Abnormalities in dopamine neurotransmission can occur at different points in the sequence from synthesis to uptake, but they can also occur at different locations in the brain. Dopamine exists as a neurotransmitter diffusely throughout the central nervous system. However, it is concentrated in four brain systems, or

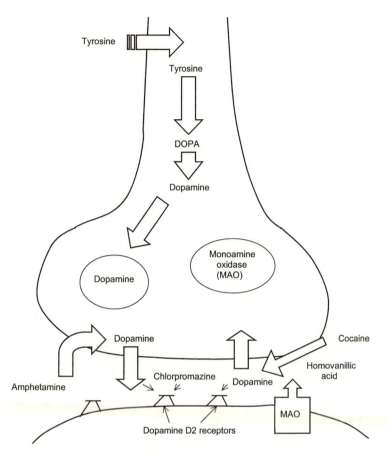

Figure 6.1. Diagram of a dopaminergic nerve terminal. Dopamine is synthesized in steps from tyrosine and stored in vesicles. Dopamine is released into the synapse to bind with receptors on the postsynaptic membrane. Monoamine oxydase is an enzyme that breaks dopamine down and yields homovanillic acid as a byproduct. Dopamine is also taken back up into the presynaptic cell. Drugs like amphetamine and cocaine induce release and prevent uptake of dopamine, thereby increasing its presence in the synapse. Antipsychotic drugs like chlorpromazine and haloperidol occupy dopamine receptors on the postsynaptic membrane, thereby blocking dopamine occupancy. This seems to be an essential aspect of the drugs' ability to reduce psychotic symptoms.

pathways, where the cell bodies are in one location and long fibers extend from these locations to terminate elsewhere in the brain (see figure 6.2). The four systems include the nigrostriatal dopamine tract, which is the most studied and best understood of the brain's dopamine systems. It ascends from the substantia nigra to the neostriatum, which is part of the basal ganglia. The basal ganglia consist of motor correlation centers that modulate movement and action, including, probably, the learning of motor skills and procedures. The importance

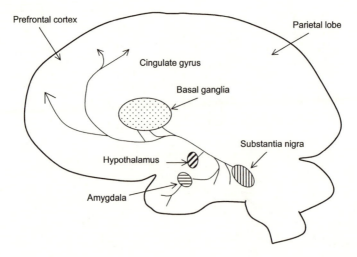

Figure 6.2. Dopamine tracts in the human brain. There are several dopamine-containing systems, but most of the neurotransmitter is concentrated in the caudate and putamen of the basal ganglia, making this region the major focus of research studies. This is despite the fact that basal ganglia functions appear to be largely motoric rather than psychological in nature.

of the nigrostriatal tract can be seen when disorders like Parkinsonism deplete the tract's dopamine. Rapid shaking or resting tremor that recedes with voluntary movement distinguishes Parkinsonism. In addition, patients show muscular rigidity, an inflexible, expressionless face, and a general slowing of motor activity that effects walking and speaking. Treatment of Parkinsonism is focused on increasing dopamine activity in remaining nigrostriatal neurons and on suppressing heightened activity of other neurotransmitter systems. Such heightened or competitive activity by other neurotransmitters occurs in response to the deficiency of dopamine action. Replacing dopamine directly is difficult, however, because, paradoxically, dopamine that is present in the blood supply is prevented from entering the brain by the blood–brain barrier. This "barrier" is really a network of cells that transports nutrients to neurons and screens out selected substances. Fortunately, dihydroxyphenylalanine, or DOPA, the immediate precursor of dopamine, can enter the brain from the bloodstream, and its administration leads to sufficient additional dopamine to improve Parkinsonian symptoms.

A second major dopamine tract is the mesolimbic pathway, which ascends from the ventrotegmental area of the midbrain to the nucleus accumbens, septum, amygdala and entorhinal cortex. A variety of functions, inferred from animal studies and human neurological cases, have been associated with these structures, including reward, fear, and anxiety and some aspects of memory (see chapter 5). There are no common diseases that preferentially deplete or enhance dopamine activity in this region. However, the important psychological functions that have been tied to the limbic region make the mesolimbic tract of special interest for researchers studying the neural basis of schizophrenia (Lidsky, 1995).

A third pathway is the mesocortical tract, which ascends from the ventral tegmental area to the prefrontal cortex, cingulate gyrus, and premotor area. As discussed in chapter 4, the prefrontal cortex has been implicated as mediating executive cognition like planning and self-regulation. Again, there are no diseases that have a special predilection for the dopamine chemistry of this tract, but it may be affected to some degree by Parkinsonism and Huntington's disease, conditions that are often characterized by executive deficits (Lezak, 1995, pp. 221–241).

Finally, dopamine neurons also occur in the hypothalamus and extend to the pituitary gland. The hypothalamus is involved in emotion, eating, drinking, sexual behavior, temperature regulation, and the secretion of releasing factors that allow the pituitary to yield steroid hormones, prolactin, and thyroid-stimulating hormone. The effects of blocking dopamine activity in this system can be seen in weight gain, lower sex drive, and excessive prolactin release and hence in lactation and breast enlargement. There may be problems with erection and ejaculation in men and altered ovulation and impaired infertility in women (Julien, 1995, pp. 356–361).

Accordingly, dopamine is a neurotransmitter that is distributed in a concentrated way in several discrete neural pathways as well as more diffusely in the brain. These pathways mediate a number of important behaviors, although no dopamine pathway has an exclusive function. Within these pathways the importance of dopamine for specifically psychological aspects of brain function is unclear. There is theory and evidence that dopamine activity influences cognition indirectly by modulating other neural systems and pathways (Cohen & Servan-Schreiber, 1993; Straube & Oades, 1992, pp. 467–468). For example, dopamine may act to adjust the signal-to-noise ratio of information flow in the brain. High levels of the neurotransmitter enhance the strength and distinctiveness of the mental "signal." Low levels make it fade into background noise. Other neurotransmitters may be responsible for generating the signal in the first place, but dopamine modulates its salience in mental activity. There is also evidence that the learning of movements and motor skills is mediated by dopamine-containing systems like the basal ganglia (see Kolb & Whishaw, 1996, pp. 137–140). And finally, the pleasure-inducing properties of drugs like cocaine that potentiate dopamine activity imply that the neurotransmitter plays a role in the reward and reinforcement of behavior.

To what extent are the cognitive symptoms of schizophrenia a logical consequence of altered dopamine activity? Two of the four dopamine systems, the nigrostriatal and hypothalamic tracts, appear to be relatively poor candidates for sites of a predominately psychological illness like schizophrenia. For example, it is known that antipsychotic medications that block dopamine receptors in the nigrostriatal tract also induce a kind of artificial Parkinsonism. Schizophrenia patients receiving such medication often develop motor slowness, rigidity, and tremor, presumably because the drug limits dopamine activity in a system that depends on it for normal function. On the face of it, therefore, this system is unlikely to be the principal cause of schizophrenia. The nigrostriatal tract is primarily motoric in function, and dopamine-blocking drugs affect it adversely rather than therapeutically.

An analogous argument can be made for excluding the hypothalamic pathway as a primary site for schizophrenia (but see chapter 8). Disturbance of the hypothalamus-pituitary hormonal system, with its eating, sexual, and bodily functions, does not suggest a direct parallel with schizophrenic disorder. Here too, antipsychotic drugs can influence normal dopamine-related activities and give rise to adverse side effects in treated patients. Therefore, it is the meso-limbic and mesocortical pathways, with their connections to psychologically significant brain regions like the medial temporal and frontal lobes, that are usually emphasized as sites for the illness. In view of these considerations, there are grounds for examining closely the mesolimbic and mesocortical dopamine tracts, insofar as they seem to be the most likely sites of therapeutic drug effects and, by implication, the most likely sites of schizophrenia itself. However, as it turns out, the most interesting dopamine systems are not necessarily the ones that are easiest to study.

The Search for Dopamine Abnormalities

The strongest support for a connection between dopamine function and schizophrenia comes from studies showing that the clinical efficacy of drugs like chlorpromazine depends on their ability to block dopamine receptors, especially the dopamine D2 receptor subtype. These studies were carried out in the 1970s using post-mortem brain tissue samples (Creese, Burt, & Snider, 1976; Iversen, 1978; Seeman & Lee, 1975). Chlorpromazine and related drugs inhibit the binding of dopamine to its receptors in direct proportion to the amount of drug required to reduce symptoms in living patients. Conversely, symptoms like delusions and hallucinations diminish to the extent that the medication displaces dopamine from postsynaptic D2 receptors.

Another line of evidence draws from the fact that various drugs, including cocaine, enhance dopamine activity rather than blocking it. This enhancement can precipitate psychotic reactions that resemble acute schizophrenic episodes. Thus high doses of cocaine may produce persecutory fears and paranoia, as well as a severely distorted sense of reality (Julien, 1995, pp. 137–138). Cocaine appears to produce these effects in part by interfering with the dopamine transporter and the process of reuptake (Cooper et al., 1996, p. 304). Concentrations of dopamine in the synaptic space are probably increased in cocaine users, facilitating the impact of the neurotransmitter on the postsynaptic neuron. In a similar vein, other drugs that enhance dopamine, including amphetamine and L DOPA, can also produce psychotic states in people who take them. Clearly there is a correlation between enhanced dopamine activity and psychosis and between blocked dopamine activity and reduced psychotic symptoms. But can this correlation be used to explain an illness like schizophrenia?

How concentrations of dopamine translate into a pleasant psychological effect like a "high" on the one hand and into a psychotic episode on the other hand is not obvious. These effects are not always related to the dose or amount of dopamine-enhancing medication. Moreover, the enhanced dopaminergic effect is believed to be inhibitory in terms of postsynaptic neural transmission. In other words, more dopamine in the synaptic cleft means an increase in the inhibition of the postsynaptic neuron. Can physiological inhibition become psychological release? Perhaps the inhibition translates into an impairment of normal mechanisms that keep thoughts and feelings within certain bounds. Yet the same increased inhibition is tied to the rewarding, pleasurable properties of external events. Does increased inhibitory action of dopamine create feelings of pleasure in the drug user but in the extreme let loose the chemistry of madness?

The problem with pharmacological evidence as an explanation for schizophrenia is the ambiguous nature of this evidence. Just because antipsychotic drugs work by blocking dopamine does not mean that the disease itself is caused by excessive "unblocked" dopamine or indeed by any dopamine-related abnormality. What is required for a neurochemical explanation of schizophrenia is direct independent evidence that something is wrong in the dopamine systems of patients with the illness. Moreover, this defect must be of sufficient magnitude to represent a clear and disease-linked abnormality. Advocates of the dopamine hypothesis agree that the neurogenesis of schizophrenia must be observed in dopamine synthesis, release, or transporter and receptor function or possibly in associated changes affecting other neurotransmitters. To what extent is dopamine transmission actually abnormal and excessive in the illness?

An Index of Brain Dopamine Activity
in Schizophrenia

Perhaps the most obvious, albeit simplistic, way of addressing the question is to measure levels of dopamine in the brain directly. However, this is difficult to do in living patients. Dopamine is not secreted intact into bodily fluids like blood plasma or cerebrospinal fluid that can be drawn and analyzed without invasive procedures. Fortunately, homovanillic acid is a major dopamine by-product or metabolite (figure 5.1), and its level of concentration probably reflects levels of dopamine activity (Amin et al., 1995). Moreover, homovanillic acid can be measured fairly easily because it is excreted into blood plasma and, to a much lesser extent, into cerebrospinal fluid. Most of the homovanillic acid in cerebrospinal fluid derives from the brain. However, the different cerebral dopamine-containing systems probably contribute disproportionately to its accumulation. It is not known to what extent cerebrospinal fluid metabolite reflects mesolimbic and mesocortical activity along with nigrostriatal dopamine function. A further problem is the perennial one that arises because most research studies are carried out on patients who are receiving antipsychotic medication. With blockade of dopamine receptors by drugs, levels of homovanillic acid tend to increase because there is more "unbound" dopamine being metabolized (Straube & Oades, 1992, pp. 470–471). Indeed, levels of homovanillic acid often fall if a patient's medication is discontinued (Bagdy et al., 1985) and increase with acute drug treatment (Lieberman & Koreen, 1993). This means that it is essential to compare patients who are drug free with normal control subjects. Yet even patients who are withdrawn from their medication may not be truly drug free, because the drug lingers in cell membranes for far longer than the normal "washout" period of a few weeks.

I searched the literature from 1980 to 1999 to assess the hypothesis that dopamine activity and therefore its major metabolite are abnormally elevated in schizophrenia. This search yielded 11 studies comparing homovanillic acid levels in the cerebrospinal fluid of drug-free schizophrenia patients and healthy people (see table 6.1). Patients had typically been off medication for about 2 weeks prior to undergoing lumbar puncture to obtain a sample of fluid from the spinal canal. The average effect size was $d = -.11$, which is not only small but in the wrong direction. Given that the margin of error for this average includes zero ($d = -.35 - d = .13$) the result can also be understood as indicating identical metabolite levels in patients and control participants. The individual studies show both moderate deficits ($d = -.62$; Lindstrom, 1985) and excesses ($d = .78$; Maas et al., 1993) in dopamine metabolite in schizophrenia. Only two studies, both by the same investigator, found substantial elevations of homovanillic acid, and these have not been reproduced by independent researchers. Moreover, only one study (Lindstrom, Wieselgren, Klockhoff, & Svedberg, 1990) examined patients who were drug naive—*never* treated with antipsychotic medication. This important study revealed *lower* levels of dopamine metabolite in schizophrenia patients than healthy control subjects. This clearly runs counter to the hypothesis of increased dopamine activity in the illness.

Overall, the findings show that homovanillic acid levels are essentially the same in drug-free schizophrenia patients and healthy people. There is also some variability, with a few studies showing relative excesses and most showing mild depletions of dopamine's major metabolite. The negative findings echo the re-

Table 6.1 Summary of neurochemistry abnormalities in schizophrenia

Finding	Mean d	Confidence Interval	N
Studies of dopamine-related abnormalities			
Excess (deficient) dopamine activity (HVA)	(.11)	−.35–.13	11
Excess D2 receptors (medicated)	1.37	.79–1.95	14
Excess D2 receptors (drug free)	.93	.28–1.58	7
Excess D2 receptors (PET, drug–naive)	.70	.16–1.24	11
Excess D4 receptors (subtraction method)	1.48	.54–2.42	5
Studies of serotonin-related abnormalities			
Excess (deficient) S2 receptors	(.72)	−.02–1.46	10
Studies of glutamate-related abnormalities			
Deficient glutamate (all regions)	.38	.10–.66	4
Deficient (excess) uptake (all regions)	(.08)	−.30–.14	5
Deficient (excess) receptors (basal ganglia)	(.85)	−1.58–.12	3
Deficient receptors (hippocampus)	.40	−.01–.81	7
Deficient receptors (frontal lobe)	.57	−.42–1.56	5

Note: The table shows effect sizes as absolute values, corrected for sample size (Cohen's d) and averaged across studies in each literature. Values in brackets indicate effects opposite to those predicted by the hypothesis. Confidence Interval is the 95% confidence interval or margin of error for the mean effect. The true population average probably lies within the range of indicated effect sizes, while intervals that include zero indicate unstable and negligible findings. Studies are post-mortem unless indicated as follows: PET = positron emision tomography; HVA = homovanillic acid index measured *in vivo* in drug-free patients and control participants. N = the number of published studies contributing to the meta-analyses.

sults of an earlier meta-analytic review of body fluid research in schizophrenia (Tuckwell & Koziol, 1993). This older review also suggested little or no difference in homovanillic acid levels between patients and controls. Hence, thus far, there is little evidence to support the hypothesis of excessive dopamine activity as a general feature of schizophrenia. The hypothesis continues to attract interest (e.g., Lindstrom et al., 1999). However, attention has also turned to the receptor side of the dopamine synthesis-release-receptor binding sequence and to the possibility that receptors hold the key to any dopamine-related abnormality in the illness.

Dopamine Receptors

Receptors are proteins that exist on the postsynaptic membrane of nerve cells. They have special properties that allow them to bind with high specificity and affinity to the dopamine molecule. Moreover, receptors mediate the physiological impact of dopamine on the postsynaptic cell. The several subtypes of dopamine receptor are distributed differentially in the brain's dopamine tracts so that one subtype may predominate in, say, the nigrostriatal pathway and another subtype may occur more frequently in the mesolimbic tract. There is evidence, for example, that the dopamine D1 receptor predominates in the frontal cortex, the D2 in the striatum, and the D3 in the limbic system. Increasingly, it is the density of different neuroreceptors that is implicated as a possible substrate for schizophrenia.

In 1976, chemical "labels," or ligands, that bind selectively with specific receptor sites in post-mortem brain tissue became available (Seeman, Chau-Wong, Tedesco, & Wong, 1976). This development gave rise to a new kind of study, the radioactive binding assay, wherein the density and distribution of various receptor subtypes are determined. Several technically sophisticated steps are involved in such studies. First, the ligand, or drug that binds to the receptor under study, is labeled with a radioactive isotope. Next, tissue samples from preserved post-mortem brains of schizophrenia patients, or healthy people who died of natural causes, are prepared in the form of slices. These slices are exposed to the ligand, which in turn proceeds to bind with receptors. Radioactivity that remains unbound is "washed" away. The tissue slices are usually prepared in the form of slides and coated with a photographic emulsion that reacts to the presence of residual radioactivity on the receptors. The result is a display that shows the location of receptors in the treated brain section. Technical considerations include the fact that the time during which many ligands bind to their receptor is very short and many ligands have an affinity for other receptors and molecules in addition to the one of interest. Hence investigators try to maximize the strength of specific binding and minimize nonspecific binding to make results as informative as possible (Lee, 1988; Pinel, 1990, p. 148).

Ligands have been found for the dopamine D1, D2, and D3 receptor subtypes (see Lee, 1988). Raclopride, for instance, is a chemical ligand that is relatively specific for the dopamine D2 receptor subtype. Many antipsychotic medications have turned out to be ligands as well. The upshot of receptor binding autoradiography, together with the discovery of selective ligands, has meant that dopamine D2 receptor densities can be measured directly in post-mortem schizophrenic and normal brain samples. A window has opened on the microscopic world of the dopamine receptor.

These important technical advances are qualified by the confounding effect of antipsychotic drugs. Medication is a major complicating factor in this research because of studies that show increases in receptor densities in response to dopamine-blocking drugs in laboratory animals. For example, MacLennan, Atmajda, Lee, and Fibiger (1988) administered haloperidol, a commonly used antipsychotic medication that blocks dopamine receptors, to two groups of rats over a period of 21 weeks. After this period a radioligand binding assay was conducted. It revealed increases in the density of dopamine D2 receptors for the medicated rats, and these increases ranged from 50% in the prefrontal cortex to 70% in the basal ganglia. Accordingly, chronic exposure to antipsychotic medications during life may cause an artificial increase in receptor numbers and distort the results of receptor assays of schizophrenic brain tissue samples.

In light of these considerations, the most valuable kind of post-mortem study is one that uses brain tissue samples from schizophrenia patients who were never treated with medication during life and compares them with healthy control tissue samples. However, since the 1950s, most patients, at least in North America, received drug treatment during life. Hence drug-naive brain samples are few in number. In contrast, there is a relative abundance of brains from medicated patients.

The Evidence for Dopamine D2 Receptor Abnormalities in Schizophrenia

To assess the strength of evidence in support of the idea that schizophrenia involves abnormally high densities of the dopamine D2 receptor, my students and I searched the published literature for post-mortem studies of medicated and drug-free patient tissue samples. The vast majority of studies report data on structures like the caudate and putamen that lie in the dopamine-rich striatum of the basal ganglia (see figure 6.2). A few report results from the nucleus accumbens, an extremely small and hard-to-find structure also considered part of the basal ganglia but with close relations to the limbic system. There were only one or two studies reporting data on the frontal cortex or hippocampus. This consistent focus on the motor striatum may seem odd because dysfunction in the limbic and frontal areas makes more theoretical sense as a basis for schizophrenia. However, ease of measurement rather than theoretical rationale appears to dictate the choice of region for study. It is simply unfeasible to measure dopamine receptors outside the basal ganglia.

Almost all of the 14 studies of medicated samples show increased dopamine D2 receptor densities in schizophrenia. The average corrected effect size for these patient–control comparisons is $d = 1.37$, with a confidence interval indicating that the average is accurate within 58 decimal points 95% of the time. This is a fairly large average effect, based on fairly consistent results. The average d suggests that less than a third of the patient and control samples overlap in terms of dopamine D2 densities. However, caution is necessary because the findings also reflect the spurious contribution of prolonged medication exposure. In addition, one study by Seeman et al. (1984) bears special mention because it yielded explicit evidence of heterogeneity. The distribution of patient dopamine D2 receptor densities was "bimodal," with the lower mode or peak showing a 25% increase in receptors and the second mode or peak showing a 130% increase. The second mode represents an effect of sufficient magnitude to achieve complete separation of schizophrenic and control samples. Although most of the tissue samples were obtained from patients exposed to medication, the receptor disparity appeared to be independent of drug exposure. Accordingly, distinctive subsets of schizophrenia patients may exist—some with normal numbers of dopamine receptors and some with abnormally high numbers of receptors.

Seven studies of "drug-free" brain tissue were also found in the published literature. It is important to point out that "drug-free" means that patients were not receiving medication for some period of time—weeks or months—before death. The term does not necessarily mean "drug-naive." Drug-naive patients are those who *never* received antipsychotic medication during life (Lee & Seeman, 1980). Clearly, drug-naive samples would provide the most convincing kind of evidence, but in most cases such evidence is unfeasible. With the exception of the report by Lee and Seeman, all of the studies in this research literature are only drug free and reflect results that may be contaminated in varying degrees by previous medication exposure. The studies yield an average effect of $d = .93$, which is accurate within 65 decimal points 95% of the time. This average effect corresponds to slightly less than 50% overlap between patient and control receptor densities. But what is most striking about this literature is the heterogeneity. One study (Mita et al., 1986) yielded a large effect ($d = 2.44$), indicating that perhaps 88% of the tissue samples from schizophrenia patients had elevated dopamine D2 receptor densities in basal ganglia. However, both Kornhuber et al. (1989; $d = -.57$) and Mackay et al. (1982; $d = -.28$) found small effects that ran in the opposite direction; namely, a small proportion of patient samples actually had *lower* receptor densities than the normal samples. Such disparate findings hint again at the possibility of different kinds of schizophrenia, only one of which may be rooted in abnormal dopamine biology.

Two recent studies are of special interest because they report dopamine receptor D2 binding in the hippocampus (Dean, Scarr, Bradbury, & Copolov, 1999; $d = .31$) and prefrontal cortex (Dean, Hussain, Hayes, et al., 1999; $d = .26$). Yet the findings are disappointingly small and provide no support for the idea that powerful evidence awaits post-mortem dopamine research when it moves outside the basal ganglia.

Imaging of Receptors with Positron Emission
Tomography in Living Patients

Positron emission tomography offers researchers the capacity to measure neuroreceptor density in living patients with schizophrenia. The general technique was described in previous chapters (chapters 4 and 5) in relation to physiological processes like blood flow and brain metabolism. Refinements have made it possible to index dopamine receptor density and receptor occupancy by drugs as well. The technique employs radiolabeled ligands that are introduced intravenously and bind to receptor sites in the brain. The positron emission camera detects these sites and furnishes data that reflect receptor density. The major limitations have to do with spatial and temporal resolution and the availability of suitable tracers. Positron emission brain images can be color coded to reflect receptor densities in dopamine-laden areas like the basal ganglia. However, small areas and those with diffuse or low concentrations of dopamine receptors are hard to detect and study. The consequence of this technical limitation is that research attention has continued to focus on the basal ganglia, a dopamine-containing "motor" region that is relatively easy to detect but hard to imagine as a primary site for schizophrenia. In addition, there are no ideal radioligands and none that bind with both high affinity and high selectivity to each individual receptor subtype.

Three different ligands have been used in positron emission studies: methyl-spiperone, bromo-spiperone, and raclopride. Raclopride is the most specific binding agent in terms of the dopamine D2 receptor. The spiperone-based ligands have a higher affinity for the D2 but at the expense of significant affinities for other neurotransmitter binding sites as well. The different binding characteristics of various ligands have to be kept in mind when evaluating findings of abnormal receptor densities in schizophrenia.

Nevertheless, the ability to measure receptor densities in the living brain at all is a great technical advance, especially when applied to acutely ill, medication-naive schizophrenia patients who have never received dopamine-blocking drugs. For the first time researchers have the ability to gather evidence while avoiding the major pitfall of medication exposure that plagues post-mortem research. Consider what this exciting approach has to say about dopamine D2 receptors in schizophrenia.

My students and I looked for positron emission studies of receptor binding in living, "drug-naive" schizophrenia patients and normal control subjects and found 11 articles (see table 6.1). The results show dramatic differences between studies. Thus Wong et al. (1986) used methyl-spiperone as the tracer and found a powerful effect of $d = 2.07$. This impressive evidence and a subsequent replication (Gjedde & Wong, 1987; $d = 1.91$) argued strongly for the existence of a dopamine D2 receptor excess in the schizophrenic brain. The potential looked good for the corollary idea that this excess might be an essential defect underlying the illness. However, soon after the exciting results were published, Farde et al. (1987) at the Karolinska Institute in Sweden reported almost no group elevation ($d = .07$) of dopamine D2 receptors in schizophrenia when raclopride was used as the ligand. Furthermore, a French team using bromo-spiperone also found only a trivial difference ($d = .11$) between patients and healthy people (Martinot et al., 1990).

It is not clear to what extent properties of different ligands contributed to the discrepant results (see Sedvall, 1992). Nonetheless, it is worth noting that the original study by Wong et al. (1986) and later studies by this research group (e.g., Gjedde & Wong, 1987; Tune et al., 1993) all employed a form of spiperone as the ligand. The Swedish group used raclopride and failed to replicate the large effect of the original report. On the other hand, Nordstrom, Farde, Eriksson, and Halldin (1995) and Okubo et al. (1997) also used methyl-spiperone. These more recent studies found deficits instead of excesses or found only trivial elevations in dopamine D2 densities in schizophrenia patients. Therefore, it seems unlikely that choice of ligand alone can explain the disappointing inconsistency of the effect sizes. However, other methodological differences between studies may have contributed as well. The scanning technology itself or the age, sex, and severity of illness in the patients may have influenced estimates of receptor densities. The overall effect size averages to $d = .70$, but this masks a great deal of dispersion, so that the bounds of accuracy around the average range from $d = .16$ to $d = 1.24$. Even if the average effect size was based on more consistent findings, it would still mean that at least half of the patients and healthy people are indistinguishable in terms of their receptor densities.

Therefore, both post-mortem and brain-imaging research on the density of dopamine D2 receptors in schizophrenia have produced moderate average effect sizes and a great deal of heterogeneity due to nonreplication. In the case of post-mortem data, the nagging issue of medication exposure is hard to resolve. The small number of studies that used tissue samples from "drug-free" patients provide some limited support for the idea that elevated densities may be characteristic of at least some schizophrenia patients. But most post-mortem findings and all positron emission studies are based on measurements taken from the basal ganglia. Many researchers hold that this is the site of unwanted drug side effects rather than of the illness itself. What does it mean to find abnormalities in a region of the brain that has been tied more to motor control than to higher mental functions? To be sure, it is conceivable that a generalized dopamine-related abnormality might manifest itself in all dopamine tracts, including the basal ganglia. In other words, what is abnormal here may be abnormal in the frontal and limbic dopamine tracts as well. Unfortunately, technical limitations in detecting receptors outside the basal ganglia mean that it is hard to examine this possibility. As a result, the puzzle of how dopamine receptors contribute to schizophrenia remains very much an open question.

Evidence for Dopamine D4 Abnormalities in Schizophrenia

The lack of compelling and consistent evidence in favor of a large abnormal elevation in dopamine D2 receptors in the illness has led to the idea that other dopamine receptors may contribute to the causes of schizophrenia. The dopamine D4 receptor subtype is a D2-like receptor that has also been implicated in the illness. The dopamine D4 is of special interest because of its putative concentration in the hippocampus and cerebral cortex rather than in the basal ganglia and because of its relation to the "atypical" antipsychotic drug clozapine (Sanyal & Van Tol, 1997). This drug helps many patients who do not respond effectively to D2-blocking drugs like chlorpromazine and haloperidol (Buchanan, 1995). Clozapine is therapeutically effective yet has an affinity for the D4 receptor that is 10 times higher than its affinity for dopamine D2 or D3 receptors (see Meltzer, 1993; Sanyal & Van Tol, 1997). Perhaps the drug works primarily by blocking dopamine D4 receptors. And perhaps these are the receptors that truly exist in abnormal numbers in schizophrenia.

Seeman, Guan, and Van Tol (1993) spurred interest in the dopamine D4 receptor as another possible basis for the illness with a powerful study that tried to measure densities of this receptor in the post–mortem brain. The researchers faced a thorny problem in that no radioligand exists that binds selectively to the dopamine D4 receptor subtype. Thus raclopride has high affinity for both the D2 and D3 receptors but not for the D4, whereas emonapride binds D2, D3, and D4 receptors. Hence the investigators adopted a subtraction method whereby the number of dopamine D4 sites was estimated by subtracting raclopride from emonapride binding data. Seeman, Guan, and Van Tol compared schizophrenia tissue samples with normal controls, Alzheimer's disease, and Huntington's disease samples. Another noteworthy aspect of the study was that many of these dementia patients had been treated with antipsychotic medication during life, albeit at much lower doses than the schizophrenia patients. This provided a way of addressing the issue of spurious medication-related influences on the binding data. If patients with different diseases but similar histories of drug treatment show different dopamine abnormalities, then the abnormalities must reflect the disease and not the medication. In addition, 6 of the 32 schizophrenia patients had drug-free treatment histories. The subtraction method of receptor estimation revealed much higher levels of dopamine D4 receptors in schizophrenia than in any of the diseased or normal brain samples. The finding corresponds to an effect size of $d = 3.07$. There was very little overlap between control and schizophrenia sample distributions. Like Wong et al. (1986), a positron emission study of the dopamine D2, this finding for the D4 was powerful enough to raise hopes that a major breakthrough was in the making.

However, as in the case of the imaging results for the D2 receptor, more recent work has cast doubt on the reality of an initially exciting finding. First, results based on the subtraction method of estimating dopamine D4 densities have weakened progressively since the initial and very powerful findings. The most noteworthy example of this weakening is a study by Helmeste, Tang, Bunney, Potkin, and Jones (1996), who failed to detect any dopamine D4 or D4-like receptors in their schizophrenia and control brain tissue. Second, when alternative methods of estimating D4 densities are used, the result is usually negative. Thus Reynolds and Mason (1995) used emonopride as a tracer and a different receptor estimation method and found no evidence of elevated D4 binding in the schizophrenic brain. They concluded that dopamine D2 and D3 receptor densities might be elevated in the illness but not the D4. Hence the preliminary reports now coexist with evidence that the dopamine D4 and possibly other dopamine D2-like sites are either undetectable in normal brains (Seeman et al., 1997; Tang et al., 1997) or are not elevated in schizophrenic brains (Helmeste et al., 1996). It will be necessary to develop more selective receptor ligands before the question of abnormally high densities of the dopamine D4 receptor or D4-like binding sites in schizophrenia can be settled (see Lahti et al., 1998).

Assessment of Dopamine

The oldest and most thoroughly studied neurochemical hypothesis of schizophrenia continues to draw its strongest support from the efficacy of antipsychotic medications that block action of the neurotransmitter dopamine. In addition, drugs that enhance dopamine activity in the brain can produce psychotic symptoms in otherwise normal people and aggravate or reproduce symptoms in stable schizophrenia patients. Yet the logical deduction from this promising evidence, that dopamine must be highly concentrated or overutilized in some way in the schizophrenic brain, has received inadequate support, despite dramatic individual studies like those of Wong et al. (1986) and Seeman et al. (1993). The basic result of post-mortem studies searching for evidence of increased dopamine neurotransmitter or receptor concentrations in schizophrenia is an inconsistent, frequently weak research literature. The same can also be said of positron emission studies, despite the great advantage that they hold in being able to study young, living, never-medicated patients. There is no consistent overall increase of the dopamine D2 receptor in these patients, only a rather modest average effect that hides inconsistency between studies. Recent findings implicating other receptor subtypes, including the dopamine D4, also resist being reproduced. There are even researchers who question the very existence of the dopamine D4 receptor in the human brain (Reynolds & Mason, 1995). Not surprisingly, the search for additional dopamine receptors is on, including a search for new ones that may exist only in the schizophrenic brain (Seeman et al., 1997; Vallone, Picetti, & Borrelli, 2000).

In any event, even with more powerful evidence, it is a major theoretical leap to understand an illness like schizophrenia exclusively in terms of elevated dopamine receptors in the basal ganglia. This region, which contains most of the brain's dopamine, seems to be a motor inhibition and control system, a system that is often effected adversely by antipsychotic medication. Where is the evidence that dopamine activity is abnormal outside the basal ganglia, in brain regions that have major influences on thinking and feeling? It is also important to point out that countervailing evidence in relation to the dopamine-based account of schizophrenia has existed for some time. For example, despite the oft-cited link between dopamine blockade and the antipsychotic potency of drugs, there has always been a substantial minority of patients who are unresponsive, or "treatment refractory," to these medications (Christison, Kirch, & Wyatt, 1991; Straube & Oades, 1992, pp. 486–489). That is, their symptoms persist despite the administration of medication that is therapeutic for other patients. This lack of benefit does not seem to be due to a lack of dopamine receptor occupancy by the drug. Indeed, positron emission studies show that treatment-responsive and unresponsive patients have about the same degree of receptor blockade following drug administration (see Sedvall, 1992). In fact, the existence of patients who fail to benefit from standard drug treatment points to the possibility of other biological causes for the illness.

A clinical example of the puzzling phenomenon of ineffective drug treatment can be seen in James, the man with delusions of external thought control and thought insertion, who was hospitalized continuously between June 16 and August 17, 1988. Despite close monitoring and adjustment of his medication (trifluoperazine, or Stelazine) he experienced persistent auditory hallucinations with increasing intensity during this period. He heard one voice, from "deep in his brain," telling him to bite off his genitals and that he was "no good." This voice seemed to recur and disappear over time in response to some idiosyncratic neurological schedule rather than to the patient's compliance with his medication regimen. Changes in the dose and type of antipsychotic drug made little difference. In marked contrast, the other two patients, Ruth, the woman with olfactory and tactile hallucinations and William, with grandiose delusions, both experienced considerable symptom reduction as long as they took their medication.

A further challenge for any dopamine-based account of schizophrenia is the fact that dopamine blockade apparently occurs rapidly, within 24 hours, following drug administration. Although patients show some benefit in step with this blockade, the improvement in psychotic symptoms like delusions and hallucinations seems to take weeks to occur. Therefore, the role of dopamine in causing schizophrenia may be indirect, and it may occur in tandem with changes in other neurotransmitter systems. Even then a dopamine abnormality might account for only a portion of what is an etiologically diverse disease (see Carlsson, Hansson, Waters, and Carlsson, 1997; Halberstadt, 1995).

Serotonin: Chemical of Sleep and Moods

In the spring of 1943 a Swiss chemist named Albert Hoffman ingested a new chemical compound as a kind of "experiment." He had extracted it from a fungus called ergot that occurs on rye plants in farmlands of Europe and North America. Hoffman described the experience as follows.

> I was seized by a peculiar sensation of vertigo and restlessness. Objects, as well as the shape of my associates in the laboratory, appeared to undergo optical changes. I was unable to concentrate on my work. In a dream-like state I left for home, when an irresistible urge to lie down overcame me. I drew the curtains and immediately fell into a peculiar state similar to drunkenness, characterized by an exaggerated imagination. With my eyes closed, fantastic pictures of extraordinary plasticity and intensive color seemed to surge toward me. After two hours this state gradually wore off. (quoted in Julien, 1995, p. 313)

Hoffman had ingested some lysergic acid diethylamide, or LSD. His scientific curiosity was aroused, and he decided to self-administer LSD to determine its properties more fully. He took a relatively high dose and experienced sensations that were even more intense than the initial one: "I felt as if I were out of my body. I thought I had died" (quoted in Julien, 1995, p. 314). This second dose seemed to bring about a kind of psychosis, an artificial, chemically created episode of madness. Such experiences of chemically induced hallucinations and delusions prompted research on LSD during the 1950s. The vivid and reality-distorting effects of the compound were described as "psychotomimetic"—an imitation of psychosis. It was found that LSD and several other "psychedelic" drugs, including psilocybin, were chemically similar to the neurotransmitter serotonin. Furthermore, LSD seemed to enhance or potentiate the effects of serotonin in the brain (Julien, 1995, p. 312). Perhaps Hoffman's "exaggerated imagination" really was a kind of drug-induced schizophrenia. If so, serotonin might be one of the neurochemical keys to the illness.

Serotonin (5-hydroxytryptamine) is a chemical that occurs throughout the body, with only a relatively small amount in the brain. The precursor or building block is the amino acid tryptophan, which derives from dietary sources and circulates in the blood. It is taken into the brain and turned into serotonin by way of a series of chemical steps illustrated in figure 6.3. Like dopamine, serotonin is unable to cross the blood–brain barrier and enter the brain directly from the circulatory system. To enhance levels of serotonin in the brain by way of the bloodstream, it is necessary to administer tryptophan or a precursor like 5-hydroxytryptophan. These penetrate the blood-brain barrier and lead to increased synthesis of serotonin just as giving DOPA eventually yields more dopamine in the brain. The serotonin that remains in the synaptic cleft after release is broken down or metabolized by the enzyme monoamine oxidase. Alternatively, the membrane transporter may return serotonin to the presynaptic cell.

Several receptor subtypes have been identified within two main receptor

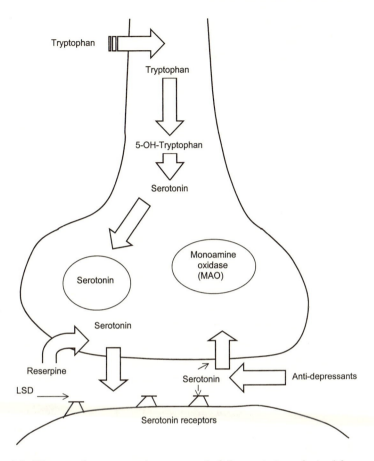

Figure 6.3. Diagram of a serotonergic nerve terminal. Serotonin is synthesized from tryptophan and released into the synapse to bind with receptors on the postsynaptic membrane. Drugs like reserpine interfere with storage and uptake mechanisms and cause depletion of serotonin. Lysergic acid diethylamide (LSD), which can induce psychotic-like experiences in otherwise healthy people, seems to reduce release of serotonin from the pre-synaptic cell but may also act on postsynaptic receptors. Monoamine oxydase (MAO) degrades serotonin in the presynaptic terminal. Antidepressants like Prozac act by inhibiting the return of serotonin from the synapse into the presynaptic cell, thus prolonging the action of the neurotransmitter. Some antipsychotic drugs, like risperidone, block serotonin as well as dopamine receptors.

families, termed serotonin S1 and serotonin S2. Generally speaking, serotonin S1 receptors have inhibitory effects in the brain and occur disproportionately in subcortical brain regions, including the basal ganglia and hippocampus. The serotonin S2 receptors seem to be excitatory and concentrate in the neocortex, especially the frontal lobes. Both receptor groupings occur more diffusely in the brain as well as in these specific regions (Cooper et al., 1996, pp. 352–409; Palacios, Waeber, Hoyer, & Mengod, 1990). Major serotonergic tracts in the brain include widespread areas of cerebral cortex, the caudate nucleus, and the hippocampus. But most of the serotonergic cell bodies are located in the raphe nucleii of the brainstem. One system of projections extends forward and reaches the cortex, basal ganglia, amygdala, nucleus accumbens, hippocampus, septum, thalamus, and hypothalamus. A second system extends back to the cerebellum and down to the spinal cord. Serotonin is more widely distributed in the brain than dopamine and occurs in higher concentrations in the cerebral cortex. From this standpoint, at least, it seems a good candidate for involvement in a psychological illness like schizophrenia.

Drug Effects and Behavioral Functions of Serotonin

Serotonin has been implicated in several behavioral functions, primarily through studies of animals. These functions include the regulation of sleep, wakefulness, mood, and sexual behavior; food consumption; temperature control; and the perception of pain (Cooper et al., 1996, pp. 376–379). For example, the drug p-chlorophenylalanine inhibits the enzyme that is involved in synthesizing serotonin. When animals are given this drug they do not sleep. Hence it is believed that serotonin is vital for normal sleep processes and may underpin sleep disorders. In psychiatric applications, drugs that increase serotonin neurotransmission alleviate mood disturbances like depression (see Julien, 1995, pp. 203–207). Thus fluoxetine (Prozac) blocks uptake of serotonin into the presynaptic neuron and therefore acts as an agonist to prolong the presence of serotonin in the synapse. This has the psychological effect of reducing anxiety and depression in psychiatric patients.

The connection between schizophrenia and serotonin derived originally from the suggestiveness of Hoffman's LSD experience and from the idea that LSD produces its hallucinatory effects by enhancing the action of serotonin in the brain. This idea quickly proved to be simplistic and only partly accurate. It is true that in animal studies small increases in serotonin and decreases in its metabolite were observed following injection of LSD. However, the mechanism of these effects was unclear because LSD did not seem to inhibit monoamine oxydase, the enzyme that destroys serotonin in the synapse. It is now believed that LSD may be a partial agonist of some serotonin receptor subtypes, thereby exerting its influence on the postsynaptic membrane rather than on uptake mechanisms (Julien, 1995, pp. 310–318). Yet the "psychotomimetic" effect of LSD remains poorly understood and may involve more neurotransmitters than just serotonin. Nonetheless, another putative link between schizophrenia and a specific transmitter substance has been raised by the interest in LSD. More recently, renewed interest in such links has been sparked by the development of antipsychotic drugs that act on serotonin receptors.

Serotonin and Schizophrenia

Interest in a possible role for serotonin in schizophrenia has rekindled with the introduction of "atypical" antipsychotic medication. Risperidone, introduced in the early 1990s, appears to work by blocking serotonin S2 as well as dopamine D2 receptors. This dual affinity distinguishes risperidone from standard antipsychotic drugs like chlorpromazine and haloperidol. The evidence from clinical drug trials shows that risperidone is an effective treatment for schizophrenia and causes fewer side effects than standard medication at low doses (Julien, 1995, pp. 291–292; Mattes, 1997; Umbricht & Kane, 1995). Intriguingly, it may be the negative symptoms of schizophrenia—the emotional flatness, disinterest, and withdrawal—that are most associated with serotonin abnormalities (Lindenmayer, 1994). These considerations are strengthening the clinical importance of serotonin-blocking drugs and also prompting a reevaluation of the serotonin hypothesis as an explanation for schizophrenia. Could schizophrenia result from an excess of serotonin-related activity in the brain?

The first and most obvious way to demonstrate serotonin-related abnormalities in living patients is to look for elevated concentrations of the neurotransmitter or its metabolites in bodily fluids like blood serum and cerebrospinal fluid. Unfortunately, it is even harder to find good peripheral indicators of brain activity for serotonin than for dopamine, and research results in this area have turned out to be relentlessly negative (see Ohuoha, Hyde, & Kleinman, 1993). Therefore, recent work has focused on serotonin receptor densities in schizophrenia. In principle, receptor estimates are obtainable post mortem or by way of positron emission techniques in living patients. Unfortunately, positron emission studies are rare, and fewer high affinity ligands exist for serotonin than for dopamine. Those ligands that are available bind rather unselectively to several neurotransmitter receptors in addition to the serotonin S2 site (Frost, 1990). In contrast, post-mortem receptor research is fairly active and provides an indication of the role of serotonin in the schizophrenic brain.

Following the general hypothesis that overactive neurotransmitters cause psychosis and the evidence that medications like risperidone work by blocking serotonin receptors, it seems reasonable to expect an excess of receptors in schizophrenic brain tissue. Therefore, consider the 10 post-mortem studies, based on 364 patient and control brains, of the serotonin S2 receptor that we found in our search. All of these studies involved tissue samples from the frontal cortex of patients who had received antipsychotic medication in varying degrees and duration during life. Ketanserin was the typical ligand employed. The average effect is $d = -.72$, but the direction of the effect indicates a receptor *deficiency* instead of excess in the schizophrenia group. An effect size of this magnitude means that about 56% of the patient and normal brain samples are indistinguishable in terms of receptor density values. Moreover, the accuracy bounds on this average are so broad that they include zero. In other words, the published results on serotonin S2 receptor densities are highly unreliable. Thus Joyce et al. (1993) found large relative excesses ($d = 1.55$), but Mita et al. (1986; $d = -2.79$), and more recently Dean, Hussain, Hayes, et al. (1999; $d = -1.37$), reported very large relative deficits. Taken together, the findings suggest that there is no overall elevation in serotonin S2 densities in schizophrenia patients. Instead, if anything, the frontal brain is deficient in these receptors in substantial numbers of schizophrenia patients. This likelihood is supported, albeit weakly, by a rare and recent positron emission study of living drug-free schizophrenia patients. Lewis et al. (1999) also found a decrease in serotonin S2 receptors in the illness, but the effect was small ($d = -.30$). The jury is still out on this topic, but the coexistence of receptor excesses and deficiencies in different patient tissue samples implies once more the presence of a chemically diverse illness or set of illnesses.

Serotonin has been investigated in relation to schizophrenia less thoroughly than dopamine. Drugs that block the action of both neurotransmitters have created interest in the idea that the pathophysiology of the illness involves abnormal dopamine or serotonin synthesis, release, uptake, transmission, breakdown, or receptor properties. However, the evidence for excessive serotonergic activity as a root cause of schizophrenia is much weaker than the evidence in support of dopamine. There is no selective serotonin antagonist that ameliorates symptoms of the illness in the way that dopamine antagonists do. All of the serotonin-linked antipsychotic drugs (e.g., clozapine, risperidone) also have some affinity for dopamine receptors. Hence the strongest piece of evidence linking dopamine with schizophrenia, the relation between neurotransmitter receptor blockade and symptom reduction, is missing or at least very equivocal in the case of serotonin. In fact, the evidence from the newer antipsychotic medications suggests an association between the two neurotransmitter systems rather than a special role for serotonin. Furthermore, the possibility that dopamine activity is mediated by still other neurotransmitter systems that lie close to the causes of schizophrenia is receiving increased attention. One of the most promising candidates in this regard is glutamate.

Glutamate: The Brain's Workhorse

How is it that strong evidence in favor of dopamine blockade as the basis for antipsychotic drug therapy can coexist with weak or inconsistent evidence for fundamental dopamine system abnormalities in schizophrenia? One way of understanding this puzzle is to propose that a second neurotransmitter system exists and is linked to dopamine in some way. It may be the second system that is abnormal in schizophrenia. A number of researchers (Carlsson & Carlsson,

1990; Halberstadt, 1995; Hirsch, Das, Garey, & de Belleroche, 1997) have pursued such conjectures and presented reasons why glutamate should be considered in the pathophysiology of the illness. First, glutamate, which is an excitatory substance in the nervous system, is the most widely distributed and essential neurotransmitter in the brain. It is the principal excitatory transmitter in the cerebral cortex. Glutamate distribution involves concentrations in several structures implicated in schizophrenia, including the entorhinal region, hippocampus, and frontal cortex. In addition, there is evidence that dopamine antagonizes glutamate, reducing glutamate release. Perhaps antipsychotic medications really work by weakening the inhibiting effect of dopamine on a depleted glutamate system, thereby promoting glutamatergic transmission and restoring balance to the ebb and flow of the chemical brain.

Once more, suggestive evidence comes from the ability of a drug, phencyclidine in this case, to induce a schizophrenia-like psychosis in otherwise normal people. Phencyclidine acts on glutamate receptors (Barchas, Faull, Quinn, & Elliot, 1994, p. 970; Halberstadt, 1995; Julien, 1995, pp. 321–326). The mechanism of action of phencyclidine is tied closely to complex receptor sites on the postsynaptic neuron, receptor sites that also recognize glutamate. It has been suggested that phencyclidine-induced psychosis is the best available neurochemical model for schizophrenia (Kornhuber, Riederer, & Beckmann, 1990). The street name for phencyclidine is "angel dust," probably reflecting the drug's ability to create feelings of euphoria in the user when taken in low doses. It is therefore not surprising that angel dust was one of the most frequently abused drugs in the United States during the early 1970s. Like the antipsychotic medications, it was developed originally as an anesthetic and pain-relieving drug. However, it dropped quickly from clinical use as severe psychiatric complications emerged. These complications include effects similar to positive schizophrenic symptoms: hallucinations, thought disorder, and intense suspiciousness. The drug also produces negative symptoms like withdrawal and unresponsiveness to external events. It is this expression of both positive and negative symptoms, along with provocative neurochemical findings, that makes phencyclidine and the glutamate system especially interesting in the search for the neurogenesis of schizophrenia (Olney, Newcomer, & Farber, 1999).

Glutamate is only one of several amino acids that occur in the brain. The others include aspartate, glycine, and gamma-aminobutyric acid. Collectively they dominate excitatory and inhibitory neurotransmission (Cooper et al., 1996, pp. 126–193; Dingledine & McBain, 1994, pp. 367–387). The two excitatory transmitters, glutamate and aspartate, depolarize postsynaptic neurons and cause them to fire. In contrast, gamma-aminobutyric acid and glycine hyperpolarize the postsynaptic neuron and reduce the likelihood that it will fire. In comparison to the pervasive amino acids, neurotransmitters like dopamine and serotonin are probably involved in only a small proportion of synapses in the brain. Yet glutamate is less understood than other transmitters, despite its ubiquity. Part of this poor understanding derives from glutamate's complex roles in the central nervous system. It is a neurotransmitter in its own right but also the precursor for gamma-aminobutyric acid. Glutamate forms the basis for other compounds as well, including peptides and special proteins. Moreover, it is not just a workhorse of neurotransmission but seems to have various roles, including detoxifying ammonia in the brain. Thus glutamate's presence in nerve cells is no guarantee that it is acting as a neurotransmitter in those cells. Glutamate's multiple roles and proliferation throughout the brain have made it hard to discern and isolate its specific neurotransmitter function. This complexity is echoed in glutamate's synthesis and metabolism.

For example, several precursors for glutamate have been identified, including glucose. Glutamine is the preliminary substance derived from glucose that interacts with the enzyme glutaminase within the nerve terminal to yield glutamate. However, a second synthetic pathway also exists. Through a process called transamination, glutamate is derived from aspartate in the nerve ending, and this occurs independently of the first process. Rate-limiting enzymes that play a role in regulating dopamine and serotonin synthesis also play a role in the case of glutamate. However, it appears that glutamate is not restricted to specific kinds of neurons and occurs even in nonglutamatergic cells. The key characteristic that distinguishes glutamatergic from nonglutamatergic neurons is the degree of concentration of glutamate neurotransmitter in the storage vesicles of the nerve terminal (see figure 6.4).

Another unusual feature of glutamate neurotransmission is that synthesis and breakdown involve interactions between nerve terminals and glial cells. Glia are not nerve cells; they perform a structural support role in the nervous system. In the case of glutamate activity, glia also take up neurotransmitter after it has been released into the synapse, convert it back to its precursor, glutamine, and then return the glutamine to the nerve cell where it acts to replenish stores of glutamate.

The complexity and distinctive properties of glutamate extend to the nature of its receptors. Speaking very broadly, receptors on the postsynaptic neuron fall into two classes: indirect and direct. Receptors for dopamine and serotonin are indirect in that they have to interact with other neurochemicals, the G proteins in the postsynaptic neuron, to effect transmission. In contrast, most receptors for glutamate are direct in that they convert chemical to electrical signals in the postsynaptic neuron directly and usually very rapidly. This class of receptors is also referred to as transmitter-gated ion, or receptor channels (Reichert, 1992, p. 68; Dingledine & McBain, 1994, pp. 367–387).

At least three "direct" receptor channel subtypes have been identified for glutamate. One of these, the N-methyl-D-aspartate (NMDA) receptor type, works like a highly regulated biological machine. For activation to occur, it is not enough for glutamate to bind with its receptor on the NMDA receptor

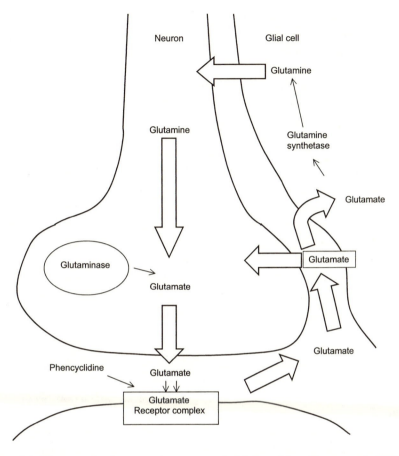

Figure 6.4. Diagram of a glutamatergic nerve terminal (adapted from Cooper et al., 1996, p. 172). Glutamate is the major excitatory neurotransmitter in the cerebral cortex. It is synthesized from glutamine and interacts with a variety of receptor types, including the NMDA (N-methyl-D-aspartic acid) family. Glutamate remaining in the synapse may be returned to the presynaptic cell by glial cell transporters as well as by neuronal transporters. Glutamate has multiple roles in the nervous system in addition to its neurotransmitter function. Phencyclidine, or "angel dust," a drug that can induce psychosis and memory loss, binds to a site on the NMDA receptor complex and appears to block action of the NMDA-glutamate receptor.

complex. Activation requires binding of another amino acid transmitter, like glycine, concurrently with glutamate. This receptor type is distributed widely in the brain but occurs with special frequency in the cortex and hippocampus. It is also the receptor where "angel dust" has its effect. Phencyclidine binds to a specific site on the NMDA complex and blocks the action of glutamate. Hence phencyclidine is regarded as a glutamate receptor antagonist. It is also believed that the analgesic, anesthetic, and psychological effects of phencyclidine all occur because of its antagonism for the NMDA–glutamate receptor and be-cause of its ability to inhibit glutamate-based transmission in the brain.

There are two other classes of "direct" receptors: AMPA (α-amino-3-hydroxy-5-methylisoxazole-4-propionate) receptors and kainate receptors. All three sub-types are activated by glutamate, but NMDA only activates its own receptor, and the same holds for AMPA and kainate. To make matters even more complex, al-though most glutamate receptors are of the "direct" type, the neurotransmitter also acts on "indirect" receptors that are coupled through G proteins.

Such descriptions illustrate the intricacy of neurotransmission. Glutamate is the most widespread excitatory transmitter in the brain. Yet beyond that fact, it can bind to not one but any of several receptor types, giving rise to different re-sponses in the postsynaptic neuron. At the same time, this principle of "diver-gence," whereby a single neurotransmitter diverges into multiple receptor sites and effector systems, is complemented by convergent influences. The same neu-ron may have different types of receptors for different neurotransmitters, which nonetheless converge on a single cell and create a joint physiological effect. Un-tangling the specific role of glutamate in schizophrenia is no easy matter in such a dynamic biological context.

The Glutamate Hypothesis of Schizophrenia

There are two basic ways of thinking about glutamate deficiency as a basis for schizophrenia. First, it is possible to conceive of an interaction between the dopamine and glutamate systems in the brain. In many brain regions, the two neurotransmitters exist in proximity, with dopamine exercising an inhibitory ef-fect on glutamate (Kornhuber et al., 1990). Thus a local deficiency in glutamate activity may lead to excessive dopamine transmission and hence bring about psychosis. However, the root abnormality is really in the glutamate system. Al-ternatively, deficient glutamatergic transmission may lie at the heart of the ill-ness and cause psychosis independently of the dopamine system.

Although hypotheses positing glutamate as a direct or indirect cause of schizophrenia have existed for some time (e.g. Kim, Kornhuber, Schmid-Burgk, & Holzmuller, 1980), they have been less systematically studied than either dopamine or serotonin-based conjectures about the illness. Moreover, research attention has not shifted completely to the postsynaptic side and to the quest for evidence of receptor abnormalities. There is still interest in determining levels of glutamate in different brain regions and in differentiating its presence as a neurotransmitter from other functions. There is corresponding interest in as-sessing presynaptic factors, including the number of sites for uptake of gluta-mate on the presynaptic membrane. At the same time, understanding glutamate receptor abnormalities in schizophrenia poses special problems because of the different forms and complexity of glutamate receptors. For example, the NMDA glutamate receptor is really a family of receptors that show a surprising degree of molecular diversity. There may be subtle functional differences among NMDA receptors, and currently available ligands cannot distinguish among them. Then there are the non-NMDA glutamate receptors. It is unlikely that ligand-binding methods and related estimates of receptor density alone will provide an adequate assessment of glutamate function in schizophrenia (see Catts et al., 1997). Therefore, techniques of molecular biology are being applied to this research area to assess the gene expression of different glutamate receptors (e.g., Porter, Eastwood, and Harrison, 1997). Thus messenger ribonucleic acid that encodes specific glutamate receptors can be quantified and evaluated in different brain regions. In the absence of highly selective ligands, this provides a way of inferring the presence of local glutamate abnormalities.

In searching the recent literature on glutamate I found that the relatively small number of studies—all post-mortem—fell into a few categories. One group of studies measures levels of glutamate or its metabolites in regional brain tissue samples. This parallels a similar but older literature that exists for dopamine and serotonin. There are also a few studies that measure uptake sites for glutamate on presynaptic membranes. The presence of such sites provides an index of glutamatergic innervation. Finally, several studies measure binding sites for NMDA and non-NMDA glutamate receptors. Taken together, this body of research provides an idea of the strength of available evidence in support of glutamate abnormalities in schizophrenia. However, there are few replications, and this means that only a preliminary and very general assessment of the field is possible.

In looking for studies of glutamate levels in schizophrenic and normal brain tissue, I limited myself to findings based on more than one study. This literature draws almost exclusively on medicated post-mortem patient samples. The three reports of data on the basal ganglia show that there is a tendency for schizophrenic tissue to have relative deficits in glutamate in this brain region. However, one study (Korpi, Kleinman, Goodman, & Wyatt, 1987) obtained a reverse effect that is very close to zero ($d = .07$). Only two relevant studies were found for assays of the amygdala, hippocampus, and thalamus, an extremely slim empirical base to evaluate an idea. The amygdala comparisons suggest nonexistent or trivial excesses in glutamate levels in schizophrenia (e.g., Korpi et al., $d = 0$). The hippocampal and thalamic comparisons are very inconsistent, perhaps revealing deficits in schizophrenia (e.g., Toru et al., 1988, $d = -.1$; Tsai et al., 1995, $d = -1.09$). Each set of comparisons demonstrates a fairly large effect and a small effect. However, the larger effects are from recent studies, which is encouraging.

Finally, I found four comparisons with tissue drawn from the frontal cortex of patient and control tissue samples. These also imply somewhat larger glutamate deficiencies in recent studies, despite considerable inconsistency between reports. Nonetheless, the two most recent studies yield effects below $d = 1.0$

(Tsai et al., 1995; Omori et al., 1997), which means that schizophrenia and normal samples overlap a great deal in terms of glutamate levels in the brain.

The studies reporting data on binding to the presynaptic uptake sites of glutamate show an average effect size for reduced binding in schizophrenia that is very close to zero. However, there is inconsistency here. For example, two studies report, alternately, modest increases (Aparicio-Legarza, Cutts, Davis, & Reynolds, 1997; $d = .35$) and decreases (Noga et al., 1997; $d = -.47$) in glutamate binding in the basal ganglia. The frontal cortex does not appear to show reduced glutamate binding on the basis of the most recent available study (Aparicio-Legarza et al.; $d = -.08$). Binding in the temporal cortex was within normal ranges in two out of three studies (e.g., Simpson, Slater, & Deakin, 1998). Overall, there is no very compelling evidence of a major reduction in binding to the glutamate uptake site in schizophrenia. Hence, this rough index of glutamatergic innervation does not suggest a primary pathology for the illness.

Studies of glutamate receptor binding have focused on the basal ganglia, the hippocampus, and the frontal cortex. However, the complexity and variety of receptors makes it hard to summarize this literature. Thus some studies address the NMDA receptor subtype and others examine the non–NMDA subtypes, like kainate and AMPA. Therefore, only the most general kind of observations can be made about this diverse field of study. The results for the basal ganglia suggest a relative excess rather than a deficit of NMDA glutamate receptors, although the finding ($d = .16$) of Noga et al. (1997) is extremely small. This runs counter to the usual argument that schizophrenia may result from local deficiencies in glutamate (e.g., Deakin & Simpson, 1997).

There appears to be a particular interest in studying receptor characteristics of the hippocampus in the glutamate literature. The articles and effects I found show that apart from an aberrant finding of excess numbers of NMDA receptors in schizophrenia (Kornhuber et al., 1989), most studies show small or moderate deficits across a variety of receptor types in the hippocampus. This is consistent with the hypothesis of reduced glutamate activity in a psychologically critical brain region. Nonetheless, the hippocampal receptor studies yield a very modest average of $d = .40$. The small size of the average effect is attributable to divergent studies like those by Kornhuber et al. (1989; $d = 1.46$), Deakin et al. (1989; $d = -.09$), and Kerwin, Patel, and Meldrum (1990; $d = -.25$) that report large and trivial receptor increases or reductions, respectively, in the schizophrenic hippocampus. The average effect size implies that at least 72% of the patient and control samples are indistinguishable from each other in terms of glutamate receptor densities.

The findings with respect to glutamate receptors in the frontal brain region are also scarce and inconsistent. On the one hand, a recent study by Sokolov (1998) reports large deficits (e.g., $d = -2.42$) in several receptor types. On the other hand, both Dean, Hussain, Hayes, et al. (1999) and Grimwood, Slater, Deakin, & Hutson (1999) found trivial differences between patient and control tissue in NMDA-glutamate receptors. Sokolov's study is of special interest because the investigator reports results from schizophrenia samples that vary in their degree of medication exposure shortly before death. The report includes tissue samples with drug-free periods ranging from a few days to about 6 months in duration prior to death. The receptor deficits are much smaller when obtained from patients who had received medication within days of death. The author suggests that antipsychotic drugs may reverse the glutamate receptor deficiencies that exist in some patients with schizophrenia.

The small number of studies and the complexity and diversity of glutamate receptor subtypes make research results very hard to evaluate and summarize. It may be premature to judge this research area. At this time, the scanty evidence on glutamate receptors in schizophrenia is too unreliable to provide any clear support for the glutamate hypothesis of the illness. The most appealing hypothesis, reduced glutamate receptors leading to increases in dopamine activity, will require much stronger findings and a replication record with tissue samples that have not been exposed to medication.

The ubiquity of glutamate in nerve cells and the difficulty in discriminating glutamate neurotransmitter from other roles, plus the complexity and number of relevant receptors, make this field of research a great challenge. Moreover, the lack of selective ligands for positron emission scanning means that there are no receptor-binding studies with living patients who have never received medication. In general, the empirical evaluation of the glutamate hypothesis of schizophrenia is still in its infancy. It remains to be seen whether evidence of convincing magnitude and consistency will accrue in support of the idea that glutamate is an essential piece in the neurochemical puzzle of schizophrenia.

General Summary and Conclusions

Is schizophrenia really a kind of biological tempest, where tides of neurotransmitter crest and recede? Do substances with cryptic and unpronounceable names play havoc with patches of protein called receptors, and do they upset chemical balances in regions of the brain that control thought, feeling, and movement? Are there other regions, poor in receptors, that are overwhelmed and silenced? Perhaps this neurochemical tempest causes contortions of mind and matter, giving birth to delusions, hallucinations, thought disorder. Then, as the tide recedes, what remains is a depleted brain and the apparent emptiness of negative symptoms.

The revolution in psychopharmacology and biological psychiatry started by the introduction of chlorpromazine in the early 1950s has provided the first genuine treatments for schizophrenia. And it has provided ideas and evidence about the neurogenesis of the illness. There is evidence for a variety of neuro-chemical abnormalities, from excessive to deficient concentrations of dopa-mine, serotonin, and glutamate and their metabolites, receptors, and uptake sites. However, apart from individual studies like those of Wong et al. (1986) or See-man et al. (1993) that show powerful differences between schizophrenia patients and healthy people, the evidence does not reach a threshold of magnitude that is convincing. Cumulatively and individually, the neurochemical effect sizes are too modest and much too variable to support causal explanations for a single ill-ness. And the evidence seldom escapes the confounding influence of medica-tion on the neurobiology of the schizophrenic brain.

This situation is illustrated by the evidence summary in table 6.1. Does a central dopaminergic index based on metabolite levels in cerebrospinal fluid re-veal strikingly large excesses in schizophrenia patients? It does not. Do estimates of the density of dopamine D2 receptors, the same receptors known to be in-volved in therapeutic drug effects, consistently yield large elevations in the ill-ness? This literature provides strands of evidence suggesting that some patients with the illness may have elevated numbers of the dopamine D2 receptor. But the evidence is colored with coexisting findings showing that when the human brain is exposed to dopamine-blocking medication it grows more receptors. And even the application of positron emission tomography to drug-naive pa-tients does not yield the needed evidence. Here is an instrument that provides receptor density estimates in living patients with schizophrenia who have never been exposed to antipsychotic medication: very exciting initial results were fol-lowed by weak results. Instead of resolving the dopamine D2 receptor issue, the neuroimaging results have added to the controversy. A conservative reading of the published literature is that there is no consistent evidence of elevated dopamine D2 receptor densities in most schizophrenia patients. Yet the dopamine D2-like group includes other receptors, including the D4, that have also generated powerful initial findings. Once again, however, these findings have not cleared the demanding hurdles of consistent and independent repli-cation that must be negotiated before evidence is convincing. Indeed, despite the fairly large average effect for dopamine D4 findings in table 6.1, this is a controversial and unstable research literature.

There have always been some doubts about the adequacy of the dopamine hypothesis of schizophrenia. An earlier literature did not support the idea that dopamine exists in excessive amounts in the schizophrenic brain. It may be that this neurotransmitter is only part of the story. Accordingly, it makes sense to ex-amine other candidates, notably serotonin, a substance targeted by a new gen-eration of antipsychotic drugs. But the serotonin findings do not fall readily into line with the idea of excess neurotransmitter activity in schizophrenia. In fact, the average effect size suggests abnormally *low* numbers of serotonin S2 receptors in the frontal cortex of schizophrenia patients. This average effect is modest in magnitude and masks too much inconsistency to suggest that an essential neurogenic mechanism for the illness has been found. Therefore, it also makes sense to consider glutamate, which is known to interact with the dopamine system. This excitatory transmitter is ubiquitous in the cerebral cortex and associates with a baffling complexity of receptor types while resisting clear delineation in terms of its multiple roles and locations in the central nervous system. The initial results are provocative and derive from psychologically important regions of the brain, regions that have already been implicated in relation to schizophrenia. Assessment is premature, but the available evidence shows the same tendency toward inconsistency or modesty that bedevils all fields of schizophrenia research.

New ideas and possibly new receptors that exist only in the schizophrenic brain may yet yield the kind of evidence that reveals the neurochemical tempest at the core of the illness. Yet there is another possibility as well. Perhaps a basic flaw exists in all of the conjectures and evidence considered thus far and in the previous chapters. Post-mortem studies reflect a brain that, in life, may have harbored schizophrenia for 50 years. Brain-imaging studies of receptor densities use adult patients who already have the illness. The average age at which people develop schizophrenia is in the early twenties for men and late twenties for women. Does schizophrenia simply erupt, full-blown, from a normal childhood in these people, with no telltale warnings, no clues as to its origins? Perhaps neuroscience has concentrated too much on studying people after they have the illness. To really understand schizophrenia it may be necessary to study the brain and the person before they become ill. It may be necessary to look back in time and development and to track the roots of madness into childhood, infancy, and beyond. And this raises the next question that must be pursued in this book. If the biology of madness is not apparent in the adult brain, can it be glimpsed in the nature of the early nervous system and early experience? Perhaps there is a twisted course that leads to madness later in life and also leads to the secrets of schizophrenia.

7

●●●●●●●●●●●●●●●●●●●●●●●●●●●●●●●●●

THE STRANGENESS OF
CHILDREN

Does madness lurk in the minds of children? Long before mental life succumbs to delusions and hallucinations, the neural seed of schizophrenia may show itself in some way. The psychological life of a child may hint at the disturbance to come. Perhaps shyness and social fear presage negative symptoms like emotional withdrawal and disinterest. Perhaps a child's empty stare, awkward movement, discomfort with affection, inconstancy of attention, or absence of empathy are early warnings of a distant but gathering illness. It is puzzling the way schizophrenia seems to erupt with little warning, early in adult life, following an apparently normal childhood. But perhaps the normality is more apparent than real. Surely there is already something different about the child who goes on to develop the illness, something that could be a clue to the whole problem of schizophrenia and the brain.

Yet neurology provides examples of diseases that do spring unheralded into existence. A rapidly expanding tumor may invade the brain and quickly push a person toward death. Other diseases insinuate themselves quietly into a seemingly healthy life. In this way multiple sclerosis arrives in young adulthood, Huntington's disease in middle age, and Parkinsonism and Alzheimer's disease in later life. Researchers do not necessarily feel compelled to inspect the early years of people with these diseases.

However, in the case of poorly understood disorders like schizophrenia, conventional neurology is an uncertain guide. When causes are obscure, when neurobiology is complicated by the effects of a disease and its treatment, and when findings lack the strength and consistency to yield secure knowledge, there are reasons to study the person before illness strikes. There are reasons to pursue the schizophrenia riddle into childhood and beyond, into birth, and even beyond birth. Indeed, there are reasons to search for the origins of madness in the evolution of the fetus and in the beginnings of life itself.

The first reason for including the study of children and their growth in schizophrenia research stems from the lack of unequivocal neuropathology in adult patients. This lack compels researchers to look for different, subtler kinds of neurological events as the basis for the illness. The neurotransmitter abnormalities and mild deficits in brain tissue volumes seen in some patients may be late products of a much earlier schizophrenic process. In other words, perhaps the way to find the neurological cause of schizophrenia is to start at the beginning and study the growth of the nervous system and behavior and attempt to find critical points where some kind of special deviation occurs that sets the course of life veering toward madness. In fact, studying infants and children may be the only way of getting an accurate picture of the schizophrenic brain. A picture of the early brain shows it before medication has changed neurochemistry. And it is a picture unclouded by long years of impoverished lifestyle, poor general health, and inadequate nutrition. Thus the neurodevelopmental strategy for understanding schizophrenia makes sense on both theoretical and practical grounds.

Possibilities proliferate once a wide net is cast in the search for biological causes of the illness. Perhaps the brain that harbors schizophrenia goes awry very early in its growth. Or the early environment may be at fault through unsuspected mechanisms. A gentle virus may creep in from the outside world through the mother's body and across the placenta, scattering blueprints for madness as it makes its way. But why stop at childhood, or even the process of fetal development? If something goes wrong with the nervous system, it may have been programmed to go wrong all along, programmed by one or more schizophrenia genes passed on through the generations. Therefore, it is with genes that the story of schizophrenia and development really begins.

Essentials of Genetics and Early Neurodevelopment

To appreciate the work on the origins of schizophrenia, it is helpful to have some elementary background information. The unit of heredity, or gene, is a sequence of DNA found in each cell of the human body. Genes are arranged in strings or chromosomes that exist in 23 pairs, with each parent contributing half of the total number that every person has. The degree of genetic overlap between a parent and offspring (50%) is the same as between two siblings, includ-

Table 7.1 Lifetime risks of schizophrenia for a patient's relatives

Relationship to patient	Risk (%)	d
Identical (monozygotic) twin	48	1.30
Fraternal (dizygotic) twin	17	.58
Son or daughter	13	.48
Brothers and sisters	9	.37
Uncles, aunts, nephews, nieces, grandchildren	3–4	.17
No relationship (general population)	1	—

Note: Adapted from Gottesman (1991, p. 96), who summarized the results of existing twin and family studies. More recent research has confirmed these findings (Cardno & Gottesman, 2000). The table shows that risk of developing schizophrenia increases progressively with the degree of genetic relatedness. However, even with complete genetic overlap, as in the case of identical twins, about half the identical twins of an ill twin remain free of the diagnosis. Risk statistics are evidence for complex genetic and environmental contributions in the causation of schizophrenia. The effect sizes (Cohen's *d*) provide a rough idea of evidential strength and are estimated by using illness frequency statistics for each relative group compared to statistics for the general population.

ing fraternal twins. However, identical twins share 100% of their genes, insofar as the twins are monozygotic, or derived from a single egg. In contrast, third-degree relatives like cousins overlap genetically by only 12.5%. On the basis of shared genes, human characteristics from eye color and height to illnesses like diabetes and heart disease "run" in families. There is evidence that most psychiatric, behavioral, and medical disorders are also under genetic influence. This applies to Alzheimer's disease, autism, major mood disorders and reading disability, as well as to epilepsy, peptic ulcer, and rheumatoid arthritis. In addition, within the spectrum of normal behavior, genes play a role in cognitive abilities like memory and intelligence and in personality traits like neuroticism. Genes even figure in vocational interests and scholastic achievement (McGuffin, Owen, O'Donovan, Thapar, & Gottesman, 1994; Plomin, Owen, & McGuffin, 1994). However, different disorders and traits are mediated by genetic factors to varying degrees. Thus hypertension, female alcoholism, and ischemic heart disease are influenced rather weakly by genetic factors, whereas genes seem to effect reading disability, epilepsy, and intelligence in a fairly strong way. At the same time, the estimated "heritabilities," or proportion of observed trait variability controlled by genes, seldom exceed 50%. Accordingly, nongenetic factors must be of roughly equal importance in determining the emergence of many psychiatric disorders and complex behavioral traits.

A familial genetic contribution to the development of schizophrenia has been assumed since the time of pioneers like Kraepelin (1919) and Bleuler (1950). Schizophrenia is observed to run in families, with a risk of about 13% to offspring of a schizophrenic parent. This compares with a general population risk of only about 1% (Gottesman, 1991). The "familiality" of the illness is summarized in table 7.1, and it shows unequivocally that the likelihood of a person developing schizophrenia is much higher if a relative also has the illness.

The risk is highest for someone with an identical or monozygotic twin, and then the risk falls off stepwise as the degree of genetic relatedness diminishes. Yet statistics like those in table 7.1 could also mean that risk for schizophrenia increases with shared family experience and not because of shared genes. But Heston (1966), Kety et al. (1968), and Rosenthal et al. (1968), addressed this possibility and argued that the familiality of schizophrenia is due to biological rather than to psychological influences. For example, in Heston's study the children of schizophrenic mothers were compared with children of normal mothers in terms of rates of developing the illness. However, the schizophrenic mothers did not raise their children. They were adopted away at birth and raised by an unrelated and healthy caregiver. Thus any occurrence of the illness in these adopted children would reflect an inherited biological predisposition and not the effect of being raised by a psychotic parent. Out of 47 adopted offspring of schizophrenic mothers, five developed schizophrenia. None of the adopted offspring from nonschizophrenic mothers developed the disorder. This rate of five in 47, or 16.6% when corrected for age, is close to the risk of illness generally seen in the offspring of schizophrenia patients. Hence adoption studies support an inherited biological liability as the key ingredient in raising the risk of schizophrenia. Noxious parenting or family experiences certainly cause trauma and suffering in children. Indeed, the child of a parent with schizophrenia is at even higher risk if raised by that parent and not given up for adoption (see Gottesman, 1991, pp. 141–142; Ingraham & Kety, 2000). However, poor parenting does not cause the illness in the first place.

But if genes contribute to the cause of schizophrenia, how strong is the contribution, and how many genes are involved? It is important to note that the risk statistics show that the vast majority (87%) of children of schizophrenic mothers or fathers will not develop the illness despite having the biological liability or diathesis. This contrasts with disorders like Huntington's disease that have a more straightforward pattern of inheritance. Defects in a single gene cause Huntington's disease, giving rise to a predictable risk: a 50% chance of developing the disease if a person has one parent with the disorder. Complex traits, including psychiatric disorders like schizophrenia, do not follow such patterns of inheritance. This can be seen if the observed risks for schizophrenia are compared with risks predicted by single gene models. For example, a single gene model predicts that risk for illness should decrease by a constant factor of 50% between different relative classes. This prediction is based on the degree of shared genetic material in relatives, which ranges from 100% in the case of identical twins, to 50% for parents, to 25% for second degree relatives like aunts and uncles. The first problem for a single-gene model is that the risk of schizophrenia for someone who has an identical twin with the illness is only about 48% instead of 100%. If all genes are in common, including the one that causes schizophrenia, both identical twins should become ill. This problem can be dealt with in theory through the concept of incomplete "penetrance." In other words, it is known that a proportion of people with a dominant gene will fail to show the effect of that gene. This may be due to the environment or to other factors in the person's genetic constitution. In any case, the penetrance of the schizophrenia gene may be much less than 100%, say only about 50%. This roughly fits the risk of illness in identical twins. However, the model still does not work for the other relative classes. Thus first-degree relatives should have a risk for schizophrenia of about 25%, but table 7.1 shows that the observed risks are much lower. Similarly, second-degree relatives should have a risk of 12.5% instead of the 3−4% actually observed. All in all, single major gene models make too many prediction errors to be acceptable, and this holds even when additional assumptions and variations of the basic model are used. As a result, the field has moved increasingly to complex multiple gene models in accounting for the inheritance of schizophrenia (see Cardno & Gottesman, 2000; Gottesman, 1991, pp. 228−232; Gottesman & Shields, 1972; Pogue-Geile & Gottesman, 1999).

Given the complexity and limits of genetic contributions to schizophrenia, it is perhaps not surprising that attempts by molecular biologists to link the illness with single genes and chromosomes have been consistently unsuccessful (O'Donovan & Owen, 1992, 1996). A series of negative linkage and association studies that examined candidate genes for dopamine receptors is especially disappointing (Coon et al., 1993; Serretti, Lattuada, Cusin, et al., 1999; Serretti, Lilli, Bella, et al., 1999). However, researchers in the field of molecular genetics are considering the possibility that more than one gene influences the development of schizophrenia. Thus there is evidence for up to 14 "risk" genes, localized on chromosomes 1, 2, 4, 5, 6, 7, 8, 9, 10, 13, 15, 18, 22, and the X. Unfortunately, the evidence has sometimes been difficult to reproduce (Kendler, 2000). Still, as the genes are cloned and researchers learn their function, the neural and developmental pathways to schizophrenia may be revealed. Moreover, with the completion of the human genome project—and its goal of finding the chromosomal location and structure of all 100,000 genes—the prospects for understanding the genetics of schizophrenia will continue to improve (see Moises & Gottesman, 2000).

In sum, twin and adoption studies have furnished convincing evidence that genetic influences are ubiquitous across a wide spectrum of human behavior and disease. This spectrum includes schizophrenia, but here, as in the case of other complex disorders, the genetic influence is not absolute, the nature of genetic transmission is unknown, and it is likely that more than one gene is involved. At the same time, the genetic evidence indirectly supplies the strongest grounds for environmental causation: many identical twins with the same genetic makeup are "discordant" for schizophrenia: one twin is ill and the other remains healthy. Hence there must be a major nonheritable contribution to etiology.

Indeed, most attempts to imagine the origins of schizophrenia involve the concepts of diathesis and stress rather than straightforward genetic causation (see Zuckerman, 1999, pp. 3–24). A diathesis is a genetic predisposition—an inherited biological vulnerability to illness. The vulnerability could take the form of an overactive dopamine system, an abnormal hippocampus, or a faulty frontal cortex. This diathesis interacts with or compounds stresses in the environment, and at some point a threshold is crossed and the vulnerable person develops symptoms. The stress component of the illness equation is often interpreted very broadly to mean almost any noxious environmental influence on the evolving person. Hence the environmental contribution to schizophrenia may involve anything from exposure to a virus during gestation, to delivery complications at birth, to psychological stresses in the family environment during childhood. On the other hand, some people may have such a potent diathesis, that very little stress is needed to push them over the illness threshold (Fowles, 1992). Conversely, other people may have so little diathesis and such good coping skills that no amount of stress will push them over the edge. In still other cases, a person may inherit adaptive personality traits along with the schizophrenia diathesis, and these traits may provide protection from the worst ravages of illness (Meehl, 1962). This broad interpretation of diathesis and stress thereby places genes into an illness equation that also includes psychological and physical environments.

But even if the general proposition is accepted that the routes to eventual schizophrenia include the inheritance of a liability for the illness *and* an environmental influence of some kind—the diathesis–stress model—how would this manifest itself in the developing nervous system and in the developing person? Some basic information follows about development and how it can go wrong.

Neural Development and Neuropathology

From a sheet of embryonic cells that deepens into a groove and then folds into a tube running the length of the fetus, the human nervous system undulates and swells into existence. During the first 3 months it is the brainstem and spinal cord that are subject to especially rapid growth, but the foundation is also laid for what will become the amygdala, basal ganglia, and cortex of the cerebral hemispheres. Toward the end of the first trimester, genetically programmed cell migration and axonal development begin to differentiate the nervous system into its major components. Cell migration is a key process whereby neurons grow and divide and move along specialized filaments to distant locations that form the basis of mature brain regions and structures. In tandem with cell migration, axons, the long processes of nerves that conduct impulses away from the cell body, develop and branch out to find their target zones elsewhere in the nervous system. Axonal development represents the groundwork of neural pathways and fiber tracts, the connective wiring of the brain. These pathways also join different components of the nervous system with the rest of the body. As axons grow, dendrites also proliferate. These are the branching, treelike projections of neurons. Dendrites end in synapses and receive impulses and information from the axons of other neurons. Dendritic development, or arborization, is a slow process that extends far beyond gestation so that growth continues well into infancy and early childhood. Paradoxically, neurons also produce excessive dendritic branching that requires periodic "pruning," or curtailment, as part of the overall maturation sequence (see Goodman, 1994).

Damage to the very primitive nervous system will effect general growth and produce severe malformations. Early-first-trimester disturbances are likely to result in small skull or brain size, complete or partial absence of key neural structures, or other gross anomalies. Later, as cell migration proceeds, a disturbed brain may take less obvious forms. Cell migration may end prematurely, resulting in neurons that distribute themselves in the wrong location. Axonal development can also go awry. Although axons seem to have the ability to overcome obstacles as they sprout, their growth can be blocked by scar tissue or altered by the effects of toxins and malnutrition. Moreover, if the target structure is damaged, axons may grow to connect with alternate but inappropriate targets, giving rise to dysfunctional fiber tracts. And dendritic abnormalities can constitute a kind of neuropathology. In such cases dendrites may be thinner, sparser, and smaller than normal. Similar abnormalities are believed to form a substrate for mental retardation (see Nauta & Feirtag, 1986, pp. 136–143). Although this is not the developmental period of primary interest in schizophrenia research, brain volume reductions in a number of structures have been observed in some patients with the illness (see chapters 4 and 5). One interpretation of these reductions is that they reflect a very early disturbance rather than adult-onset events or neurodegenerative changes later in life (Lyon & Barr, 1991, pp. 135–136).

The fourth through sixth months of development bring rapid change at many levels in the developing brain. Cell migration proceeds apace to produce the basal ganglia, and psychologically important brain regions and structures form and grow. They include the thalamus, which has connections with the frontal cortex, limbic, and striatal regions. These brain structures are implicated in behavioral functions like mental flexibility, memory, emotion, and movement control. Patterns of cortical sulcii and gyrii, the convolutions and fissures of cerebral gray matter, are also laid down in the second trimester. Myelination, the insulation of nerve cells, proliferates at this time (see Gilbert, 1997, pp. 253–339). In addition, the development of layers of neurons, one of the most distinctive features of the mature cerebral cortex, takes place at this juncture. In contrast, development of structures like the hippocampus is more stable and gradual throughout this period. The slow growth means that processes like cell migration and axonal and synaptic connectivity are still taking place in the hippocampus after other structures have developed more permanent form. Hence the vulnerability of the hippocampus may also continue over a correspondingly prolonged period of time.

In addition to maturation of key neural structures, there is indirect evidence, obtained from animal studies, that neurotransmitter systems of importance to schizophrenia begin to evolve during the second trimester (Lyon & Barr, 1991; Nauta & Feirtag, 1986, pp. 26–33). Thus the first dopaminergic cells are detectable at this point, and it is believed that serotonin tracts follow suit and begin to emerge, with development continuing into the postnatal period. Not surprisingly, the second trimester is the focus of speculation about the origins of schizophrenia. For example, as the germinal mass recedes within the ventricles, bleeding and cell death may occur in the periventricular region. It has been speculated that such a mechanism might underlie findings of lateral and third ventricle enlargement in schizophrenia (Lyon & Barr, 1991; Lesch & Bogerts, 1984). For the most part, however, disturbances at this point compel researchers to look for more subtle brain pathology: altered cell distributions, abnormal cell densities, and unusual cell positions (see Bunney, Potkin, & Bunney, 1997).

The last 3 months of gestation are remarkable for particularly rapid growth and differentiation of the cerebral cortex into its sulcii and gyrii and for ongoing synaptic development. It is believed that synapse numbers increase at this point and then peak soon after birth before undergoing a gradual pruning in early life. There is also extensive loss of neurons and retraction of axons during this time as the nervous system is cut back as well as expanded. This combination of neural accretion and reduction seems to be a normal feature of development. When brain lesions occur during the third trimester they leave signs that microglia have been at work in response to tissue injury. Because gliosis is often absent in post-mortem schizophrenic brain tissue, it is theorized that the key pathological events underlying the illness must occur before the third trimester (Falkai et al., 1999; Roberts et al., 1986).

Pregnancy, Birth, and Their Complications

Numerous influences may affect the fetus as it prepares for life outside the womb. These influences include the mother's age, diet, and general health, use of drugs, and exposure to environmental toxins. One of the great insulating and protective factors in prenatal life is the uterus itself. The placenta acts as a selective filter to screen out at least some of the toxins that might damage the fetus. Nonetheless, certain poisons, termed teratogens, negotiate this screen to interfere with neural and general physical development. Diseases like smallpox, measles, venereal disease, and the AIDS virus can pose a threat to the fetus and cause brain damage and mental retardation. Similarly, certain drugs, from aspirin to the nicotine in cigarettes, may influence the fetus. The disorder of fetal alcohol syndrome is an example of how a teratogen can induce a variety of physical and psychological deficits in the developing fetus and ultimately, in the infant and child (Jenkins & Culbertson, 1996, pp. 409–451). Additional examples include toxins from the environment like industrial chemicals ingested in food, water, or air. Thus, maternal consumption of fish containing polychlorinated biphenyls (PCBs) is related to low infant birth weight, head size, length of gestation, reflex functioning, and autonomic nervous system activity (Fein, Jacobson, Jacobson, Schwartz, & Dowler, 1984).

Pregnancy complications and many teratogenic influences tend to occur in multiples. Thus smoking, alcohol abuse, poor nutrition, and the ingestion of contaminants may coexist in a mother's life. Therefore, it is often hard to isolate the specific influence of particular teratogens on the mental and physical maturation of the child. Moreover, teratogens are often insidious in nature, with a capacity to cause both short- and long-term, or "sleeper," effects in the growing child. Streissguth, Barr, and Martin (1984) found a relation between maternal smoking and alcohol consumption during the first trimester and attention-related difficulties in the offspring. However, these difficulties did not appear until the children were 4 years of age. It is perhaps not surprising that the concept of a sleeper effect is of special interest in relation to schizophrenia. The long latency between birth and the onset of psychotic symptoms in young adulthood makes the concept an attractive way of thinking about the timing of the illness.

The birth process itself is also a source of possible trauma and damage to normal development. During birth, the fetus is forced out of the mother through involuntary uterine muscle contractions. The narrowness of the birth canal can give neonates a damaged appearance as they negotiate their way into the world. However, the real dangers come from other events, like reduced oxygen supply when the umbilical cord is restricted or misplaced around the baby. The baby's position in the birth canal may be abnormal and pose hazards. Oxygen deprivation, or anoxia, can damage the brain if it is protracted enough to cause neuronal death. In addition, anoxia can increase blood pressure and lead to intracranial bleeding. Minor anoxia seldom has chronic effects, but severe cases yield numerous neurological deficits, including seizures and cognitive impairment (Lamb & Bornstein, 1987). Premature deliveries are a special case of obstetrical complications. They are documented routinely, and therefore this information is available to researchers examining birth records. Marked prematurity is associated with respiratory, sucking, and swallowing problems. Moreover, a significant percentage of preterm infants, up to 25%, experience a range of lifelong impairments, including mental retardation and blindness, as well as less severe disabilities (see Gilbert, 1997, pp. 805–841).

Neurological Development in Infancy,
Childhood, and Adolescence

Having survived the normal trauma of birth, brain development continues in the form of irregular spurts that increase brain mass. There appear to be spurts in brain growth during the first year and a half of life and between 2–4, 6–8, 10–12, and 14–16 years (Kolb & Whishaw, 1996, p. 99). Yet neuron numbers, dendrites, and synapses are also being reduced even as remaining cells increase in size. The density of synapses provides a good example of how the nervous system seems to proliferate and then prune its internal connections. Synaptic density increases after birth until the second year of life, when it is about 50% higher than in the adult brain. Thereafter, synaptic density declines until roughly the age of 16, at which point it remains constant well into old age. In a way, the brain seems to have an excess of synapses until the late teenage years (see Lewis & Volkmar, 1990, pp. 3–13).

Neurochemistry also ebbs and surges in the developing nervous system of the infant and child. Thus dopamine levels appear to be at their peak in the cortex around the seventh year of life. At the same age, levels of dopamine beta hydroxylase, the enzyme that turns dopamine into norepinephrine, another neurotransmitter, are low. However, enzyme levels increase tenfold by the second decade of life, and this probably effects levels of both dopamine and norepinephrine (Lewis & Volkmar, 1990). Accordingly, neurotransmitters, including those implicated in schizophrenia, are organized into developmental phases and sequences. These phases and sequences probably build and recede well into adolescence, just the time when psychotic symptoms are first experienced.

Hence, neural development is not a simple process of rapid cell growth in the womb and early period of childhood. It is a dynamic process, and cell death as well as cell growth is essential to neural maturation. The nervous system has been likened to a sculpture whereby material is added and removed selectively and in staggered phases to build a complex structure. This complexity can be seen in the brain's varied and specialized regions, regions that in concert regulate the body's functions and, in ways not yet understood, produce mental life and mental illness.

Unfortunately, it is hard to tie the phases of neural growth precisely to behavior and to psychological development. There is a close correspondence between maturation of the sensory and motor systems in the brain and basic motor skills like crawling and walking during infancy. The same period corresponds roughly to the sensorimotor stage of cognitive development. Here the young child is concerned with exploring, manipulating, and forming mental representations of the environment (Case, 1985; Kolb & Whishaw, 1996, p. 499). Similarly, the development of "object permanence" occurs at about the same time that metabolic activity increases in the prefrontal cortex (Goodman,

1994, pp. 49–78). Object permanence means that mental images of objects in the environment become more durable and no longer vanish from the child's mind following shifts in attention. However, such biology–behavior correspondences are not always present, and there is no clear lock-step relation between mental and neural growth.

Similarly, understanding how a damaged or arrested nervous system effects psychological maturation is a challenge. It is known from primate studies, for example, that early brain lesions do not always have an immediate impact on behavior. The impact may not occur until much later if the damaged brain system is not essential for immediately emergent behaviors. The early lesion may only cause a deficit when the effected brain system comes "on-line" in the course of normal growth. Suddenly the damaged system is needed to support a new cognitive or behavioral skill, and it fails. Alternatively, a seemingly dormant lesion may, in the course of maturation, be "unmasked" by normal events like myelination or by the reduction of synapses. Thus behavioral defects are sometimes postponed until adolescence or adulthood even though the key neurological defect occurred much earlier (Goodman, 1994, pp. 64–65).

Could something akin to a "sleeper effect" or "dormant" lesion account for the fact that schizophrenic symptoms emerge so much later than any possible insult to the brain during gestation or early life? Perhaps the onset of illness signals the crossing of a fateful threshold, the culmination of many years and many interactions between inherited vulnerabilities and the stresses and strains of early adulthood (Gottesman & Shields, 1982). People are not suddenly struck with madness; it is a gradual descent, or perhaps a final collapse, after flagging resilience, as one of life's many obstacle courses takes its toll.

Neurodevelopmental Evidence and Schizophrenia

Suppose that some kind of pathology occurs early in the growth of the brain and then stops occurring, also early in development (Breslin & Weinberger, 1991). This pathology then interacts and interferes with subsequent maturational or environmental events to cause schizophrenia. The mechanisms that cause the pathology in the first place may be genetic, environmental, or both. But whatever the original cause, there should be evidence of the pathology. Neurological abnormalities of some kind should be detectable very early in the lives of people who go on to develop schizophrenia. And the evidence for these abnormalities should be behavioral as well as biological in nature. This is the neurodevelopmental hypothesis of schizophrenia. But is it true?

There are indeed a large number of indirect findings that support the idea that the brain disorder in schizophrenia is an early, even prenatal, life event. For example, the hippocampal abnormalities seen in some schizophrenia patients may reflect second-trimester insults (see chapter 5). The hippocampus is most vulnerable to selective damage during this period. Such glimmers of evidence are suggestive. However, much more direct evidence of prenatal and perinatal abnormalities is required to provide a really compelling neurodevelopmental explanation for schizophrenia.

If it were possible to design an ideal study to find what is wrong in the early brain that leads to madness, it would mean monitoring the biological growth of a preschizophrenic fetus from conception through childhood to symptom and illness onset. This ideal study would observe microscopic neural processes and compare the data with information from healthy children and adolescents. It would be possible to see when and where a pathological deviation occurs. In practice, however, most studies have to make inferences about the growth of neural systems with evidence that is several steps removed from ideal conditions. Detailed knowledge of human developmental biology is usually obtained from post-mortem studies of fetuses, infants, and children who died prematurely through disease or accident. Post-mortem tissue analysis offers the best opportunity to examine neuroanatomy at the microscopic level of observation. However, there is no way of knowing if brain specimens obtained post mortem come from infants or children who were on the road to schizophrenia. Opportunities to examine directly the immature preschizophrenic brain are almost nonexistent. Yet researchers have found a way of looking for clues about how brain growth goes wrong prior to the illness.

Inferring Developmental Disturbances from Post-Mortem Brain Tissue

It is perhaps ironic that the best available method for studying the roots of schizophrenia in the beginnings of life involves brain tissue from deceased older people and adult patients and not from infants or children. Nonetheless, very early disturbances in development leave enduring marks in the brain, and these marks can be observed with post-mortem analysis of adult tissue. For example, cytoarchitectural anomalies—alterations in the arrangement of cells within biological tissue—may point to abnormal patterns of cell migration during development (Arnold & Trojanowski, 1996; Bunney, Potkin, & Bunney, 1997; Cannon, 1996; Chua & Murray, 1996; Stefan & Murray, 1997). The density of neurons in different cortical layers, along with their position, orientation, arrangement, and distribution, are all aspects of cytoarchitecure that can be studied with post-mortem techniques. High densities of neurons in "deep" cortical layers adjacent to white matter may indicate that cell migration stopped prematurely. The spatial orientation or misalignment of neurons in their columns may also suggest that migration was unsuccessful, even if cell densities are normal. These two possibilities are illustrated in figure 7.1.

Normal cytoarchitecture   Abnormal cytoarchitecture

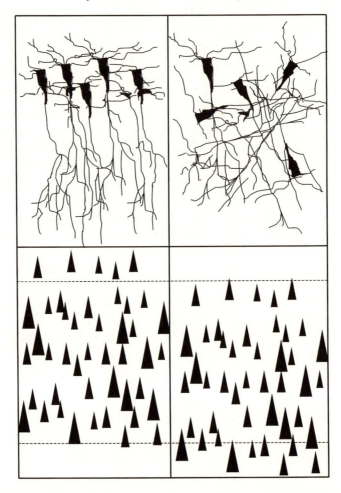

Figure 7.1. Cytoarchitecture and neural development. The upper diagram shows examples of normal and abnormal pyramidal cell orientation in the hippocampus. (After Kolb & Whishaw, 1996, p. 599). The lower diagram is a schematic representation of stained neurons and the "downward-shift" phenomenon. Premature arrest of cell migration during development may underlie the high frequency of cells in lower regions close to white matter and their relative paucity near the cortical surface. (After Arnold & Trojanowski, 1996, p. 227). Both cell disorientation and maldistribution may occur in the presence of normal cell counts and densities and in the absence of scar tissue (gliosis). Microscopic cytoarchitecture can only be observed in detail with post-mortem tissue analysis and may be complicated by exposure to antipsychotic medication during life.

Table 7.2 Neurodevelopmental abnormalities in schizophrenia

Finding	Mean d	Confidence Interval	N
Neurobiological abnormalities			
Hippocampal cell disarray and disorientation	.90	0–1.80	8
Hippocampal cell size reduction	.36	−.08–.80	4
Prefrontal cell decrease in upper layers	1.12	.25–1.99	6
Prefrontal cell increase in lower layers	.87	.24–1.50	10
Birth-related influences on schizophrenia			
Pregnancy and birth complications	.32	.20–.44	15
Maternal exposure to influenza	.02	0–.04	4
Excess winter births	.05	.02–.08	17
Behavior in high-risk and pre-illness populations			
Motor abnormalities	1.35	−.95–3.65	5
Intellectual deficit	.26	.07–.45	6
Attention deficit	.85	−.35–2.05	9
Language deficit	.68	.27–1.09	4
Learning and memory deficit	3.23	−1.98–8.44	2
Social and emotional withdrawal	.37	.14–.60	15
Behavior problems	.42	.15–.69	13
Parenting, family, and life experiences	.33	.13–.53	8

Note: The table shows effect sizes (Cohen's d) as absolute values, corrected for sample size and averaged across studies in a research literature. Confidence Interval is the 95% confidence interval for the averaged d. The true population average probably falls in the range indicated. Intervals that include zero represent unstable literatures where the true effect may be negligible. N = the number of studies contributing to the meta-analysis.

Now consider the evidence for cytoarchitectural abnormalities in schizophrenia. My students and I searched the literature and found a variety of studies that examine different aspects of cytoarchitecture in normal and schizophrenic brain tissue (table 7.2). The schizophrenic tissue samples were generally obtained from patients who had been exposed to antipsychotic medication during life. There were eight studies reporting data on cell disarray and disorientation in the hippocampus. Abnormal cell positions in the neuropil—the mass of axons, dendrites, and embedded cell bodies—are possible signs of defects in brain maturation. Thus Kovelman and Scheibel (1984) studied pyramidal cells in the anterior and middle hippocampal regions. They defined disorientation as cells rotated 35 degrees or more from a reference axis. As in most post-mortem studies, the sample size was small, only 10 patient and 8 control brains. However, the effect size, averaged across sectors, is large (d = 1.56), with an implied schizophrenia–control overlap of only about 28%. Hence a substantial majority of the schizophrenia brain samples showed abnormal cell orientation. However, most of the other studies found much smaller differences or no differences at all between patient and control tissue. Christison, Casanova, Weinberger, Rawlings, and Kleinman (1989) measured orientation in the CA1 sector of the hippocampus and found no statistically significant patient–control differences. Because no descriptive statistics were reported, only the lack of significance, I set the effect size at zero. This study is unusual in that it employed fairly large sample sizes, with 17 schizophrenic and 32 control brains. However, the researchers included tissue from patients who had undergone brain surgery during life, and it is doubtful whether all would have met standard diagnostic criteria for schizophrenia. Two more recent studies differ dramatically from each other in their estimates of hippocampal cell disorientation in schizophrenia. Jonsson, Luts, Guldberg-Kjaer, and Brun (1997) studied the average deviation from the perpendicular in 100 pyramidal cells in three sectors of the hippocampus. These researchers obtained a very large effect size ($d = 4.25$), suggestive of complete separation of patient and control samples. However, this impressive result was based on only four cases, and these were all "treatment refractory" patients who did not respond well to antipsychotic medication during life. Perhaps they were an atypical group. In any case, Zaidel, Esiri, and Harrison (1997) obtained no significant differences between patient and control tissue samples in their much larger set of 14 patient and 17 control brains.

The average effect size across studies for disorientation of hippocampal neurons is substantial at $d = .90$. However, the margin of error, or 95% confidence interval, is equally large, reflecting the great variability in the magnitude of findings. Further caution is in order, because investigators often report results on different parts of the hippocampus. It cannot be assumed that the cytoarchitecture of different sectors is exactly the same. Moreover, the reliance on tissue samples from patients who were exposed to antipsychotic medication during life almost always creates problems. For example, Benes, Sorensen, and Bird (1991) report a strong relationship between medication dosage during life and altered cell orientation at the time of post-mortem study. Such relationships seriously undermine the confidence that can be placed in post-mortem findings.

It is conceivable that, apart from their orientation, the size or shape of hippocampal neurons reflects a developmental abnormality. However, the four studies that report results on neuronal size are split between effects that approximate zero and those that report moderate or large effects. The study by Zaidel et al. described earlier (1997) reports a large effect ($d = -1.13$) for reduced neuronal size in schizophrenia, despite no findings for neuronal orientation. This effect size corresponds roughly to 44% patient–control overlap and reflects an average across two sectors of the left and one sector of the right hippocampus. Yet in some ways the study by Arnold et al. (1995) is more informative because it reports results for each sector of the hippocampus. This second study yields a very modest effect ($d = -.49$) whereby about two-thirds of the patient and control samples of hippocampal tissue are indistinguishable in terms of neuronal size. And the same pattern of variable evidence is apparent in the two reports of cell shape irregularities. Christison et al. (1989) reported no differences between patients and controls. Yet Zaidel, et al. (1997) again found a large difference ($d = 1.13$), showing abnormal cell shape in the CA1 and CA3 sectors of the schizophrenic hippocampus.

Overall, it is only the research on cell orientation that permits any kind of real evaluation. There is great inconsistency in the findings, and this inconsistency may reflect reporting and technical differences between studies. It could also reflect the existence of subgroups of patients with and without disturbed neuronal migration patterns.

However, these results only reflect the state of the hippocampus in the schizophrenic brain. Perhaps studies of cytoarchitecture in the frontal system provide evidence of a more homogenous defect in neural development. The postmortem literature on the prefrontal cortex has focused on the distribution patterns of neurons instead of on their spatial orientation and columnar organization. The idea here is that if neuronal migration is arrested early, there will be fewer neurons in upper cortical layers, their final destination, and more neurons in lower layers, close to white matter (see figure 7.1). White matter, comprising connective fibers rather than cell bodies, is the descendant or remnant of the embryonic subplate where prenatal nervous system growth began.

A variety of different cell populations have been investigated with a focus on finding evidence that upper cortical layers are abnormally low, and deep layers close to white matter are abnormally high in cell numbers. This hypothesis of a "downward shift" in neuron distribution is quite different from traditional expectations in neuropathology, where the goal is often to find net losses in neuron numbers. Yet it must be said that there is occasional evidence for conventional neuropathology in schizophrenia. Thus Benes, Davidson, and Bird (1986) reported net reductions of large pyramidal neurons, the most common cells in the cortex, in both superficial and deep layers of prefrontal cortex. This is *not* what a hypothesis that posits arrested cell migration would predict. There should be relative deficits of neuron numbers in superficial layers and relative excesses in the deep layers. Benes et al. (1986) also measured glial cell numbers and concluded that the ratio of glia to neurons did not support degenerative adult-onset brain damage as an explanation for their findings. Still, the neuronal distribution pattern did not fit the expected "downward shift" needed for a developmental explanation.

On the other hand, more recently Benes, McSparren, et al. (1991) have reported findings conducive to the neurodevelopmental hypothesis of schizophrenia. Thus pyramidal neurons occur more frequently in a "lower" layer (V) of the schizophrenic cortex than in the same layer of normal cortex ($d = .64$). Moreover, small connecting interneurons appear to be remarkably scarce in layer II, a "higher" region of schizophrenic prefrontal cortex ($d = -3.01$). Benes, McSparren, et al. (1991) also found an overall trend for greater neuron densities close to white matter—exactly what a failed migration hypothesis would predict. Unfortunately, this study is beset with shortcomings. Most of the layer comparisons are not statistically significant; the values are presented in graphs, making it hard to obtain accurate effect sizes; and several aspects of the neurobiology vary with study features like sample age and the length of time between death and tissue fixation.

Akbarian et al. (1993, 1996) focused on a special cell population and also found the pattern of superficial deficit–deep layer excess that a developmental account requires. The NADPH-d (nicotinamide-adenine dinucleotide phosphate-diaphorase) cell is much less numerous than pyramidal cells in the prefrontal cortex. However, the NADPH-d cells play an important role in establishing connections between neurons. Moreover, these special cells are resistant to a variety of acute and degenerative events that occur in adult life. This resistance means that NADPH-d numbers probably reflect developmental events more than they reflect adult-onset pathology. If these cells are abnormal, the abnormality probably has very early origins. In the first report, NADPH-d neuron numbers were reduced in upper ($d = -1.07$) and increased in lower cortical layers ($d = .75$), and this held up to some degree in the second report, which was based on more patients. Unfortunately, the effect sizes are estimates based on graphs because the articles do not report statistics. Nevertheless, the same research group went on to report large excesses of neuron numbers in compartments of white matter. Excesses were found for two other interstitial cell types, the MAP2 ($d = 2.04$) and the SMI-32 ($d = 1.94$) types. These findings are based on cell counts in white matter far from the cortical surface. The presence of "deep" excesses in cell numbers could reflect either abnormal migration of neurons or failed "pruning," whereby unneeded cells are eliminated in the course of maturation. These interstitial cells may have survived the elimination process and remained and functioned where they did not belong.

In a different line of work, Kalus, Senitz, and Beckmann (1997) examined the density of Cajal-Retzius cells (CRCs) in the uppermost layer (I) of the prefrontal cortex. The CRC population is interesting because it is the main type of neuron in this layer of cortex during the prenatal period. The Cajal-Retzius cell type establishes synapses with migrating neurons and plays an important role in the growth of other cortical layers. Moreover, during the second half of pregnancy, CRCs decrease in number, and very few remain in the top layer of the normal adult cortex. Hence, unusual densities of CRCs within layer I could signal altered neuronal migration patterns. Kalus et al. (1997) found that CRCs were much denser ($d = 2.28$) in the lower region of layer I in schizophrenia than in control samples and less dense in the upper region ($d = -2.07$). This kind of distribution difference also suggests a very early deviation from normal neurodevelopment in schizophrenia.

When generic counts are made of all cells in upper and lower layers of cortex, the results are less supportive of a "downward shift" hypothesis or early migratory arrest in the schizophrenic brain. Thus Rajkowska, Selemon, and Goldman-Rakic (1998) looked at layer II of a circumscribed area of the prefrontal cortex and found virtually no difference between schizophrenic and control cell densities ($d = .02$). The deepest cortical layer showed a modest excess in the patient samples ($d = .57$). The same group (Selemon, Rajkowska, & Goldman-Rakic, 1998) also reported on another small region of prefrontal cortex and found a moderate deficit ($d = -.47$) of cells in the uppermost cortical layer of the schizophrenia sample. However, the deepest layer showed a much larger deficit ($d = -1.34$) instead of the excess that the "downward shift" idea predicts. This kind of finding of overall cell deficit fits with arguments for conventional neuropathology in schizophrenia and contradicts the idea of an early arrest in neural development.

In general, it is hard to characterize the results of the post-mortem studies on the prefrontal cortex. The most promising findings seem to stem from work on specific cell populations. However, researchers do not always report data from both upper and lower layers when they look at these special cells. Nonetheless, the average effect size for upper cortical cell loss is $d = 1.12$, and for deep or white matter cell excess it is $d = .87$. These are moderately large effects, suggesting that at least half of the schizophrenic tissue samples have anomalous cell distributions. Unfortunately, the findings are also extremely variable between studies, and this results in large margins of error (.87, .63) for the average effect sizes (see table 7.2).

If the post-mortem studies from both hippocampus and frontal cortex are considered together, it is evident that no findings are large and consistent enough to argue for a single cytoarchitecural anomaly in schizophrenia. Current thinking in the area is considering the role of neurotrophins, which are important determinants of cell survival and migration. Programmed cell death, an essential process as the nervous system is "sculpted" into final form, may not work normally in schizophrenia. And there may be subtle shifts and alterations in cortical "wiring" in the frontal lobe. All of these processes might figure in a brain that harbors schizophrenia (see Bunney et al., 1997; Harrison, 1999; Selemon & Goldman-Rakic, 1999). However, no neurological "smoking gun" has been found so far, and post-mortem samples are hard to gather and tend to be small in size. Therefore, less biologically direct means of assessing the developing brain and mind must also be considered. If the developmental brain defect itself is elusive, perhaps its causes and circumstances can be found. Perhaps infections or environmental insults are early events that lay the biological groundwork for faulty neural development and eventual schizophrenia.

A Schizophrenogenic Virus from the Environment?

Consider the possibility that some of the events that cause schizophrenia are external. Part of the answer to understanding the illness may lie outside the brain in the biological environment that surrounds the fetus, infant, and child. An example of research in this area concerns health factors during pregnancy and birth in mothers who have children that develop schizophrenia as adults (see table 7.2). Of particular interest are studies examining specific environmental agents like viruses and whether maternal exposure to such agents associates with an increased risk of schizophrenia in the offspring.

In the fall of 1957 the city of Helsinki, Finland, suffered an epidemic of influenza. Mednick, Machon, Huttunen, and Bonnett (1988) proceeded to study and monitor children born during or shortly after this time. The question was asked whether these children would develop schizophrenia at an abnormally high frequency. Indeed, an abnormally high rate of the illness was observed in children of mothers who had been in the Helsinki area during the epidemic. The increased incidence of schizophrenia did not appear to be part of a broad increase in mental health problems at this time but seemed specific to schizophrenic illness. Could it be that an agent like the influenza virus enters the mother during her pregnancy and then enters the fetus to wreak subtle havoc in the nervous system, the kind of havoc that increases the likelihood of psychosis?

In searching the literature on this topic, my students and I found that the number of useful articles is quite small. A useful article is one that compares the rates of schizophrenia in offspring of mothers who were exposed to the virus with rates in offspring of mothers without exposure. It also makes sense to compare the maternal health records of schizophrenia patients with the records of healthy people. However, such research designs are few and far between. Often there is no healthy comparison group at all, and there is a frequent lack of basic statistics like sample sizes and standard deviations that are needed to compute effect sizes. Most studies simply show that schizophrenia births increase slightly over base rates when diseases like influenza are rampant in the population (e.g., Kendell & Kemp, 1989; Takei et al., 1994). Many studies do not provide information on whether mothers were actually exposed to the virus, only that their children were born in a year when influenza was prevalent in the population.

I was left with just four well-designed studies to consider. However, they provide a consistent indication that a mother's exposure to influenza barely figures in the incidence of schizophrenia in her children. Thus Susser, Lin, Brown, Lumey, and Erlenmeyer-Kimling (1994) studied birth cohorts in the Netherlands and compared the risk of schizophrenia among children of mothers exposed and not exposed to influenza. The effect size for increased risk and exposure was $d = .06$. Sacker, Done, Crow, and Golding (1995) studied British mothers and children and found an effect size of only $d = -.02$. Moreover, this result was for influenza exposure and *lower* rates of schizophrenia in the offspring. Cannon et al. (1996) followed up on their Finnish study and also obtained results that yield an effect size close to zero ($d = .02$). And Selten et al. (1999) reported an effect size of zero for influenza exposure in their Dutch sample. With such consistent and negligible findings, the argument that the influenza virus is a culprit in the environmental story of schizophrenia seems indefensible.

Nonetheless, exposure to viral and other infections has also been invoked to explain one of the earliest epidemiological findings in schizophrenia, the relation between the season of the year during which a child is born and the child's subsequent risk of developing the illness. As early as the studies of Tramer (1929) and Huntington (1938), it was noted that more schizophrenia patients than healthy people were born in late winter months. To evaluate this line of thinking, we searched for studies and found 17 articles that allowed for comparisons of winter birth rates in schizophrenic and healthy people. The results consistently approach a zero effect. The average effect size for winter births and schizophrenia is $d = .05$, and almost all of the studies had effect sizes below $d = .1$. There is simply no compelling evidence for the "seasonality" effect in schizophrenia. And there is too little heterogeneity in the findings to argue for the existence of a subset of children with increased risk for illness due to winter births.

One indirectly related study is worth mentioning. Rantakallio, Jones, Moring, and Von Wendt (1997) looked at the association between infections in Finnish children and adolescents and subsequent schizophrenia. They considered a variety of central nervous system infections, not just influenza viruses, and obtained an effect size of $d = .25$ in support of the hypothesized association. Although this is a small effect, it suggests that infectious agents may have a role to play in some cases of schizophrenia. However, it appears to be the child and not the developing fetus that is vulnerable to infections that raise the risk of psychotic illness.

Even proponents of viral hypotheses for schizophrenia, like Torrey, Bowler, Rawlings, and Terrazas (1993), suggest that any viral contribution to illness must occur in conjunction with other biological influences. These influences include genetic predisposition, immune system factors in the fetus during viral exposure, and the nature of the viral strain itself, as well as the severity, site, and timing of infection during gestation. On reflection, the specifics of any viral hypothesis need to be described and analyzed much more fully. An influenza virus must survive in the mother's circulatory system, cross the placenta into the fetus, and negotiate the blood–brain barrier to disturb the nervous system (Lyon & Barr, 1991). Although some researchers, like Conrad and Scheibel (1987), provide a theoretical basis for such viral actions, empirical support is required and thus far the support is lacking.

Birth Complications and Schizophrenia

Medical and delivery-related problems at birth may be key environmental and biological events that interact with any genetic diathesis and predispose a person to schizophrenia later in life. If this idea is correct, it is reasonable to expect high rates of birth complications in children who go on to develop schizophrenia. Birth complications can be studied by interviewing adult patients and their relatives with respect to obstetrical events and by examining birth and health records, if these are available. To what extent do schizophrenia patients have abnormal births?

Early evidence in this field was reviewed by Parnas et al. (1982), and there were grounds for a link between complications like premature delivery or extended labor and eventual schizophrenia. To assess the recent literature, I looked for relevant studies published since 1980 and found 15 articles. These studies vary widely in the way they define and measure obstetrical complications. Thus length of labor, breech delivery, term, low birth weight, evidence of asphyxia, and fetal distress are all potential obstetrical complications. Some studies combine everything into a single index (Jacobsen & Kinney, 1980). Some focus on one or two specific complications (e.g., perinatal bleeding; see Sacker et al., 1995), and still others report results using scales and composite indices (McNeil, Cantor-Graae, & Sjöstrom, 1994). Given such diversity between studies, it is perhaps surprising to find a considerable degree of consistency in the results. The only exception to consistent findings of increased complications in schizophrenia births is a study by Gunduz, Woerner, Alvir, Degreef, and Lieberman (1999). With an average effect of $d = .32$, there is a modest tendency for schizophrenia to be associated with more frequent birth complications. The average effect size suggests a hypothetical overlap of about 76% between schizophrenia and healthy distributions. Accordingly, there is no reason to believe that obstetrical complications are necessary for the development of schizophrenia. Still, with a confidence interval for the average of only 12 decimal points, this is one of the more consistent findings in the schizophrenia research literature.

A perspective on obstetrical events and schizophrenia can be gained from studies of twins who are concordant or discordant for the illness. Recall that monozygotic twins are siblings with identical genetic endowments, yet one twin may develop schizophrenia while the other remains healthy. Such "discordant" twins provoke an important question. If all genes are shared, what makes both twins develop the illness in some cases and not in others? Perhaps noxious environmental and biological birth events that effect only one of the twins are the missing ingredient. Pregnancy and birth complications might cause subtle neurological damage and compound the genetic liability that already exists. Perhaps the twin who sustains the most complications is also the twin who develops schizophrenia by the time adolescence arrives.

Unfortunately, the evidence does not support any special role for pregnancy and birth complications in the etiology of schizophrenia. Torrey, Bowler, Taylor, and Gottesman (1994), in an important study, found that obstetrical problems are about equally frequent in healthy and ill monozygotic twins. To be sure, all twin pairs with at least one psychotic sibling had more birth problems than did completely healthy twin pairs. But some of the twins of schizophrenia patients experienced obstetrical problems and still remained free of illness. Hence the evidence argues against any simple notion that biological and environmental insult compounds a genetic diathesis to cause schizophrenia. Pregnancy and birth complications probably make the illness slightly more likely, and that is about all that can be said.

Abnormalities of Children Vulnerable to Schizophrenia

It is difficult to observe brain development directly in the fetus, infant, and child who go on to suffer from schizophrenia. This difficulty reflects the technological limitations of brain imaging, as well as the challenge of identifying pre-schizophrenic children. However, behavior provides another valuable kind of information in the search for the developmental secrets of schizophrenia. After all, mental and behavioral change reflects the growing nervous system in action. Perhaps children with a genetic liability for schizophrenia differ from normal children in terms of evolving competencies and abilities. The life histories of adult schizophrenia patients may reveal evidence that the illness effected psychological life before symptoms actually struck. Researchers like Fish (1975, 1977; Fish, Marcus, Hans, Auerbach, & Perdue, 1992) have argued for the existence of neurointegrative defects in children who go on to develop schizophrenia. If such defects exist, they should be observable in the basic motor and neurobehavioral features of children who are vulnerable to the illness (table 7.2).

Motor Abnormalities in Children and Adolescents at Risk for Schizophrenia

If genetics are a key factor in raising the likelihood of schizophrenia, do children with schizophrenic relatives show defects in movement and motor development early in life, defects that presage the illness? This seems a straightforward question, but the small number of relevant studies suggests that it is hard to answer. I found an assortment of high-risk research reports, but some of these examined adult relatives of schizophrenia patients rather than children. Five studies were more to the point and considered both older children and adolescents or studied genuinely "preschizophrenic" children. Thus Schreiber, Stolz-Born, Heinrich, Kornhuber, and Born (1992) compared high-risk and control children on a motor task that is sensitive to the erroneous repetition of movements. This comparison yielded a moderate effect of $d = .66$. Yet it was the high-risk children and not the normal children who had the fewest errors. In contrast, Marcus, Hans, Mednick, Schulsinger, and Michelsen (1985) reported data on Israeli adolescents' motor coordination and found that children of schizophrenic parents displayed a slight disadvantage when compared to normal children ($d = -.34$). The same research group replicated this finding in a mixed sample of Israeli and Danish adolescents with an effect size of $d = -.35$. But these studies beg the question: Are the children with motor defects the children who grow up to suffer from schizophrenia?

The best way to answer this question would be to roll back time and look for behavioral evidence of brain dysfunction in the childhood histories of diagnosed schizophrenia patients. This kind of strategy is usually undermined by the insecurity of knowledge obtained from retrospective interviews. However, Walker and associates (Walker, Davis, & Gottlieb, 1991; Walker, Grimes, Davis, & Smith, 1993; Walker, Savoie, & Davis, 1994) provide a fascinating approximation to an ideal "follow-back" method with their "archival-observational" studies. These researchers collected and analyzed old home movies that showed the everyday behavior of infants and children. Some of these children grew up to develop psychiatric disorders. Thus home movies were obtained from a schizophrenia sample, a mood disorder sample, and a mentally healthy comparison group. In many cases the movies began as early as the first months of life and continued into adolescence. Some of the children showed behavioral abnormalities in the film clips, and trained observers could identify children who were "preschizophrenic" about 78% of the time. Moreover, Walker et al. (1994) reported data on the prevalence of motor abnormalities like abnormal posture, strange facial movements, and tremors in their preschizophrenic and normal siblings. The combined effect size is $d = .26$ for the study's two measures of motor dysfunction. This is a very modest finding, suggesting that perhaps only 20% of preschizophrenic children have abnormal motor abilities.

However, the jury is still out on this question of early motor defects. Erlenmeyer-Kimling et al. (1998) report much stronger and more encouraging findings from a group of 51 high-risk children who have now entered adulthood. A small number (10) of these grown children of a schizophrenic parent have been diagnosed with schizophrenia or a closely related psychosis. Motor tests carried out previously during childhood and adolescence show that the same 10 children were severely impaired relative to the normal group. The effect size ($d = 6.48$) is large enough to separate completely the motor performance of preschizophrenic and healthy children. It is puzzling why the finding is so much stronger than the results obtained by Walker et al. (1994). Nevertheless, it is one of the most powerful single findings in the schizophrenia literature. If both the result and strength of Erlenmeyer-Kimling et al. (1998) are reproduced, researchers will have confirmation that schizophrenia first shows itself not in delusions or hallucinations but in the movements of children.

Cognitive Abnormalities in Children and
Adolescents at Risk for Schizophrenia

In some ways movement, posture, and manual dexterity are the most observable reflections of a developing nervous system. However, cognitive functions, including intelligence, attention, and learning and language skills are equally dependent on the brain. As a case in point, consider James, the man who became convinced that a parasite had entered his brain and was controlling him. Long before he developed schizophrenia, James showed cognitive and learning problems. These were sufficient to slow his schooling and lead to a diagnosis of learning disability.

How prevalent are such problems in children who harbor the schizophrenia diathesis? My students and I found six studies that report intelligence data in high-risk children who ranged in age from birth to midadolescence. The average effect size is $d = -.26$, indicating a small intellectual disadvantage in children and adolescents who had at least one schizophrenic parent. However, one study (Schreiber et al., 1991) found the opposite—a slight intellectual advantage for the high-risk children. More important, a recent and extensive Israeli study of 9,724 army draftees and their adolescent health records found only a trivial ($d = -.12$) intellectual deficit in those who went on to develop schizophrenia (Davidson et al., 1999).

Studies of attention, employing primarily variations of the Continuous Performance Test and dichotic listening tasks, also reveal small (Friedman, Cornblatt, Vaughn, & Erlenmeyer-Kimling, 1986) or contradictory (Hallett, Quinn, & Hewitt, 1986) findings. The noteworthy exception to this in nine published studies is Cornblatt, Lenzenweger, Dworkin, and Erlenmeyer-Kimling's (1992), which yielded an effect size ($d = -5.82$) large enough to indicate attention deficit in all of the study's high-risk 10-year-old children. Unfortunately, the effect size had to be derived by estimating values from graphs. Still, if such a large effect could be reproduced, convincing evidence would be at hand that the faulty nervous system of schizophrenia shows itself in problems of attention. Yet no other research group using any measure of attention has managed to approximate such a large effect size. In fact, the other studies suggest only small or modest differences between high-risk and normal children. Indeed, the weakness of attention deficit as a characteristic of preschizophrenic children is exemplified by recent data from the study by Erlenmeyer-Kimling et al. (1998). This study differs from most in reporting results on high-risk children who actually developed the illness. The small effect size ($d = -.25$) for attention suggests that the vast majority of healthy and preschizophrenic children do not differ from each other in terms of attention-related performance. Therefore, it is likely that the finding of Cornblatt et al. (1992) is a chance aberration.

A handful of studies examining language functions in high-risk children and adolescents also reveals one large effect ($d = -1.4$; Hallett & Green, 1983) amid generally small findings. And the disparity between studies is even larger in the two articles reporting memory-related results. An older study by Klein and Salzman (1981) found essentially no differences in learning skill between high-risk and normal children at two age periods. However, the recent publication by Erlenmeyer-Kimling et al. (1998) reports a very large effect size ($d = -9.72$) for verbal working memory deficits. These deficits occurred in the 10 children who were followed into adulthood and received a diagnosis of schizophrenia. Working memory involves the ability to keep information in mind while manipulating or using it in some way. The extremely large deficit in these pre-illness children is impressive and awaits the acid tests of replication and larger samples that always challenge exciting findings in schizophrenia research.

Social and Emotional Behavior in Children and Adolescents at Risk for Schizophrenia

James, who had learning problems in childhood, was emotionally withdrawn and unresponsive to affection according to his mother. Moreover, William engaged in antisocial behavior and was a member of a gang that ran afoul of the police by the time he was 12 years old. Could it be that the neurological dysfunction underlying schizophrenia manifests itself in the emotional and social behavior of children and adolescents?

I have cast the available evidence into two categories. First, there are studies of emotional withdrawal and social isolation in normal and high-risk children; second, there are studies of antisocial behavior and aggression. Consider the evidence for emotional withdrawal in these vulnerable children. Several studies indicate more withdrawn and isolated behavior in the offspring of schizophrenic parents than in normal children. The average effect is $d = .37$ for the 15 published studies that were found. This suggests a mild overall tendency—and perhaps 75% group overlap—for withdrawn behavior in high-risk children. However, there are exceptions, and some of the studies have special features that should be mentioned. Naslund, Persson-Blennow, McNeil, Kaij, and Malmquist-Larsson (1984) studied fear of strangers and found that infants at risk for schizophrenia were *less* fearful than normal infants. Yet perhaps distress in response to an unfamiliar face is a normal reaction during infancy. Therefore, its absence in high-risk children makes sense if fear of strangers is part of normal social development (Lewis & Volkmar, 1990, pp. 70–73). Several other studies are also of interest because the researchers had access to adult outcomes for their high-risk children. Thus Done, Crow, Johnstone, and Sacker (1994) studied teachers' ratings of social adjustment in children at the ages of 7 and 11. Some of the children eventually developed schizophrenia, and their social adjustment was compared retrospectively with the normal children. The pre-schizophrenia group was more "underreactive" socially than the normal group. However, with an effect size of this magnitude ($d = .47$), about 70% of the preschizophrenic and normal children remain indistinguishable from each other in terms of social adjustment. Cannon et al. (1997) used a less objective but still valuable approach. Mothers of schizophrenia patients retrospectively rated their children's social functioning by recalling behavior prior to the illness. Here there was a substantial effect ($d = -1.01$), indicating that the preschizophrenic children were deficient in social behavior. But Davidson et al. (1999), an important study of pre-illness adolescent health records, yields a small effect ($d = .38$) for similar behavior. Finally, Walker, Baum, and Diforio (1998) provide an unusual report on withdrawal in adolescents with schizotypal personality disorder. These adolescents, rather than the children of patients, represented the high-risk group in this case. And indeed, when compared with normal adolescents, the schizotypal group was rated as withdrawn, anxious, and depressed ($d = .82$).

Against the trend for increased withdrawal and isolation in children and adolescents at risk for schizophrenia, a few studies report only very small and even contradictory findings. Thus Dworkin et al. (1993), Weintraub (1987), Bagedahl-Strindlund, Rosencrantz-Larsson, and Wilkner-Svanfeldt (1989), and Bergman and Walker (1995) all failed to find evidence in support of the idea that children and adolescents at risk for schizophrenia are abnormally withdrawn and isolated.

Yet withdrawal and lack of social response are limited aspects of emotional behavior. Some children, including William, who felt connected to Christ, engage in antisocial and criminal behavior by the time they enter adolescence. The 13 studies in this second category of social behavior show that there is a moderate tendency (average $d = .42$) for high-risk children to have abnormally frequent behavior problems. A couple of studies report large effects (e.g., Amminger et al., 1999). But a few studies also show that children at risk for schizophrenia have slightly *fewer* behavior problems than normal children (e.g. Bergman, Wolfson, & Walker, 1997; Weintraub, 1987).

It is always difficult to interpret small and medium effect sizes in studies of high-risk children, because those who actually develop schizophrenia are in the minority. The true pre-illness children may or may not show the abnormality or deficit in question. It is hard to tell whether these children or others in the high-risk sample are the source of the statistical result. And there is no way of clarifying this uncertainty without an adult diagnosis of schizophrenia. On the other hand, diagnostic uncertainty does not afflict Done et al. (1994), a study of behavior problems in "true" preschizophrenia children ($d = .79$). Moreover, the use by Walker et al. (1998) of schizotypal adolescents as the high-risk group also yielded a large d (1.36) for disturbed behavior. Studies like these will keep the idea of abnormal childhood emotional functioning in schizophrenia alive, despite the weakness and variability of most findings in high-risk populations.

Drawing conclusions from the high-risk literature as a whole is a challenge. Neurobehavioral and social measurements obtained on these children may reflect to some degree the influence of a genetic liability for schizophrenia. Some children with this liability show a variety of psychological problems early in life, but most show normal psychological development. Solid replicated evidence that behavioral abnormalities precede schizophrenia in even a consistent minority of these children is still lacking.

In some ways it is hard to escape the conclusion that too much attention has been paid to finding abnormalities in the children themselves. Perhaps not enough attention has been paid to finding abnormalities in the environment, especially in the psychological environment. After all, most versions of the diathesis-stress model hold that a genetic or acquired central nervous system defect is not sufficient to cause schizophrenia. Therefore, it is important to address the "stress" component of the model. Surely stress must play a role in the illness. Perhaps parenting, family, and life events are crucial if neglected influences on the road to schizophrenia.

Psychological Perspectives on Development

Environmental stresses, including those that are psychological or social in nature, may be necessary before a genetic predisposition or defect in brain maturation manifests itself in psychosis. The first psychological environment for the child comprises relations with parents, usually beginning with the mother and later including father and siblings as well as other caregivers. Under the influence of psychoanalytic thinking, researchers and clinicians have tried to find evidence that schizophrenia results from pathological parenting or from disturbed family life. Thus one early view was that maternal behavior could be "schizophrenogenic," taking the form of intrusiveness and dominance coupled with overprotectiveness and rejection (Fromm-Reichmann, 1948). The support for such a hypothesis was always modest and open to varying interpretations. For example, disturbed parenting behavior might be a result rather than a cause of a child's psychopathology. A mother or father with good intentions might see strange and frightening signs of disturbed behavior emerging in a child and respond poorly, inadequately, to the child's needs. But the parent did not induce the psychopathology in the first place. Are there really grounds for believing that the opposite is true and that parenting itself might be a causal factor in schizophrenia?

An old literature has shown only small differences in childhood parenting and family experiences in healthy people compared with schizophrenia patients. For example, Schofield and Balian (1959) found that about 65% of their schizophrenia sample reported receiving affection from their mothers during childhood. This proportion was somewhat lower than what the control sample experienced (81.3%). Yet it is hard to assign a causal role to inadequate affection on the basis of such results. In some instances, involving reports of rejection experiences, the same researchers found almost identical rates in healthy and ill people (i.e., 6.0 vs. 6.2%). Still other comparisons revealed disparities between the groups, but the overall prevalence of the abnormal parenting behavior was still low. Thus memories of "domination" occurred more frequently in patients with schizophrenia (10.9%) than in healthy people (.7%). But the vast majority (almost 90%) of patients did not report such memories.

At the same time that research on maternal behavior was being conducted, interest shifted to the entire family as a source of inconsistent or contradictory communication patterns. It was felt that such patterns might mediate the development of schizophrenia (Bateson, Jackson, Haley, & Weakland, 1956; Jacob, 1986). This research was weakened by the inaccuracies inherent in asking people to remember their childhood experiences and also by the modest findings. Studies of adopted children further undermined the importance assigned to early social factors and their role in the illness. Having a psychotic adoptive parent does not in itself induce later psychosis in an otherwise healthy child (Gottesman, 1991, pp. 146–147; Wender, Rosenthal, Kety, Schulsinger, & Welner, 1974). Still, the idea that specific kinds of parenting behavior or family interactions influence the development of illness does not depend on parents being schizophrenic themselves. Therefore, it makes sense to reconsider environmental contributions to schizophrenia, contributions that are psychological in nature, while steering clear of dubious concepts like the schizophrenogenic mother.

I looked for recent evidence on links between parenting, family, and life stresses and increased incidence of schizophrenic illness and found a very small number of useful studies. Goldstein's (1985) report is remarkable in showing that disturbed patterns of communication in the family predate the illness in a substantial number of cases. This implies a causal link, although the effect is moderate, with probably less than half of the patients' families actually showing the deviant communication. In addition, the effect ($d = .65$) has not been reproduced. Then there are several studies that look at life events—changes in circumstance and situation that may be stressful to a person. A stressful life event might be something as mundane as a change of address but might also include changes in financial support, work, schooling, and personal relationships. For example, Chung, Langeluddecke, and Tennant (1986) looked specifically at threatening events and found moderate support ($d = .54$) for the idea that such events are prevalent in the month before illness onset. The studies on life events prior to illness are also of interest because they include findings from diverse cultures like Saudi Arabia (Al Khani, Bebbington, Watson, & House, 1986) and Nigeria (Gureje & Adewunmi, 1988) as well as from Britain (Bebbington et al., 1993). Nonetheless, there is no consistent picture here of environmental stress as a precipitant of psychosis. The effect for the Saudi Arabian study is extremely small ($d = .12$), and the Nigerian data actually ($d = -.48$) suggest a somewhat *lower* incidence of life events in the month before schizophrenic illness. The other studies show moderate effect sizes.

Finally, there are three studies that deal with parenting experiences or with memories of these experiences. McCreadie, Williamson, Athawes, Connolly, and Tilak-Singh (1994) report moderate findings ($d = .60 - .73$) in support of the notion that schizophrenia patients remember their parents as being relatively cold emotionally. Skagerlind, Perris, and Eisemann's (1996) report yields small effect sizes ($d = .32 - .35$), indicating a tendency for patients to have childhood memories of rejecting parents. Perhaps most telling is a Finnish study that examined family type and experience in a birth cohort of 11,017 people (Makikyro et al., 1998). Children who went on to receive a diagnosis of schizophrenia as adults hardly differed from those who remained healthy in a variety of experiences, including the death of a parent ($d = .08$), a divorce ($d = .1$), or just growing up in a single-parent family ($d = .1$).

All of this research on the pre-illness psychological experience of schizophrenia patients can be criticized on the grounds that the effect sizes are small or moderate and somewhat inconsistent. Moreover, the studies rely on methods like retrospective interviews and on the perceptions of the patients themselves—methods that may yield distorted results. Yet it is also worth pointing out that the effect sizes themselves are not out of line with what is obtained in many of the more popular areas of schizophrenia research. Given the potential importance of environmental contributions to the onset of the illness, the role of early—and late—psychological experience requires much more attention from researchers.

Summary and Conclusions

How different are children who grow up to develop schizophrenia from children who remain free of the illness? If there is a genetic diathesis for the illness, how does it show itself in the growing nervous system, in the evolving person? If environmental stresses push people who have the diathesis over some terrible threshold, what are these stresses?

The evidence summarized in table 7.2 indicates that some proportion of people with the illness—it is hard to be precise—have cellular abnormalities in prefrontal or hippocampal brain regions. And these abnormalities are the kind that might have originated early in fetal development, perhaps during the second trimester. They do not comprise the usual hallmarks of neuropathology like reduced neuron numbers or the presence of scar tissue. Instead, they comprise unusual neuronal organization and distribution patterns—faults in the microscopic biological architecture of the brain. It is this altered architecture that points the finger at the growing nervous system because the organization and distribution of nerve cells are laid down very early in life. Yet the number of studies that look at the same brain region and at the same cell population is small, and they are based on very small numbers of patients and healthy people. Moreover, technical problems in tissue analysis can lead to erroneous conclusions about what is really "abnormal" in a post-mortem brain. In addition, the effect sizes are not large or consistent enough to suggest the existence of a single uniform anomaly in all schizophrenia cases. There is great variability within and between studies. The most logical conclusion from current evidence is that a subgroup of schizophrenia patients exists and these patients probably have neurobiological abnormalities that stem from prenatal origins.

Yet even if the illness is embedded partly in developmental biology, the question arises of what noxious events or influences precipitate, aggravate, or interact with early central nervous system abnormalities. One class of potential illness-promoting events is pregnancy and birth complications. These complications include everything from premature delivery to length of labor. It is difficult to assess the specific importance of any individual complication because they are usually reported as aggregated totals or frequencies. Still, the average effect size in table 7.2 indicates that a small but consistent minority, perhaps 24%, of schizophrenia patients endured pregnancy and birth complications not seen in the records of people without the illness. It seems likely that these complications contribute in some general and modest way to the risk of schizophrenia in adulthood.

There are other candidates for the role of the environmental influence that pushes the immature nervous system further down the path to schizophrenia. It is conceivable that exposure to a virus during pregnancy raises the probability of giving birth to a child who develops psychosis. This possibility can be measured by examining maternal health records or can be inferred by finding the month of a patient's birth. Viral exposure is implied if the patient's birth was during winter months when, presumably, viruses are prevalent. This is a very tenuous inference, but there are many studies, based on literally millions of cases, that try to address it. In contrast, there are very few good studies of documented maternal infectious exposure and psychiatric outcomes in the offspring. In either case, however, the average effect sizes for well-designed studies are close to zero. It is extremely unlikely that exposure to common viruses like influenza during a mother's pregnancy is an important influence on whether a child goes on to develop schizophrenia in adult life.

Aside from physical insults, what happens to the vulnerable child as he or she endures, resists, or falters in the face of the unknown environmental dangers that promote mental illness? Perhaps it is in the developing mind and in behavior that the early schizophrenic nervous system reveals itself. And perhaps the psychological environment is as important as the physical environment in stressing the child or adolescent who is at risk for the illness.

The question of early behavioral signs of nervous system disorder seems a simple one, but there are many difficulties involved in answering it. The most serious difficulty is the absence of a dependable, accurate way of identifying in advance who will go on to have symptoms of full-blown schizophrenia. Nevertheless, researchers have useful if imperfect ways of identifying children who have a greater than average likelihood of developing the illness. One strategy makes use of the fact that the child of a parent with schizophrenia has at least 10 times the normal risk of developing the disorder. Yet even with a large sample to maximize the number of eventual patients, a researcher may have to wait for 20 years to discover which children actually become ill. To counter this problem, some researchers use the "follow-back" approach, which begins with known schizophrenia patients in adulthood. Developmental histories, archival documents like hospital records, and interviews with living relatives are all employed to find evidence of disturbed mental life and behavior during infancy and childhood. The main disadvantage of the follow-back method is the limited availability and variable accuracy of old records and old memories.

Nonetheless, despite procedural obstacles, evidence has accumulated that the inherited liability for schizophrenia does manifest itself, albeit weakly and variably, in a spectrum of early neurobehavioral abnormalities. A few studies suggest that a proportion of children at risk for schizophrenia show early signs of impaired movement and fine motor skills and have intellectual and language-related limitations not shared by normal children. The average effect sizes for motor and attention-related disturbances in high-risk children seem substantial, suggesting that at least half have difficulty in these areas. However, the average effects in table 7.2 are inflated spuriously by large and anomalous findings. For example, the singularly powerful results of Cornblatt et al. (1992) unduly influence the average effect size. Without the inclusion of this one effect size ($d = 5.82$), the magnitude of the attention average drops to a much more modest value of $d = .23$. Recent work by Erlenmeyer-Kimling et al. (1998) suggests that high-risk children who go on to receive a diagnosis of schizophrenia show only a very mild group deficit in attention. On the other hand, severe deficits in motor skill and working memory may yet prove to be a flag for the presence of a schizophrenic nervous system.

At the same time, it may be a mistake to look for nervous system abnormalities exclusively in the form of cognitive and motor deficits. Social and emotional behavior can also reveal neurodevelopmental problems. Thus some children who are vulnerable to schizophrenia are also more withdrawn, socially reclusive, or antisocial and aggressive than normal children. Here again, this probably applies to a small minority of high-risk children. Moreover, the evidence is both modest and variable, and some studies find less problematic behavior in high-risk subjects than in normal children.

Finally, it must be that experience in some way shapes the mind and behavior of those children who become ill, and this experience is partly psychological and social in nature. The importance of psychological experience in the development of schizophrenia is an old and somewhat discredited notion, and it has attracted little research attention in recent years. A handful of studies tie the illness to patients' memories of parenting experiences in childhood and to stressful family and life events. The differences between patients and healthy people are small and inconsistent, and the research is plagued with the uncertainty of relying on memories of childhood and life experience, memories that may be contaminated by the distortions of psychiatric illness. Still, every field of research has limitations, and these limitations do not detract from the potential importance of environmental contributions to liability. This is a contribution that behavioral geneticists consider essential, if neglected, in the study of schizophrenia.

Overall, the idea of a cumulative liability for schizophrenic illness that increases with genetic and environmental "hits" over the course of childhood and adolescence is very appealing from a theoretical vantage point. Such a perspective can make up for the causal weakness of individual stresses and vulnerabilities. However, the empirical findings do not amount to a very powerful collection of illness-promoting hits and risks at the present time. Too many vulnerable children are indistinguishable from their peers and siblings and still go on to suffer from schizophrenia as young adults. Thus, to the question whether children who become schizophrenic are already different from their peers in childhood, the answer is that some are but most are not, at least not in terms of the characteristics studied to date.

Hence, unfortunately, there are no quick answers to the schizophrenia puzzle in the study of childhood and early development. To be fair, this field of research is itself nascent. Neurobiological investigations are considering new questions that relate to the formation of the nervous system and to how it may deviate from normal maturation to yield psychotic illness. But as it stands, there are still no replicated biological or behavioral abnormalities shared by even a consistent majority of high-risk children or patients with schizophrenia.

Perhaps the solution to the puzzle of schizophrenia and the brain does not lie entirely in more empirical data gathering. Perhaps it is possible to account for existing findings, their strength and degree of consistency, by approaching schizophrenia in a more conceptual way. Perhaps there are theoretical models and analyses of the illness that go beyond the general diathesis-stress model. Perhaps the theoretical imagination can make sense of the disparate, negative, and variable findings encountered so frequently in this book. Schizophrenia has fascinated theorists in psychology and psychiatry since the illness was described formally at the turn of the century. What theories of schizophrenia exist, and what do they say about its cerebral basis? Can theory make sense of an illness that has defied empirical analysis?

8

● ●

FLIGHTS OF THEORY

The science of schizophrenia is a parade of questions. What is wrong with the brain in the illness? Is it in some way "damaged," and if so, where is the damage, and how extensive is it? If the brain that produces the schizophrenic mind is free of obvious pathology, what is the nature of the abnormality that underpins the illness? Is the infantile nervous system at fault, as chapter 7 suggests? And does schizophrenia arise through the influence of biological inheritance—one or more genes, through the influence of biological or social environments, or through a hybrid of causes? How do nature and nurture merge into the grim equation that yields madness?

When such questions are not answerable fully by clinical and laboratory research they can be answered by disciplined imagination in the form of theory. In the absence of empirical truth, researchers can imagine the truth—what it could be, what it should be—and this imagined truth may provide a temporary answer to the schizophrenia puzzle. And a good theory may do more. It may tie together the puzzle pieces that have been discovered, none of which make sense in isolation, and thereby yield insight. Theory can also lead to scientific breakthroughs by proposing new ideas and predictions and by analyzing the illness from previously unexplored perspectives. Furthermore, theory can spur progress by criticizing and exposing errors in current thinking and evidence. In many ways, therefore, theory can advance schizophrenia science and provoke the development of new knowledge.

Neither Kraepelin (1919) nor Bleuler (1950) provided a comprehensive theory of schizophrenia. Kraepelin drew attention to the "hereditary taint" of dementia praecox and to the frontal and temporal lobes of the brain as possible neural sites for the illness. However, his contributions were primarily descriptive and observational rather than explanatory and theoretical. In contrast, Bleuler was influenced by psychoanalytic ideas about the primacy of early experience and the role of the unconscious in mental life. He theorized about psychological processes involved in symptom formation. Yet he did not develop a theory of what causes the symptoms and the illness in the first place. Several other psychoanalytic thinkers were drawn to schizophrenia, including Bleuler's associate Carl Jung (1939, 1956, 1960), as well as followers of Sigmund Freud, such as Tausk (1948), Fromm-Reichmann (1959) and Reichard and Tillman (1950). Early theorists postulated regression or return to an infantile state of ego development as a key psychodynamic mechanism in the illness. It was argued that, like an infant, the person with schizophrenia could not distinguish wishes and fantasies from real experience. However, the psychoanalysts were uncertain of the causes of this regression. It might result from biological events and the influence of a genetic predisposition. Alternatively, the regression might be rooted in early traumas and psychological conflicts.

Jung (1956) had considerable clinical experience treating schizophrenia patients with psychotherapy. He regarded the content of hallucinations and delusions as interpretable in psychological terms. Power and divinity, fear and sexuality—these were universal themes in psychosis and in Jung's concept of a collective unconscious. He liked to tell the story of an elderly schizophrenia patient at the Burghölzli Psychiatric Hospital who once told him that the sun had a penis that swung back and forth producing the wind. This seemed like just another idiosyncratic delusion until Jung came across a striking parallel in ancient religious symbolism. In the Persian religion centered on the god Mithras it was believed that a tube hanging down from the sun produced the wind. Therefore, Jung came to believe, the content of the patient's delusion was no coincidence, no empty product of a disturbed mind, but evidence for the existence of universal symbols and meanings. The same images appeared in both religious mythology and in psychotic symptoms (see Ellenberger, 1970, p. 705). Accordingly, the madness of schizophrenia could be understood as a kind of unrestricted eruption of symbols and meanings out of the collective unconscious and into everyday mental life.

Thinking back to the patients described in the first chapter (see chapter 1), it is easy to see how the dramatic content of psychosis lends itself to elaborate theoretical interpretations. William believed that he had divine powers and was recapitulating the life of Jesus Christ. This might represent an attempt to repair a damaged self-image by invoking one of the oldest and most powerful archetypes of the Self—the divine, glorified, perfect man, in the form of Jesus Christ (Jung, 1958, pp. 35–60). The symptoms of the other patients, tactile hallucinations of a creature draped around Ruth's neck and James's delusion of being controlled by a parasite, have less obvious meanings. However, a good Jungian psychologist would search the inventory of cultural and historical symbols and discover that these symptoms also have significance and are not simply random products of a disordered brain and mind.

Yet even Jung was uncertain about what caused this incursion of the collective unconscious into waking life. He suggested that a more basic psychological defect underlay symptoms like delusions and hallucinations (Jung, 1939). The primary defect comprised the same kind of "associative" disturbance or disconnected thinking and feeling that Bleuler (1911/1950) had proposed as a "fundamental" symptom of the illness (see chapter 2). Psychological conflicts and emotional experiences might give rise to the associative disturbance, but organic causes were also plausible explanations, in Jung's view. In contrast, Freudian psychoanalysts eventually proposed a very specific psychological cause for schizophrenia in the form of a rejecting but controlling "schizophrenogenic mother" who created the conditions for weak ego development and regression (see Diamond, 1997).

In contemporary research, almost no one believes that inadequate parenting causes schizophrenia. Few psychotherapists even treat people with the illness, let alone bother to interpret the symbolism of delusions and hallucinations (see Karon & Widener, 1994, for an exception). The combination of inadequate empirical support and the growth of biological psychiatry has brought about the demise of psychodynamic theories of schizophrenia. Family influences are still regarded as important stresses and mediating forces in the life of the schizophrenia patient (Butzlaff & Hooley, 1998). But they are not regarded as causes of psychotic illness. On the other hand, the interpretation of symptoms in psychological if not mythological terms continues in the cognitive science approach to delusions, hallucinations, and thought disorder (see chapter 2). For the most part, however, current theoretical accounts of schizophrenia are grounded in neuroscience and genetics.

Root Problems for Theories of Schizophrenia

There are several key puzzles or problems that any comprehensive theory of schizophrenia must address. First, there is the problem of *neurogenesis*. What is the nature of the neuropathology, the brain disorder that causes schizophrenic illness? The neural cause may take the form of a specific neurotransmitter abnormality, an excess or deficit of receptors, an excess or deficit of neurons in different layers of the cortex. Perhaps neurogenesis inheres in a dysfunction of neural circuitry whereby different brain regions interact in an abnormal way. A good theory will broach these possibilities and propose an answer to the neurogenic puzzle.

Second, there is the corollary but distinct problem of how *symptoms* and the schizophrenic mind are generated by the brain. The microscopic plaques and tangles of Alzheimer's disease occur disproportionately in the medial temporal lobe, thereby affecting structures involved in memory formation (Bauer, Tobias, & Valenstein, 1993). Hence, the typical early signs of dementia like rapid forgetting of recent events make sense in light of the location and distribution of pathological changes in the brain. Similarly, the tremor, rigidity, and slowed movements of Parkinsonism make sense because dopamine depletion takes place in neurons that project to the basal ganglia, a region known to mediate these aspects of motor control (Cooper, Bloom, & Roth, 1996, pp. 346–349). Can the origin of schizophrenic symptoms be explained in a similar way?

It is tempting to assume that a theory of neurogenesis automatically takes care of symptoms at the same time. Yet this temptation should be resisted. A theory about brain pathology in schizophrenia does not automatically serve as a theory of symptom formation. For example, dopamine and the basal ganglia are implicated in both schizophrenia and Parkinson's disease. In the case of schizophrenia, however, an abnormally high density of dopamine receptors rather than depletion is the proposed neurogenesis (see chapter 6). But do delusions, hallucinations, and disordered thought make sense as consequences of a disturbance in the basal ganglia? After all, most of the functions ascribed to this region have to do with control of movement and not with thought and feeling. It requires complex theorizing about neural networks and transmitter interactions to provide an account of symptoms that locates the essential defect of schizophrenia in the basal ganglia (e.g., Gray, Feldon, Rawlins, Hemsley, & Smith, 1991). Or consider the fact that completely different kinds of pathology sometimes lead to similar symptoms because the same brain region is effected. Thus a cancerous tumor and contusions due to traumatic head injury can both produce the same kind of memory impairment—if the medial temporal lobe is the effected brain region. Hence it would also be a mistake to reason backward and to assume that similar symptoms always reflect similar pathologies. Finally, recall that symptoms are subjective states of illness. They are psychological as well as physical in nature, and their relation to tissue damage is seldom straightforward or obvious (see chapter 2). For all of these reasons, explaining the symptoms of schizophrenia is a root problem in its own right.

An ideal theory also proposes mechanisms that explain how and why an illness takes place in effected individuals. In other words, theories should provide explanations of *etiology*. Does schizophrenic neuropathology stem from genetic influences, from the physical environment, or from some weighted combination of origins? Many diseases are the outcomes of complex etiologies. Thus one or more genes probably influence cerebrovascular disease or stroke. But strokes are also influenced by general health status and by smoking and diet—factors that in turn interact with other genetic influences (Plomin, Owen, & McGuffin, 1994). Many risk factors may come together and provide the conditions for the evolution of a disease. Something similar must take place with respect to schizophrenia.

The illness has two additional puzzles that challenge the theorist. Schizophrenia has a characteristic *onset* in late adolescence and early adulthood, although some liability for illness remains into middle age. What determines the timing of the disorder? Why is schizophrenia so rare in childhood and so much more common in the third decade of life? Many illnesses are age-linked in some way. Alzheimer's disease and stroke seem to be extremes of normal biological changes that occur with aging (Ball, 1983; Walton, 1985, pp.183–225). Huntington's disease tends to strike in middle age, whereas there are cystic tumors that disproportionately afflict teenagers (Walton, 1985, pp. 165–166). What noxious combination of events causes such a high incidence of schizophrenia just when a person has negotiated the changes of puberty and adolescence and entered physical maturity?

Finally, *heterogeneity*, that nemesis of the schizophrenia researcher who is bent on studying one disease state, also has a claim on the theoretical imagination. Does a single disease state really underlie the diversity of symptoms and biological findings that characterize the illness? Consider once more the case of stroke, an example of a neurological condition whereby a set of events interrupts cerebral blood supply and leads to losses of functional brain tissue. Yet these interruptions may occur in different locations of the brain, thereby yielding the great variety of behavioral deficits seen in stroke syndromes (Lezak, 1995, pp. 194–202). Moreover, stroke is really a loose term for several different pathological events, including thrombosis, aneurism, and embolism, that share the property of compromising the brain's blood supply. Hence it is possible to account for apparent illness heterogeneity by proposing a number of different pathological events that share key physiological features. On the other hand, medicine suggests that this is not always the case. There are several distinct kinds and causes of dementia, mental retardation, visual loss, and movement disorder. Sometimes clinical diversity does translate into different diseases—what does it mean in the case of schizophrenia?

A truly comprehensive theory provides explanations for each of the root problems of neurogenesis, symptom formation, etiology, onset, and heterogeneity. Yet a theory may address only some of these questions and still be helpful. Indeed, scientific theories often vary in their ability to explain phenomena comprehensively. The most famous example of this is probably Darwin's (1958) theory of evolution by natural selection. It explained why evolutionary processes occur, but Darwin did not address the mechanisms underlying variation in species and individuals or tackle the means of inheritance. Hence, all-embracing comprehensiveness may be too much to expect of a theory, and failure to explain everything is not grounds to reject a theory. On the other hand, theories can be so narrow and specific in focus that they do not explain the illness as a whole. For example, it is possible to imagine a theory of delusions that has little to say about hallucinations and nothing to say about neurogenesis or onset. But is this a theory of schizophrenia?

A careful look at the scientific literature on the illness shows that there are few truly comprehensive theories. There are theories that address aspects of neurogenesis and positive symptoms but have nothing to say about negative symptoms, etiology, onset, or heterogeneity (e.g., Gray, 1998; Gray et al., 1991). There are theories of dopamine function and how it causes cognitive deficits in schizophrenia (Cohen & Servan-Schreiber, 1992, 1993). Still other theories focus on genetics and etiology (e.g., Gottesman & Shields, 1972; 1982). Conversely, there are diathesis–stress theories that are so general that they apply across the spectrum of psychopathology, including schizophrenia. Such inclusive approaches are helpful in organizing existing evidence and in providing a general framework for thinking about an illness (e.g., Zuckerman, 1999, pp. 3–23, 319–411). However, the diathesis–stress model is really just a first step, a working assumption, that by itself does not offer new or detailed answers to the root problems of schizophrenia research. In the end I was left with only three theories, all based on the diathesis–stress notion, that address neurogenesis, symptoms, etiology, onset, and heterogeneity directly or indirectly. These theories are the subject of the rest of this chapter.

Schizotaxia, Schizotypy, and Schizophrenia

Meehl (1962, 1990b) formulated a diathesis–stress theory that schizophrenia arises from a single gene and from a pervasive neurological defect (see table 8.1). However, full-blown symptoms and psychosis do not always develop. The gene creates a vulnerability to illness that is influenced by numerous other genes, as well as by rewards and punishments that stem from the social environment. The inherited diathesis, independently inherited traits, and the influence of the social world jointly bring about schizophrenic illness. Consider Meehl's position on each of the root problems of schizophrenia science.

The original and most recent version of his theory describes the neurological diathesis of schizophrenia as "hypokrisia"—an abnormality of nerve conduction wherein neurons fire too readily and too frequently in response to incoming stimulation. The concept is short on details, but Meehl holds that hypokrisia is ubiquitous, represented in every neuron throughout the central nervous system. Yet this defect is also too subtle to interfere with basic, ele-

Table 8.1 Meehl's (1990b) theory in relation to key problems of schizophrenia research

Problem	Theoretical Concepts
Neurogenesis	Hypokrisia (reduced selectivity of neuronal firing)
	Integrative defect (defective sensorimotor processing)
Symptoms	Cognitive slippage (associative loosening)
	Subjective interpretation of slippage (hallucinations)
	Aversive social experience and normal capacity for irrational thought (delusions)
	Aversive experience, temperament (withdrawal)
Etiology	Single dominant gene for schizotaxia (neural basis of schizophrenia)
	Multiple genes for potentiating and protective traits (intelligence vs. introversion)
	Social reward and punishment of traits (schizotypy)
Illness Onset	Unspecified, cumulative effects in adolescence?
Heterogeneity	True schizophrenia (schizotaxia)
	Phenocopies

mentary nervous activities. The brain is still able to regulate bodily processes, register, and store and retrieve information. Nor does the hypokrisia produce mental retardation or other gross disorders of brain function. Still, the affected child and young adult carry this vulnerable, quietly aberrant neurology into the tumult of social experience. And under certain conditions the combination will lead to symptoms. But the symptoms that emerge are rather different from most current descriptions of schizophrenia and psychosis.

Years before schizophrenia actually erupts as an overt illness, the person with hypokrisia must endure its psychological consequences, "cognitive slippage" and "aversive drift." Cognitive slippage echoes Bleuler's (1950) descriptions of "associative loosening." Information is differentiated poorly, and cognitive signals are "scrambled" and lack integrity. All systems in the brain are involved, but some are especially impaired. Sensory integration of different kinds of information is highly sensitive to synaptic and cognitive slippage. Integrative functions might include, for example, positioning the body in space, wherein vision, balance, and touch have to be coordinated. In contrast, and perhaps surprisingly, intelligence and reasoning abilities are not regarded as functions that are vulnerable to cognitive slippage. In Meehl's theory, even high intellectual ability can coexist with hypokrisia and cognitive slippage.

Yet the neurological defect underlying schizophrenia does distort thinking in certain ways by causing associative loosening—an exaggerated and rather unselective tendency to form haphazard connections among ideas, emotions, and events. Associative loosening resembles symptoms like thought disorder and incoherence (described in chapter 2). Moreover, the exaggerated neuronal firing that causes cognitive slippage also causes a gradual increase in punitive, aversive social experience. The brain amplifies pain and attenuates pleasure. This aversive "drift" is related to negative symptoms like social withdrawal and disinterest. As the brain scrambles and distorts rewarding and punitive emotional associations, the person who is vulnerable to schizophrenia begins to find social contact more and more unpleasant. Increasingly, such a person withdraws from social intercourse and comes to be viewed as strange and subject to disapproval by other people. This in turn accelerates the process of withdrawal and creates a vicious circle.

Meehl's position on positive symptoms like hallucinations and delusions is somewhat difficult to pin down. On the one hand, they are "accessory" symptoms and rather indirect by-products of the neural defect. Positive symptoms occur because the person with schizophrenia experiences strange sensations due to synaptic slippage. "Explanations" are developed in the form of delusions to account for these sensations. But the true schizophrenic abnormality lies more in the sensory-integrative defect than in the irrational explanations. After all, strange, crazy thoughts, biased judgment, and cognitive errors are widespread in humans. They have no specific tie to schizophrenia. Consider, for example, the widespread belief in astrology or the pervasive purchasing of lottery tickets against enormous odds of winning. Elsewhere, however, Meehl regards delusions like those with persecutory content as gross forms of cognitive slippage. Perhaps it would be fair to say that positive symptoms can arise in a number of ways that have only weak links to schizophrenia. Associative loosening and primary aversive drift are the most direct consequences of the inherited neural defect that underlies the illness.

If Meehl is correct, the symptoms of the patients described in chapter 1 might be understandable in the following ways. Ruth, the woman who smelled and felt a creature around her neck, experienced sensory slippage caused by hypokrisia, and she developed the "creature" as an explanation for the experience. James, who was controlled by a parasite that had entered his brain, also experienced the hypokrisic sensory integration disorder. Perhaps he felt bizarre internal sensations in his head and explained this in terms of a theory of alien control. William, who reexperienced the life of Christ, is less easily understood in Meehl's terms. His grandiose delusions and hallucinations of speaking to famous people are harder to interpret as by-products of the hypokrisia defect. However, William also showed signs of thought disorder and incoherence. Perhaps he was effected by the associative thinking disturbance that both Bleuler and Meehl regard as an essential symptom of schizophrenia. But in each case, the symptoms are by-products of the synaptic and cognitive slippage that creates unusual linkages between ideas and prevents the integration of sight, sound, touch, and smell into normal experience.

Meehl (1962, 1990b) goes on to argue that a single major gene contributes to the etiology of schizophrenia. However, the gene is so weakly penetrant that it is expressed overtly in only about 10% of the offspring of schizophrenic parents. This risk for offspring of a single ill parent corresponds very roughly to observed statistics and is much lower than the rate (50%) that is expected from a gene with full penetrance (Gottesman, 1991, pp. 96–97). Hence it is not surprising that only one of the three patients (William) previously described actually had a parent with schizophrenia.

In most life circumstances, Meehl theorizes, the expressed "schizogene" reveals itself in a schizotypal personality rather than in schizophrenia. People with the gene suffer from "primary" cognitive slippage and difficulty feeling pleasure. They endure social fears and other aspects of aversive drift. However, numerous "moderator" genes that influence everything from intelligence to shyness can prevent or facilitate the eruption of a person's schizotypal constitution into full-blown schizophrenic psychosis. Moreover, the environment plays a role in shaping, or in restricting, the malignant inheritance. For example, a number of temperament traits are under genetic influence. Schizophrenia becomes more probable when a schizotypal person also inherits tendencies toward introversion, anxiety, low energy, passivity, and a lack of ability, talent, or physical attractiveness. However, these "polygenic" characteristics still have to combine with the influence of a social world that punishes such traits before a person crosses the threshold into schizophrenic illness. Conversely, different polygenes may combine in such a way that a person becomes a "compensated schizotype," someone who is able to function in the world, although usually at a cost to himself or herself or to other people. Adolf Hitler and the philosopher Ludwig Wittgenstein are mentioned as examples of compensated schizotypes.

Recall again the clinical cases and that Ruth, the woman with olfactory hallucinations, had her first psychotic episode after experiencing rejection in an intimate relationship. The rejection did not cause the schizophrenia, but it reflected one facet of an increasingly aversive social environment that moved her along the continuum from schizotypy to schizophrenia. William, with delusions of divinity, had a schizophrenic mother who attempted suicide when he was a teenager. In addition, he was in trouble with the police at an early age. And James, the man with delusions of alien control, had his first hospitalization following marital breakdown. Moreover, during childhood James was already emotionally troubled and avoided touch and displays of affection. He adjusted poorly to school and had learning problems. In each case there are signs of a negative relationship with the social environment or signs of maladaptive temperament characteristics. Moreover, none of the three patients had special talents or valued traits like high intelligence that might compensate for their vulnerability to schizophrenia. According to Meehl, the development of the illness is understandable only as the product of all of these influences: primary schizotaxia (genetic), personality influences (genetic), and aversive, stressful social environments.

On the other hand, the theory has little to say about the characteristic onset of schizophrenic illness early in the third decade of life. Meehl's conjectures imply that the interaction of schizotypy and the social environment takes place over a period of years. Late adolescence and early adulthood represent an intensification of a person's transition from the family to broader social life. This time period corresponds to major life events, including sexual relationships and intimacy and educational and occupational choices. These events bring the schizotypal person into close contact with the rewards and punishments of the social world. At the same time, the actual liability for schizophrenia encompasses about 2 decades. Yet Meehl would probably argue that this large window of vulnerability is due to the way people differ in their polygenic traits and to how these differences interact with social reinforcement. The illness is not due to a single event but to the accumulation of many aversive experiences within an increasingly punitive and unsupportive social and life situation. In this light, the potential for schizophrenia seems likely to persist for many years and remain subject to individual variation. But it also makes sense that illness onset peaks during the emotional fragility, the stresses and strains, of late adolescence and early adult life.

Finally, Meehl's theoretical view of heterogeneity is that there is one "true" schizophrenia, a product of the schizotaxic brain, and one or more "phenocopies" of the illness. Phenocopies are disorders that resemble schizophrenia from a clinical standpoint but differ in their etiology and neurogenesis. These false schizophrenias occur because there are several genetic and environmental influences on the development of the illness. For example, there must be people who carry only the undesirable temperament "polygenes" and not the primary "schizogene." In addition, many people are exposed to unfortunate or punitive environments. Hence, there will be people whose behavior superficially resembles schizophrenia but without schizotaxia and primary cognitive slippage. Such people will not show psychophysiological or cognitive abnormalities that are linked with the neural defect of hypokrisia. However, a person with a phenocopy of the illness may still be prone to delusions and to other cognitive distortions, albeit in a more fluctuating, inconsistent way than is seen in genuine schizophrenia. It stands to reason that this mixture in the patient population, a mixture of true schizophrenia and its phenocopy, will yield diverse symptom profiles and an equally diverse and inconclusive body of biological findings.

Evaluation

Meehl has provided an explanation that addresses several of the root problems in schizophrenia research. But how valid is the theory? Meehl (1990a) has written extensively on theory evaluation in science, and he stresses the importance of a theory's "track record" and its ability to survive "risky" and precise tests as criteria for evaluation. Yet in terms of the neurogenesis problem and the inter-related concepts of hypokrisia and cognitive slippage, there are no explicit tests or studies available. Hypokrisia theory lacks neurobiological detail. The idea is that neurons fire more readily, more frequently, and perhaps more persistently in the schizotaxic brain than in the normal brain. But how does this differ from situations where enhanced synaptic transmission is regarded as beneficial? For example, long-term potentiation is also a kind of lowered neuronal firing threshold, yet it underpins important aspects of normal learning and memory (see Cooper et al., 1996, pp. 468–473; chapter 6 of this book). Meehl (1990a) argues that single nerve cell stimulation and recording in living patients is needed to assess hypokrisia. However, this is technically and ethically unfeasible at present. As it stands, hypokrisia theory is simply not testable.

A related consideration is the testability of Meehl's concept of cognitive slippage. Cognitive slippage is the functional consequence of hypokrisia. There should be no major ethical or methodological problems in applying tests of cognitive slippage to living patients and healthy people. However, notwithstanding the allusions to Bleuler's (1950) notion of associative loosening, this concept also needs articulation and more detailed description. What exactly is cognitive slippage, and how can it be measured? Clinical ratings of symptoms like "marked loosening of associations" often reveal prevalence rates of only 17–19% in schizophrenia patients (Andreasen & Flaum, 1991). This seems very low for a symptom that is supposed to reflect cognitive slippage—the hallmark of the illness. But then how many of these patients have the "true" schizophrenia? Perhaps people with the true schizophrenia are in the minority in many research studies, and perhaps this leads to underestimations of rates for symptoms like associative loosening. Meehl also argues that hypokrisia creates disadvantages on tasks that require simultaneous processing of more than one type of sensation. These tasks require integration of stimuli—something that the hypokrisic brain, with its unselective and enhanced synaptic transmission, finds hard to accomplish. But is this *cognitive* slippage, and if so, how can it be captured with readily designed and applied tests and instruments?

One possible candidate for cognitive slippage that lends itself to objective measurement is semantic priming (see chapter 2). Semantic priming is the cognitive process whereby prior experience with a meaningful stimulus, like a word, facilitates subsequent perception of semantically related stimuli—other words. In this way, a subject who is exposed briefly to the word "stripes" finds it easier to perceive subsequent words like "tiger" (see Spitzer, 1997). Perhaps cognitive slippage manifests itself in increased but less discriminating priming of associations and connections between words and ideas. There is a small number of studies (see chapter 2) that report abnormally enhanced semantic priming in schizophrenia patients. Further work is needed to develop this and other cognitive tests as indicators of cognitive slippage and the hypokrisic brain.

A reasonable assessment of Meehl's treatment of neurogenesis may be to say that hypokrisia and cognitive slippage are interesting concepts that require much more detailed description and specification. They also require an empirical literature of risky, accurate, and successfully replicated predictions. At present all of these requirements are lacking, so there are insufficient grounds to reject or accept this aspect of Meehl's theory of schizophrenia.

In explaining the formation of positive symptoms, Meehl argues that delusions and hallucinations often reflect a patient's interpretation of an abnormal sensory experience. This view is echoed by a number of researchers who suggest the existence of a defective sensory filter in schizophrenia (e.g., Maher, 1974; see chapter 2). In such a view, the reasoning of the person with schizophrenia is not abnormal or impaired, but sensory-perceptual experience is disturbed or unusual. This in turn gives rise to delusions and hallucinations, which are nothing more than explanations for strange "feelings." Unfortunately, the sensory-deficit hypothesis has always lacked consistent, strong evidence to support the twin principles of altered sensation and preserved reasoning (Frith, 1987; Heinrichs & Zakzanis, 1998). But the issue is not decided completely. A separate literature on sensory "gating" and the P50 evoked potential shows that most schizophrenia patients fail to dampen their response to a repeated sensory event like a sound (see chapter 3). Could this be synaptic slippage in action? There is fertile ground here for future exploration.

On the question of etiology, Meehl acknowledges that most contemporary genetic researchers reject single gene explanations for schizophrenia. According to Gottesman (1991, 1994), the evidence from population genetics, the data on incidence and prevalence of schizophrenia in families, identical and fraternal twin studies, and studies of adopted children of schizophrenic parents all fail to support a single major gene theory. Meehl defends his position on the grounds that most single gene theorists do not include genetic moderator and environmental variables in their models. He also suggests that his ideas may be more testable in the future as instruments and technologies improve.

One way of testing Meehl's views on etiology might be to focus on the "potentiating" traits and to predict an inverse relationship between socially valued traits and the development of schizophrenic illness. In other words, patients with schizophrenia should be low in intelligence, talent, and physical attractiveness. The lack of these positive traits exposes the person to the full force of the schizophrenic diathesis and also makes aversive drift more likely. At the same time, a direct relationship should exist between devalued traits, like introversion and anxiety-prone behavior, and the illness. This is not a very precise prediction or a very risky one, because these valued and disparaged traits probably influence many kinds of social adjustment and psychopathology to some degree. Therefore, a riskier prediction would be to hold that the polygenetic traits have a much stronger relation with schizophrenia than with any other form of mental illness. Yet, as Meehl points out himself, it is difficult to achieve precision with this kind of theory, and alternative explanations are possible for any observed relationships. For example, patients with schizophrenia do have lower intelligence quotients on average than healthy people (Heinrichs & Zakzanis, 1998); however, this may reflect reduced educational achievement caused by early stages of the illness. Low intelligence may not be an independent "potentiating" trait at all; it may be not a cause of schizophrenia but an effect of it. The same relationship may apply to the other potentiating traits. They may be consequences rather than causes of the illness. Even if Meehl is correct about the importance of these traits, testing his etiological ideas will be difficult.

It seems to be the case that testing schizotaxia theory depends in part on finding people with "true" schizophrenia who can be distinguished from people with the illness phenocopy. But how does a researcher find the real illness? According to Meehl, identifying the schizotypal person in the general population can be achieved through application of statistical techniques called "taxometrics." People with schizotypy have the true schizophrenic diathesis. Potential indicators of schizotypy include anatomical abnormalities like facial asymmetries, skull shape and size, and various perceptual and cognitive disturbances. Most of these abnormalities and tests have not been validated, and they are proposed as candidates for research rather than as evidence for the theory. However, Meehl does mention smooth pursuit eye movements and the P50 component evoked potential as two of the strongest candidates for indicators of schizotypy. These psychophysiological variables have been researched extensively, and they offer another perspective on the difficulties involved in testing a theory of schizophrenia.

Eye movement abnormalities and evoked potentials were analyzed in some detail in chapter 3. The effect sizes derived from comparisons of schizophrenia and normal subjects' performance are sometimes substantial, but they are still too small to represent markers for a single disease entity. Yet perhaps there is an alternative to such interpretations, one that also incorporates Meehl's ideas on phenocopies and heterogeneity. It would not be surprising that base rates for eye movement abnormalities seldom exceed 50% in schizophrenia samples, if too many of these putative schizophrenia patients represent phenocopies of the illness and not the true disease. Moreover, the finding that rates of eye movement dysfunction in healthy people are often as high as 10% would make sense. After all, the illness gene and hence schizotypy are relatively common in the general population. Most of the "normal" schizotypal people in the general population will remain healthy. But they still show the indicator trait that reveals their schizotypy and genetic liability for illness.

The problem with such speculations is that there is no way of knowing if the patients who show abnormalities on one or more of Meehl's candidate indicators also have the gene for schizophrenia. There is no way of knowing if

Table 8.2 Weinberger's (1987) neurodevelopmental theory

Problem	Theoretical Concepts
Neurogenesis	Prenatal or perinatal lesion (fronto-temporal tracts)
	Depleted prefrontal dopamine (due to lesion)
	Excessive medial temporal dopamine (unregulated)
	Maturation and stress (potentiation of dopamine)
Symptoms	Reduced prefrontal dopamine function (negative)
	Enhanced limbic dopamine function (positive)
Etiology	Genetic and polygenetic
	Environmental (perinatal trauma, adolescent stress)
Onset	Maturational increase in dopamine activity
	Maturation-linked stress (adolescence)
	Interaction of old lesion and brain maturation
Heterogeneity	Multiple etiologies with single common neuropathology
	Severity continuum of neuropathology

the large number of diagnosed patients who fail to show such abnormalities lack the gene. And there is no way of knowing if those who lack the major illness gene possess some or all of the potentiating genes that produce the schizophrenic phenocopy. Independent evidence of the schizophrenia gene is missing, and without it Meehl's theory is hard to test (Gottesman, 1991; O'Donovan & Owen, 1996). Even if Meehl is successful in identifying healthy people with schizotypy in the general population, more is needed. It has to be shown that these "compensated" people nonetheless have hypokrisia and primary cognitive slippage. It must also be shown that they lack the potentiating genes and social histories that would otherwise propel them beyond mere schizotypy and into schizophrenia. Such are the complexities of trying to derive and test predictions from this theory.

As Meehl points out, he cannot be faulted for the absence of instrumentation that is capable of bringing his theory to prediction and empirical test. However, the fact remains that critical aspects of Meehl's theory of schizophrenia are either at variance with existing evidence or do not meet the requirements for a good theory that he has laid out in his own very helpful writing on theory evaluation in science.

Neurodevelopmental Diathesis-Stress Theories

Meehl's (1962, 1990b) formulation of schizotaxia, schizotypy, and schizophrenia remains the most comprehensive theory of the illness. However, a number of additional viewpoints have emerged that differ from his general model in important respects. These differences include a greater interest in specific subregions and systems of the brain, avoidance of single major gene concepts of etiology, and greater attention to the onset and timing of the illness. Yet these more recent viewpoints still fall within the framework of the general diathesis-stress model. Two examples of such approaches are Weinberger's (1987, 1995, 1996, 1997) formulation of the illness and Walker and Diforio's (1997) model.

Weinberger's Neurodevelopmental Theory

In general terms, Weinberger (1987) argues that schizophrenia is a disorder that reflects the existence of a brain lesion or maturational failure of some kind. However, the lesion occurs very early in life and thereafter it does not progress and change. Moreover, the lesion, on its own, is not sufficient to cause clinical schizophrenia. Instead, the early pathology interacts with normal biological and behavioral events and stresses over the course of growth and development, and it is through this interaction that the illness springs to life. Weinberger holds that the etiology of the perinatal lesion may be environmental, in the form of a traumatic or toxic congenital event, or it may reflect genetic influences, abnormal neural maturation, and hence "hypoplasia." In all cases, it is the inability of the compromised brain to deal adaptively with the stresses and strains of emergent adulthood that causes schizophrenia.

In approaching the question of neurogenesis, Weinberger argues that most of the available neurological evidence points to medial temporal and prefrontal lobe pathology in schizophrenia. He acknowledges that healthy people and patients typically overlap in measures of brain volume and function and that it is hard to pinpoint how selective or diffuse the brain damage is in schizophrenia. Nonetheless, he regards the fronto-medial temporal system as the basis for schizophrenic symptoms, and he specifically links the temporal lobes to positive and the prefrontal system to negative symptoms. Yet the lesion or dysplasia effecting these systems is "old" and probably reflects neurological events that occurred before or during birth. That is why few studies have found reactive gliosis, a kind of scar tissue, in post-mortem schizophrenia brain samples. Gliosis tends to occur in response to cerebral insults after birth and is most evident in adulthood following injuries like brain trauma and focal destruction of tissue. Its relative absence in schizophrenia samples implies that the illness must involve very early forms of pathology. There is also little to suggest that brain pathology increases over the course of schizophrenia. The common finding of enlarged cerebral ventricles, for example, does not appear to be linked to length of illness and may predate the onset of symptoms. Overall, there is no justification for arguing that the schizophrenic brain lesion occurs at the same time as positive and negative symptoms. There is also little to indicate that the pathology progresses in step with the illness. Therefore, the evidence indirectly implies a schizophrenic lesion that is old and stable.

Yet there is more to the neurogenesis of schizophrenia than a static lesion that effects the executive and semantic systems of the brain. After all, other ill-nesses with pathology in these systems do not closely resemble the symptom picture of schizophrenia. There must be something else in the progression of events that lead to madness. In Weinberger's view, the additional ingredient stems from the normal course of brain growth and maturation. He notes evi-dence that the dorsolateral prefrontal cortex reaches physical maturity in early adulthood. In healthy people it is also about this time that the frontal executive region begins to play an increasingly important role in behavioral adjustment to the environment. The same maturation process occurs in the preschizophrenic person, but it is maturation within the context of a partially defective, or lesion-compromised, frontal brain rather than within the context of a normal brain. But still more is involved in the neurogenesis of schizophrenia. The interplay between preexisting pathology and maturational events gives rise to an unbal-anced dopamine system. On the one hand, the old lesion alters dopamine con-nections between the midbrain and the executive frontal system. Hence there is an abnormal reduction in dopaminergic innervation of the frontal brain. On the other hand, while the prefrontal area is underactive, the midbrain medial temporal dopamine system is overactive. This overactivity arises from a stress-linked response that occurs normally in late adolescence. Ordinarily the frontal brain increases its own dopamine activity and controls the maturational surge in limbic dopamine activity, but the compromised prefrontal system is unable to carry out its regulatory function in the case of the preschizophrenic person. Thus normal environmental stress causes enhanced medial-temporal dopamine activity, but this overwhelms the damaged prefrontal system. Acute schizophre-nia is the result.

Accordingly, Weinberger's concept of the neurogenesis of schizophrenia in-volves the idea of a "sleeper effect," in that an early lesion has relatively little behavioral importance until its associated brain regions are faced with matura-tional challenges. He also places heavy emphasis on the importance of dopa-mine, proposing a deficit of this neurotransmitter in the prefrontal region due to the early lesion and an excess of it in the temporal lobe due to normal mat-uration. Regulatory failure of the semantic brain by the executive brain is the spur for psychosis. In concert this amalgam of pathology and normal develop-ment causes schizophrenia.

Weinberger holds that positive symptoms like hallucinations and delusions are direct consequences of excessive dopamine activity in structures like the amygdala and hippocampus. He cites studies showing that electrical discharges or lesions in medial-temporal areas can produce psychotic-like experiences. Thus an overactive semantic brain is responsible for positive symptoms. In con-trast, negative symptoms of the illness, including social withdrawal, emotional "flatness," loss of motivation, and poor insight, reflect diminished prefrontal brain activity. Weinberger maintains that the same symptoms are seen in neurological patients with prefrontal lobe lesions. They are consequences of an ineffective executive brain. Then, over the course of illness, excessive temporal lobe dopamine activity slowly declines as maturation proceeds. What remains is the diminished frontal executive system. Hence negative symptoms predominate increasingly in later adulthood, as schizophrenia becomes more chronic.

Thus for Weinberger local brain disturbances cause schizophrenic symptoms in a fairly straightforward way. This differs from Meehl's (1990b) theory, in which positive symptoms reflect cognitive elaboration and subjective interpretations of disturbed sensory experience. In Meehl's analysis, the biological aspects of the illness are tied more closely to impaired sensory integration than to disturbed reasoning. Moreover, Meehl regards the content of symptoms as a reflection of the schizophrenia patient's social environment. Weinberger has a fairly strong "reductionist" view, wherein hallucinations, delusions, bizarre behavior, and emotional withdrawal simply mark the surge and ebb of abnormal brain activity in the illness.

A further contrast with Meehl's position is that Weinberger's theory takes a neutral stance on the question of etiology. Weinberger raises several possible causes for the early lesion or dysplasia that underlies schizophrenia. Hereditary brain disease, a susceptibility to environmental traumas or toxins, or a failure of normal maturation due to genetic influences could all be involved in the etiology of the illness. His theory has little to say about whether one proposed etiology is more likely than another one.

On the other hand, Weinberger's conjectures allow for a specific explanation of the timing of illness onset. Schizophrenia occurs most frequently early in the third decade of life because of the convergence of normal maturation, stress experiences, and existing pathology. As dopamine activity heightens normally in response to the stresses of young adulthood, the defective executive brain is unable to control the overactive semantic brain, and florid psychosis erupts. Presumably, if this dopamine surge does not take place, schizophrenia remains dormant. It is this temporal convergence of biological and environmental changes that makes schizophrenia an illness of young people. Weinberger is also able to account for gender variation in age of onset by suggesting that dopamine activity peaks later in women than in men. This leads to a later average age of illness onset in women, a long-observed finding in the epidemiology of schizophrenia.

The theory also involves a rather complex view of heterogeneity and what it means about the nature of schizophrenia. Thus Weinberger maintains that variable combinations and weightings of genetic and environmental influences may cause the illness. He even raises the possibility that there is more than one lesion or lesion location involved in schizophrenia. However, he also insists that the neural mechanism, wherein an underactive prefrontal system interacts ineffectively with an overactive medial temporal lobe system, is common to all cases

of schizophrenia. What appears to be clinical and biological diversity in the patient population is really a difference in severity between people who all fall on
the same neurogenic continuum. To support this idea, Weinberger argues that
neurobiological findings obtained from groups of schizophrenia patients do not
have the kinds of irregularities that imply the existence of discrete subtypes of
illness. Instead, patients overlap with healthy people at one end of the scale and
then range completely outside normal values at the other end of the scale. In
other words, all schizophrenia patients share the same basic neurobiological abnormality, but they share it in different degrees. For example, patients with pronounced abnormalities like enlarged brain ventricles have a poorer long-term
outcome and prognosis than patients with normal ventricles. Perhaps ventricular enlargement is a continuum, with greater degrees of dilation associated with
greater pathology in the underlying neural mechanisms of the illness.

More recently (Goldberg & Weinberger, 1995), this school of thought has
used findings from studies of monozygotic twins discordant for schizophrenia
to support the single illness neurodevelopmental model. The affected twins are
almost invariably deficient in cognition and brain measurements when compared with the healthy twin. Yet this deficiency may not reach statistical significance thresholds or exceed the range of normal values. Nonetheless, the twin
with schizophrenia shows consistent, albeit subtle, inferiority on many behavioral and biological comparisons. The theory holds that the multiple etiologies
of schizophrenia nevertheless converge on a common neural mechanism for
the illness. This mechanism is abnormal in varying degrees in different people,
which accounts for the clinical diversity of patients and for the tendency for
large amounts of overlap between patient and control group values on many biological and behavioral measurements.

Evaluation

Weinberger suggests that at least two aspects of his theory could be developed
into predictions and tested. First, the theory holds that illness onset is governed
by biological maturation. People who are prone to early maturation should also
be prone to early onset of schizophrenia. Testing this idea requires an independent index of maturation like, perhaps, the onset age of puberty. If puber-
tal development is linked with brain maturation, then people with early puberty
should be the first to develop schizophrenia. To make this a meaningful prediction, the presumed tie between sexual and brain maturation would have to be
unequivocally established. Still, it is worth noting that Cohen, Seeman, Gotowiec, and Kopala (1999) found early puberty to be associated with later, not
earlier, illness onset in women, while no relationship was found for men. This
does not augur well for at least one aspect of Weinberger's theory.

Another prediction has to do with the role of dopamine in schizophrenia onset. Can a very early lesion lie dormant for many years and then erupt to deregulate dopamine activity in late adolescence? This aspect of Weinberger's (1987) theory was not fully articulated in the original paper. However, in more recent reviews, Weinberger (1996,1997; Lipska & Weinberger, 2000) has cited animal research to argue that neonatal lesions of the hippocampus can interfere with cortical connections without creating major behavioral and neurobiological changes until the animals reach sexual maturity. These changes eventually include "hyperresponsiveness" of dopamine systems to environmental stresses and to drugs. From a behavioral standpoint, the animals engage in exaggerated exploration of their environment. Animals who receive brain lesions in adulthood do not show this hyperresponsive pattern. At least in principle, the idea of a sleeper effect for psychopathology makes sense and can be mimicked with animals.

Further empirical support for delayed behavioral and neurochemical defects would enhance the credibility of a neurodevelopmental theory of schizophrenia. However, as Weinberger (1996) has pointed out himself, the behavioral disturbances seen in rats do not constitute a convincing analogue for human schizophrenic illness with its myriad of psychological symptoms. In addition, recall the findings on temporal lobe abnormalities reviewed in chapter 7. There is little evidence that people with schizophrenia sustain the kind of hippocampal lesions that have been produced experimentally in animals.

Of course Weinberger's neurological conjectures do not end with the early fixed lesion. It is the interaction of the lesion with normal brain changes that is pathogenic for schizophrenia. Specifically, it is argued that the early prefrontal-medial temporal lesion disrupts and disconnects the mesocortical and mesolimbic dopamine systems, making normal modulation of dopamine activity impossible. The disruption remains largely unnoticed until it is "unmasked" by the surge of dopamine activity and stress in early adulthood. Then, in vulnerable individuals, an underactive prefrontal system and an overactive limbic system yield the first psychotic episode. This part of the theory also implies predictions even if they are not stated outright. First, any structural lesions or cytoarchitectural anomalies in schizophrenia should effect the brain's major dopamine tracts. Indeed, given Weinberger's views that heterogeneity in schizophrenia is more apparent than real, disruption of the dopamine system should occur in all cases of the disease. There must be evidence of reduced and excessive dopamine activity specifically in the prefrontal and limbic areas during the illness, and this must correspond to the relative prevalence of positive and negative symptoms. Furthermore, there must be data showing that increased dopamine activity occurs in response to stressful events in both normal and schizophrenic cases in late adolescence and early adulthood. This follows from the idea that stress and dopamine surges are normal parts of maturation in all people, but with the schizophrenic brain unable to handle the increased activity.

At this time the available data do not support directly any hypothesis of a disconnection of neural systems or any fixed lesion in every case of schizophrenia. As the review of evidence on prefrontal and temporal lobe abnormalities in chapters 3 and 4 revealed, most patients with the illness do not have reduced tissue volumes, let alone direct evidence of a lesion. In addition, the biological evidence bearing on developmental anomalies is sparse (see chapter 7). In Weinberger's (1996, 1997) own words, neurodevelopmental findings are "circumstantial" with respect to the possibility of arrested cell migration or failed maturation in the schizophrenic nervous system. How such findings relate to dopamine abnormalities is also uncertain. Speculations about stress and dopamine are based on animal studies that may or may not hold for humans.

It is also troubling that so much theorizing rests on a dubious interpretation of existing evidence for the role of dopamine in schizophrenia. This evidence, reviewed in chapter 6, is simply not strong or consistent enough to carry the weight of Weinberger's conjectures. The relationship between dopamine blockade and symptom reduction is well established. But independent reproducible evidence of a dopamine abnormality in all cases of schizophrenia remains elusive. It is not surprising that his more recent writings (Weinberger, 1996, 1997) suggest a role for other neurotransmitter systems in the illness.

On the question of whether psychotic symptoms are direct consequences of local disturbances in brain activity, it is true that metabolism and blood-flow changes in the left temporal lobe correspond to at least some positive symptoms in schizophrenia patients (e.g. Cleghorn, Garnett, et al., 1990). Similarly, there are reports that reduced activity in prefrontal regions accompanies negative symptoms (e.g., Liddle, et al. 1992). However, these data do not necessarily mean that local increases or decreases in dopamine, or any other neurotransmitter, cause the symptoms in the first place. There is no damaged or stimulated brain region that will reliably produce the symptoms of schizophrenia. As Meehl (1990b) argued, the neurobiology of the illness may create conditions for symptom formation. But the nature of schizophrenic symptoms suggests that social and psychological processes, not just an abnormal brain, are involved in the formation of delusions, hallucinations, and disordered thought. After all, a person cannot have a delusion about Jesus Christ unless religious images and concepts are first learned and represented in the brain. In this more psychological respect, schizophrenia research has moved away from Weinberger's simple reductionism to more elaborate models of symptom formation (e.g. Gray, 1998; Gray et al., 1991; Hoffman & McGlashan, 1993; Ruppin, Reggia, & Horn, 1996).

What of the single illness—continuum view of schizophrenia and the heterogeneity puzzle (Goldberg & Weinberger, 1995)? The evidence summoned in support of this view includes a study of brain ventricle enlargement in pooled samples of schizophrenia patients (Daniel, Goldberg, Gibbons, & Weinberger, 1991). This study used a statistical technique called mixture analysis to search for signs of more than one patient group in the data distributions. The authors concluded that there was little support for the idea of separate groups of patients with and without abnormal ventricles. Instead, the data seemed to fit a continuum interpretation. However, this can hardly be regarded as a convincing or "risky" test of single versus multiple illness views. In the first place, the statistical technique used to search for multiple distributions is not considered completely reliable, even by the authors of the report. Moreover, ventricular enlargement is a poor candidate for being a neuropathological marker of schizophrenia. It is an aspect of brain structure influenced by many conditions, including normal aging. Indeed, the degree of enlargement seen in normal aging over decades is much more pronounced than the mild changes seen in schizophrenia (Raz & Raz, 1990). Brain ventricle size is almost certainly very "distant" from the neural basis of the illness. Moreover, studies looking at other aspects of neurobiology have found explicit evidence of subgroups. For example, dopamine receptor densities have distributed themselves into subgroups in some studies (see Seeman et al., 1987). In other cases, putative genetic "markers" of the illness, like eye movements, have shown distributions that also suggest the presence of discrete patient subgroups (see Clementz, Grove, Iacono, & Sweeney, 1992; Iacono, Moreau, Beiser, Fleming, & Lin, 1992). In the final analysis, the testing of heterogeneity predictions requires systematic analysis and cannot rise or fall on the basis of a single study or a single aspect of neurobiology.

Weinberger (1996) is an astute critic of neurodevelopmental theorizing about schizophrenia. In his assessment, the evidence of a very early lesion or neural dysplasia is weak and circumstantial. However, the basic neurodevelopmental premise continues to guide conceptual models of schizophrenia. Its continuing influence can be seen in a recent attempt to integrate developmental views with the biology of stress as an explanation for the illness.

Walker and Diforio's (1997) Neural Diathesis-Stress Theory

For Walker and Diforio, stress-related neural and behavioral mechanisms are the neglected elements in schizophrenia theory. It is not enough to posit a basic neurochemical defect in neurotransmission or an early brain lesion. Such defects must be coupled with abnormal biological responses to stress. These stress-linked responses augment and interact with neurotransmitter functions to cause schizophrenic symptoms in late adolescence and early adulthood. Building on Weinberger's (1987) sketch, Walker and Diforio provide a more detailed argument for how stress and dopamine combine to yield schizophrenia. They propose a dynamic relationship between three aspects of neurobiology as the neurogenesis of schizophrenia. First, there is an overactive neurotransmitter system,

Table 8.3 Walker and Diforio's (1997) neural diathesis-stress model

Problem	Theoretical Concept
Neurogenesis	Dopamine-related abnormality, possible glutamate defect
	Hypothalamic-pituitary-adrenal stress system dysfunction
	Defective hippocampus (glucocorticoid receptors)
	Interaction among elements
Symptoms	Excessive dopamine activity (positive)
	Coping with stress of positive symptoms (negative)
Etiology	Multiple (genetic, environmental)
	Prenatal maternal stress
	Perinatal trauma, insults
	Psychosocial stress
Onset	Adolescent increase in stress hormone levels
	Hippocampal stress hormone regulatory failure
	Dopamine potentiation
	Increased psychosocial stress in adolescence
Heterogeneity	Unspecified (different weightings of neurogenic elements)

probably centered on dopamine but with glutamate as a second component. This overactive system represents the biological diathesis or vulnerability in people who develop the illness. Second, the hypothalamic-pituitary-adrenal system of the brain is involved. This system secretes glucocorticoids and other hormones that normally constitute the body's response to stress. However, in schizophrenia hormonal activity is excessive, and it exacerbates the defect in neurotransmission. Third, it is known that the hippocampus has numerous glucocorticoid receptors. Normally the hippocampus plays an important role as part of a feedback system that modulates the hormonal system. However, prenatal or perinatal insult can impair its modulating role in the stress system. Impaired modulation results in excess release of glucocorticoids, and this in turn propels dopamine neurotransmission to abnormal levels.

It is the reciprocal relationships between the three neural elements of the theory that really comprise the neurogenesis of schizophrenia. Thus, enhanced release of glucocorticoids due to hippocampal damage creates an abnormal sensitivity to stressful events in the environment and also enhances dopamine activity to the point where psychotic symptoms develop. At the same time, the reverse holds true, so that increased dopamine activity stimulates activation of the hypothalamic-pituitary-adrenal system. These are interlocking dynamic systems that cause and then perpetuate schizophrenic illness.

Although Walker and Diforio accept prevailing views that abnormal dopamine activity is a major substrate of schizophrenia, they acknowledge the possibility that other neurotransmitters may be involved in the illness. Thus the excitatory amino acid transmitter glutamate is also believed to interact with the hypothalamic-pituitary-adrenal stress system. Reduced activity of receptors that bind glutamate, like the N-methyl-d-aspartate (NMDA) receptor complex, increase cortisol levels and therefore enhance the behavioral response to stress. Conversely, from the other direction, increased stress, leading to greater glucocorticoid release, can stimulate increases in glutamate activity. Moreover, glutamate interacts with dopamine, so that on the one hand increased dopamine activity contributes to reduced NMDA receptor function and on the other hand, in response to stress, NMDA receptors in the frontal brain inhibit dopamine activity in other regions of the brain like the basal ganglia.

Walker and Diforio have little to say about the formation of positive and negative symptoms, although they maintain that stress makes them worse. Like Weinberger these theorists appear to accept the idea of psychotic behavior as a direct consequence of excessive dopamine activity, with little discussion of how this excess actually yields delusions, hallucinations, withdrawal, or thought disorder. They do suggest that positive symptoms are themselves stress inducing. Therefore negative symptoms, like withdrawal and emotional "blunting," may reflect the patient's attempt to reduce the stress caused by the psychotic experience. However, the theory does not describe detailed ideas about symptom formation.

Walker and Diforio's view of etiology holds that the environment plays a crucial role in moving the person who is vulnerable to schizophrenia into a state of psychotic crisis. The normal stress-inducing events of life and the interpersonal behavior of family members are important influences on the stress-sensitive person who also has a dopamine abnormality that predisposes him or her to schizophrenia. Extraordinary or traumatic events may not be necessary to stimulate the vicious circle of stress hormone release and dopamine overactivity that gives rise to illness. In addition, there are earlier and less direct environmental contributions to etiology. Thus animal studies are cited to support an argument that maternal stress during pregnancy influences hypothalamic-pituitary-adrenal hormone activity in the mother's offspring. Moreover, many of the obstetrical and neonatal complications studied in relation to schizophrenia are capable of causing hippocampal damage. Such damage also implicates stress hormone activity, given the existence of glucocorticoid receptors in the hippocampus. Hence prenatal and perinatal insults along with normal but stressful experiences during psychological development are environmental contributions to the etiology of schizophrenia.

On the question of genetic influences, Walker and Diforio seem to accept the idea of an inherited liability to schizophrenia, perhaps in the form of a basic defect in dopamine transmission. However, their primary interest is in establishing a role for the environment in the prenatal and postnatal experience of the preschizophrenic infant, child, and adolescent. Indeed, their argument that environmentally induced hippocampal damage and stress hypersensitivity influence the dopamine system begs a corollary argument. Is it possible that environmental influences are sufficient in themselves to set the stage for schizo-phrenia in the complete absence of an inherited vulnerability?

In terms of illness onset, Walker and Diforio maintain that the eruption of acute schizophrenic psychosis in late adolescence and early adulthood makes sense in light of the biology of stress. Thus there is a gradual increase in hypo-thalamic-pituitary-adrenal activity during childhood and then a rapid rise in cortisol release during adolescence. Therefore, during late adolescence the per-son with an abnormal dopamine system is also abnormally sensitive to stress. Stress hormones are released at higher rates, and in the vulnerable person they are not modulated by the damaged hippocampus. The result is an escalation of dopamine activity past the threshold for symptom formation, and the initial psychotic episode takes place. Among the evidence cited is the finding that early treatment with antipsychotic medication leads to better long-term out-come in schizophrenia. Walker and Diforio argue that this is because antipsy-chotic drugs dampen activity in the hypothalamic-pituitary-adrenal system, in turn reducing the effect of the hormonal system on dopamine transmission. In a sense, early drug treatment serves a protective function by retarding activity in biological stress mechanisms that would otherwise accentuate the severity of symptoms.

The theory also alludes to the possibility of etiological heterogeneity, and the authors suggest that their model may only account for "some" cases of schizo-phrenia. However, they do not have an explicit position on the existence of multiple illnesses or an interpretation of the great clinical diversity of the illness. Instead, they acknowledge heterogeneity issues by suggesting that glutamate as well as dopamine may be involved in some cases of schizophrenia. And they as-sert that dopamine is effected by factors other than the hypothalamic-pituitary-adrenal system. It is possible, therefore, to extrapolate from their basic model and to imagine different variations of schizophrenic illness. For example, some people may have normal dopamine systems but abnormal stress systems. Con-versely, other people at risk for schizophrenia may have a dopamine abnormal-ity but a normal stress system. Still others may have neither but sustain subtle hippocampal damage in the womb or at birth, which leads to abnormal stress sensitivity and excess dopamine transmission by a different route. These alter-nate variations of illness might have contrasting symptom and outcome profiles that translate into the clinical diversity seen in the illness.

Evaluation

In principle, several predictions follow logically from Walker and Diforio's diathesis-stress model of schizophrenia. Preschizophrenic adolescents should have abnormally high cortisol responses to stressful experiences. Such experi-ences might include social events or critical communication and hostility from family members. Another prediction is that the rise and fall of symptoms should parallel stress hormone biology, including glucocorticoid levels in the brain. Moreover, by monitoring stress biology during childhood and adolescence it should be possible to predict which high-risk offspring of schizophrenic parents will develop the illness.

Some of these predictions are difficult to test. For example, it is hard to identify preschizophrenic adolescents with a high degree of confidence (see chapter 7). However, the high-risk study strategy, where children of schizophrenic parents are followed over time, is workable, if time consuming. Moreover, stress hormones are readily detected in saliva and blood plasma, if not in brain. On the other hand, the lack of a valid central dopamine activity index makes it hard to track the hypothesized relations among glucocorticoids, dopamine, and environmental stresses suggested by the authors. Clearly, a longitudinal high-risk research strategy using sensitive biochemical measures would be required to test Walker and Diforio's ideas.

Walker, Baum, and Diforio (1998) have recently published results that provide partial support for their theory. They studied teenagers with schizotypal personality disorder and compared them to adolescents with other personality disorders and to normal subjects. Schizotypal personality was defined by formal criteria in the *DSM-IV* (1994). In this diagnostic scheme people with schizotypal personality have few close social relationships and experience cognitive and perceptual distortions, illusions about their bodies, suspiciousness, and other peculiarities that fall just short of psychosis. Walker and associates measured cortisol levels with a simple saliva test and found an elevation in the schizotypal participants relative to controls ($d = .84$). In addition, the authors had longitudinal data on the adolescents' behavior at several points in time. Not only did cortisol release increase with age, it increased in step with behaviors like withdrawal, physical complaints, anxiety, and depression. Therefore, in keeping with the theory, stress hormone release does accelerate as children move into late adolescence and is higher in those at risk for schizophrenia than in normal teenagers. However, it must also be noted that although adolescents with schizotypal personality disorder are vulnerable to a range of psychiatric problems, most of them do not develop schizophrenia. In addition, the schizotypal subjects in Walker et al. (1998) did not differ in cortisol release from teenagers with other kinds of personality disorder. It is also noteworthy that a report by an independent group (Jansen et al., 1998) suggests abnormally weak rather than abnormally strong cortisol responses to stressful situations in schizophrenia patients. It could be argued that stress hormone increases have no tie to schizophrenia at all, just possible ties to a variety of other behavioral or psychiatric problems.

Several other facets of the neural diathesis-stress model are questionable from the standpoint of available evidence. First, like Weinberger's theory, Walker and Diforio rely heavily on the idea of a major defect in dopamine activity in schizophrenia. The evidence in favor of this possibility is not convincing at present, at least not in terms of a basic defect that underlies every case of the illness. Even more evidential weakness applies to the possible link with glutamate. The published evidence reviewed in chapter 6 does not support the existence of a basic glutamate deficiency in all cases of the illness. This emergent research area is afflicted by the great problems involved in the study of a substance that is ubiquitous in the central nervous system. Glutamate has multiple roles in addition to neurotransmission, and it binds to a bewildering array of receptor types. It may be that Walker and Diforio are correct in arguing for a link between glutamate and schizophrenia, but this is very much an ongoing research question in its own right rather than a solid finding that is capable of supporting a theory.

Another problem has to do with the nature of the literature review that is used to support the developmental neural diathesis-stress theory. In narrative literature reviews, it is never clear whether the authors have considered all relevant evidence, whether they are overemphasizing findings that support their viewpoints, or whether they ignore or downplay contradictory findings. These are general problems that are not unique to Walker and Diforio's article, but they are certainly in evidence here. For example, in their review it appears that not all studies show that schizophrenia patients have higher baseline cortisol levels than healthy people and a few studies even indicate that patients have lower levels. Yet the authors seem to emphasize the studies that support their theory. At other points as well they appear to accept nonsignificant trends and very weak differences between patient and control groups as evidence in support of their model. This reliance on weak and inconsistent findings occurs in relation to some of the most important aspects of their model, including, for example, the size of the cortisol change that occurs in response to stress in patients and healthy people. The authors rely on findings that are clearly questionable and inadequately replicated. The same applies to the idea that hippocampal abnormalities exist in schizophrenia that may contribute to deregulation of the biological stress response. These abnormalities are very modest in magnitude and are not characteristic of a majority of patients (see chapter 5).

Nonetheless, Walker and Diforio's model is an advance over Weinberger's (1987) theory in the detail and suggestions it provides on mechanisms linking neurotransmission, perinatal, and postnatal events, the stress system, and the puzzle of illness onset. Moreover, stress-related hormone abnormalities are more testable than vaguer concepts like Meehl's (1990b) notion of hypokrisia. Finally, although scant attention is paid to the mechanisms of symptom formation or to heterogeneity and multiple illness models, the groundwork is laid for further exploration of these problems. Thus it is suggested that one type of schizophrenia may involve an abnormality in dopamine receptors in the basal ganglia, coupled with impaired regulation of the hypothalamic-pituitary-adrenal stress system. Although dopamine receptor density effects are too small or inconsistent to support the idea that they represent the primary diathesis for all forms of the illness, it is possible that patients with one kind of dopamine-based illness are interspersed with patients suffering from other kinds of schizophrenia. This might also account for the inconsistency and modesty of the dopamine findings for the illness as a whole.

Summary and Synthesis

Diathesis-stress theories have arisen to explain schizophrenia in light of the accumulation of knowledge in neuroscience and genetics. But how successful are these theories? Do they organize the accumulated results of schizophrenia research and provide potential solutions to the root problems of neurogenesis, symptom formation, etiology, onset of illness, and heterogeneity?

Paul Meehl (1990a) has argued that scientific theories should be evaluated in terms of their ability to generate "risky," precise predictions and in terms of their "track records" in surviving the outcomes of such predictions. With these evaluative criteria in mind, it is disappointing to find that the diathesis-stress theories of schizophrenia actually make very few testable predictions. Moreover, the predictions that do flow from the theories generally lack precision or have track records that seem sparse and spotty. Where evidence is available, it does not support many of the ideas advanced to explain the root problems of schizophrenia research. Where evidence is missing, it may not be forthcoming until major advances in measurement and technology are achieved. Yet there are some concepts of value, as well, and some that can be translated into predictions in the near future.

With respect to the neurogenesis of schizophrenia, Meehl (1990b) is the only theorist to eschew dopamine-based explanations and to propose a defect that occurs in every neuron in the schizotaxic brain, a defect that causes synaptic "slippage" so that neurons fire less selectively than in the normal brain. On the face of it, this seems a risky and even an unlikely prediction, because hypokrisia is held be present in all nerve cells. Meehl also briefly describes predictions that follow from hypokrisia theory. However, he regards the theory as untestable and the predictions as technically and ethically unfeasible at this time. Therefore, there is no track record to appraise, and this aspect of his theory remains unevaluated.

To some extent, technical limitations also figure in Weinberger's ideas about neurogenesis. His formulation includes the concept of depleted prefrontal dopamine function as one of the abnormalities that underlie the illness. However, turning this idea into a testable prediction requires a means of measuring dopamine activity in living patients. Currently available positron emission tomography and spinal fluid biochemistry technologies do not possess the resolving power to detect the relatively diffuse dopamine activity of the prefrontal cortex. The same technical limitation applies to the other aspect of Weinberger's neurogenic hypothesis, the putative excess of activity in medial temporal dopaminergic regions.

Walker and Diforio's (1997) formulation of neurogenesis also posits a dopamine-related excess in the illness, and this raises the same technical questions about the feasibility of detecting neurotransmitter activity in living subjects, especially during childhood and adolescence prior to illness onset. Thus, it is one thing to suggest a prediction, risky or otherwise, but it is another matter to actually test the prediction. At the same time, predictions may run afoul of existing evidence. Walker and Diforio posit damage to the hippocampus in their theory of schizophrenic neurogenesis. In this case, there is an extensive neuroimaging literature on hippocampal volumes in schizophrenia patients and a smaller post-mortem literature (see chapter 5). A risky and fairly precise prediction would propose hippocampal damage in every case of schizophrenia. However, the available evidence, reviewed in previous chapters, indicates that this prediction is wrong. On the other hand, research has not focused on stress hormone receptor sites in the hippocampus and the relation of these sites to activity in the hypothalamic-pituitary-adrenal stress system. It may be that abnormalities at the receptor level do not manifest themselves in overall volume reductions. Still, the immediate future will not resolve the issue. Research at microscopic levels in human subjects will be limited to post-mortem study until much higher degrees of spatial resolution and more selective receptor ligands are available for use with living patients.

Perhaps the most useful idea for neurogenesis developed by Walker and Diforio is the connection between stress hormone activity and dopamine. Several aspects of this proposition are probably testable in humans or in animals. For example, their theory predicts reciprocal enhancement between stress hormones and dopamine activity. These hormones are relatively easy to measure, although it is more difficult to determine whether they are active in brain regions implicated in schizophrenia. Hence, one approach is to measure glucocorticoids in high-risk subjects during adolescence and to hypothesize that those with the highest levels will develop schizophrenia. The major practical limitation in such an approach is the time that has to elapse between initial measurement of stress hormone levels and the period of peak liability for schizophrenia in the third decade of life. Yet Walker et al. (1998) have already provided data that tie cortisol levels to psychopathology, if not to schizophrenia. In addition, animal research may be helpful on this question. In animals it should be possible to look in detail at predicted relations between, say, dopamine receptor densities, the hypothalamic-pituitary-adrenal system, and the hippocampus. This kind of basic research can determine whether the neural components proposed as substrates for schizophrenia make biochemical and behavioral sense.

On balance, therefore, it appears that the model proposed by Walker and Diforio offers the most opportunities for developing testable predictions and workable research strategies for the neurogenesis problem.

Each of the three diathesis-stress theories also has something to say about symptom formation, although this is minimal in the case of Walker and Diforio's model. Both Weinberger and Walker and Diforio rely on dopamine-based accounts of symptoms, and they have little that is new to offer in this regard. Weinberger invokes the popular notion that negative symptoms reflect diminished prefrontal activation and positive symptoms reflect enhanced temporal-limbic activation. Walker and Diforio depart somewhat from a complete reliance on dopamine, in that they raise the possibility that negative symptoms like withdrawal and disinterest may be responses that occur as the person at risk for schizophrenia tries to cope with high stress levels. However, they do not suggest predictions to test this idea, and it does not seem to be central to their model. Accordingly, the view of symptom formation represented in these two theories rises or falls on the basis of the existing evidence relating to the role of dopamine in schizophrenia. The adequacy of this evidence has already been criticized (see chapter 6), and its track record is inconsistent at best. On the positive side, new ideas continue to emerge regarding the involvement of dopamine in the neurogenesis and symptoms of the illness, and some of these may bear fruit in the near future (Cohen & Servan-Schreiber, 1992, 1993).

Meehl's (1990b) view of how symptoms develop in schizophrenia is markedly at variance with the dopamine-based accounts. In the first place, he rejects the primacy given to positive symptoms in the *DSM-IV* (1994). He resurrects Bleuler's (1950) ideas concerning associative loosening as a "fundamental" symptom and delusions and positive symptoms as "accessory" symptoms. He also argues that delusions and some hallucinations, like hearing voices, are extreme forms of irrational mental processes that occur in healthy people. Other aspects of symptoms can be understood as the result of the schizophrenia patient's attempt to explain strange sensory experiences that derive from integrative deficits and hypokrisia. If there is a primary symptom of schizophrenia in Meehl's view of the illness, it is probably cognitive slippage, the mental consequence of indiscriminant and exaggerated neural activity.

Is it possible to propose a risky and precise prediction based on Meehl's ideas about symptom formation? Probably not. First of all, given his views on etiology and heterogeneity, not every patient in a schizophrenia research sample will have "true" schizophrenia. Therefore, the underlying hypokrisic defect, along with cognitive slippage, will occur in only a proportion of such a sample. Even if his rough estimates regarding the relative proportions of schizophrenia and its phenocopies are used as guidelines, there is no "gold standard" test for cognitive slippage. Although technical inadequacy does not invalidate a theory, it can prevent the development of predictions based on the theory and prevent an evaluation of the theory itself. This appears to be the case at present with respect to Meehl's ideas about symptoms.

Meehl takes a much more detailed position on etiology than either Weinberger or Walker and Diforio. Instead of simply arguing for the importance of both environmental and genetic influences on schizophrenia, he takes a strong position on a single major gene for the illness. He also argues for the existence of many genes that can aggravate or compensate for the basic predisposition toward schizophrenia. Moreover, the environment is essential to Meehl's view of the illness, in that it punishes most of the peculiar behavioral features of the schizotypal person. Without this increasingly aversive relationship with the social environment, schizophrenia does not develop. Conversely, the environment may provide support and positive reinforcement if the schizotypal person is fortunate enough to possess socially valued traits like high intelligence or physical attractiveness. In this way the environment helps prevent the emergence of the illness in some people who carry the gene for schizophrenia.

This is an imaginative account of etiology, but deriving testable predictions from the theory is again a challenge. Meehl acknowledges that single major gene theories have not been supported and indeed are regarded as incorrect by much of the research community. However, he maintains that the role of mitigating polygenetic factors must also be considered in evaluating his theory. This idea is also very hard to test. Many behavioral and temperament traits may influence each other, as well as influencing the development of a spectrum of disorders. Finding the schizophrenic needle in this psychiatric haystack will require a major interdisciplinary research effort.

If Meehl provides the most detail on questions of etiology, he provides the least on the question of why schizophrenia has a characteristic onset in late adolescence and early adulthood. It may be that the various genetic and environmental influences he describes have their greatest impact at this time, but the case is not made clearly. Weinberger uses the concept of increased stress and maturational changes to account for the timing of schizophrenia. Walker and Diforio provide the most explicit description of a mechanism that joins environmental stress with the biology of the illness. Their model introduces stress hormones and maturational changes in the hypothalamic–pituitary–adrenal system to explain not only the neurogenesis of schizophrenia but also the timing of illness onset. The theory predicts that young untreated patients experiencing their first episode of illness should have very high levels of glucocorticoids. To some extent high stress hormone levels reflect normal maturational changes, but in the person with vulnerability for schizophrenia they exist in synergy with abnormal dopamine activity. If stress hormones are important in determining when the illness strikes, it should be possible to assess this importance by studying high-risk, patient, and healthy samples in terms of life-span changes in these hormones.

Unfortunately, Walker and Diforio make no real contribution to the debate on heterogeneity and what it means about schizophrenia. In contrast, both Meehl and Weinberger take the position that there is one fundamental disease state with a common neural diathesis underlying schizophrenia's apparent diversity. However, Meehl argues for the existence of phenocopies that do not share the neural basis for schizotaxia. These phenocopies present superficially like schizophrenia, but they are qualitatively different. Weinberger holds that a common neural diathesis for schizophrenia exists in all patients, but in varying degrees, giving rise to a misleading impression of multiple disease states.

Meehl's theory certainly has implications for solving the heterogeneity puzzle. His theory predicts that only a proportion of patients in a sample of *DSM-IV* (1994) schizophrenia will demonstrate cognitive slippage—the hallmark of hypokrisia and "true" schizophrenia. The remaining patients will have the polygenic features that aggravate the expression of schizotaxia—traits like social introversion and passivity—but not the schizotaxia trait itself. Unfortunately, in the absence of sensitive measures of cognitive slippage or hypokrisia, it is hard to parse the true illness from its phenocopies. Moreover, the effects of medication, hospitalization, social stigma, and chronic mental illness may frustrate looking for the polygenic traits in a patient population. Therefore, this is another aspect of Meehl's theory that has explanatory value but must await improvements in psychometrics, cognitive science, and neurophysiology before it can be tested in a meaningful way.

Weinberger and his associates (Goldberg & Weinberger, 1995; Daniel et al., 1991) are strong advocates of a single disease model for schizophrenia. They have argued that a continuum model of the schizophrenia neural diathesis predicts data distributions that have a single mode or "peak" when studied with techniques like mixture analysis. If there is more than one schizophrenic neural mechanism, it should reveal itself in complex, multipeaked distributions. One test of this idea considered a rather unlikely candidate for the neural diathesis of schizophrenia—ventricular enlargement. However, the technique of mixture analysis used in this study (Daniel et al., 1991) could be applied to many other findings with extensive databases, including eye movement abnormalities, evoked potentials, and tissue volume densities. To be sure, there are some doubts about the reliability and validity of mixture analysis in uncovering complex distributions and subpopulations. Moreover, some of the research areas of greatest value for understanding schizophrenia, including post-mortem receptor and cytoarchitectural studies, have very small cumulative data pools. Still, the prediction of single distributions seems to be an idea that is more testable than many conjectures in schizophrenia theory.

In considering all three theories, it seems fair to say that they often rely on existing evidence that is of questionable validity to build their arguments. The most obvious example of this is the continuing reliance on dopamine abnormalities in relation to neurogenesis, symptom formation, and onset, despite the often weak and inconsistent evidence in support of such abnormalities. On the other hand, the introduction of more novel or alternate concepts, like hypo-krisia, neural dysplasia, and maturational processes, entails ideas and variables that are hard to test and measure. While the future may remedy technical limi-tations, it is not possible to evaluate theories based on promissory notes. Still, some recent ideas, like the hypothesized role of stress hormones in schizophre-nia, may lead to predictions and insights that can be implemented with cur-rently available research strategies.

But where does this leave the present understanding of schizophrenia? The track record of diathesis-stress theories is often inadequate. There are interest-ing, provocative, and perhaps helpful ideas that require examination in future re-search. Yet theoretical work is enormously difficult. The theorist has to stay true to what is known about the illness but also propose new concepts that lead to predictions that can be tested. None of the diathesis-stress theories are really successful in this regard. Therefore, it is necessary to return a final time to the evidence and to reconsider it comprehensively and in light of what the difficult task of theory construction has revealed about the nature of schizophrenia and its science.

9
●●●●●●●●●●●●●●●●●●●●●●●●●●●●●●

THE END OF THE
BEGINNING

Now this is not the end. It is not even the beginning of the
end. But it is, perhaps, the end of the beginning.
—Winston S. Churchill, 1943

Sober words from the past and from a different kind of war. But they may also
apply to the scientific war on schizophrenia: a war that uses questions as weapons;
a war where victory will mean understanding and hope. How and why does the
brain make the mind of madness? How can schizophrenia be defined, grasped,
encompassed, and bound to neuroscience? These are the questions that have
dogged schizophrenia researchers since the turn of the century. They are also
the questions that have followed the course of this book through the study of
symptoms, disease markers, the frontal and temporal brain systems, through
neurochemistry and neurodevelopment, and through diathesis-stress theories of
the illness. Yet the book also asks its own more reflective and critical questions.
There is a story within the story of schizophrenia science. How much do we
really know about the mind and brain of madness, how strong and consistent
is the evidence, and what does it tell us about the nature and the future of the
illness? In this chapter I will try to answer these questions.

The Neuroscience Sweepstakes

The first challenge for this chapter is descriptive: to outline in general terms
what the accumulated research findings say about schizophrenia, its outstanding
biological and psychological features, its scientific anatomy. It is important to assess what is known and not known about the illness. And it is important to as-

sess the security of this knowledge. The second challenge is imaginative. Chapter 8 provided some theoretical views of schizophrenia. Yet these theories were developed without the benefit of a quantitative synthesis of findings, a synthesis that spans 2 decades and many fields of research. The synthesis begs the question: What kind of illness produces a body of neuroscience findings like those summarized in this book?

To meet the descriptive challenge, I first cast 54 research literatures from the previous chapters into a ranked order of average effect sizes. In other words, I ranked findings on the basis of their evidential strength, their ability to distinguish people with schizophrenia from healthy people. Each average d describes the magnitude of difference between schizophrenia patients and healthy control participants in terms of some aspect of behavior or biology. However, I included only literatures based on at least 100 patients and healthy subjects and those based on more than a single study. In addition, I excluded findings that did not focus on diagnosed schizophrenia patients. This meant eliminating studies that compared high-risk or preschizophrenia children and adolescents to normal children and adolescents (see chapter 7). I also excluded studies of cognitive processes in patients with very specific symptoms, like persecutory delusions or thought disorder (see chapter 2). These patients cannot be considered representative of the patient population as a whole, and that is what I wanted to represent—patients with the schizophrenia diagnosis, not just those with a particular symptom. The summaries include 33 averaged effect sizes that reflect the strength of neurobiological differences between patients and healthy people, 13 that reflect primarily cognitive differences, and 8 that represent psychophysiological differences. Neurobiological differences include neurochemical, and neuroanatomical abnormalities. The cognitive differences include memory, perception, language, and related processes. Psychophysiological findings comprise eye tracking, evoked potentials, and cognitive activation conditions from functional brain scanning studies.

These compiled findings, or research literatures, accumulated since 1980 from thousands of patients and healthy research participants, represent a body of evidence that can be used to answer questions about schizophrenia and its science. For example, is there any biological or behavioral abnormality that is shared by all people with the illness? Research on disease causes and etiology carries with it expectations for large effect sizes. Moderate and weak effects may indicate the discovery of risk factors, secondary and contributing causes, or what Meehl (1990a) calls "nuisance" correlation (see also chapter 1). So consider the effect sizes of the individual literatures. None of the literatures in any of the chapter summaries even approach values like $d = 3.0$, which would indicate a powerful (93%) separation of patient and healthy distributions. Thus, to make a long answer short, there are no abnormalities that occur in all people with a diagnosis of schizophrenia.

However, there are some large effects. The most powerful replicated neuroscience finding in schizophrenia research involves the P50 evoked potential waveform. Recall from chapter 3 that when healthy people are presented with two "clicks" separated by an interval of half a second, a positive evoked potential waveform is produced by the brain in response to each click, and the amplitude of the second response is normally smaller than the first. Perhaps this reflects the brain's ability to "gate" or dampen the effect of identical sensory events when they are repeated within a very short time span. From a psychological, learning-based perspective, the reduced second waveform indexes habituation to the click. Yet many patients with schizophrenia respond almost as strongly to the second click as to the first. Therein lies the abnormality. It is as if the brain does not realize that the sound has already occurred or as if the second sound is perceived in isolation from the first. Adler and associates (Adler et al., 1998) have speculated that the causes of the P50 abnormality are rooted in receptors for the neurotransmitter acetylcholine. A deficiency of one receptor subtype in learning-related regions like the hippocampus might underlie the brain's inability to gate successive sounds. Adler and associates also argue that a deficit in the same receptor could effect neural cell growth and development, as well as sensory and information processing. This in turn ties in with neurodevelopmental conjectures about schizophrenia. An effect of the magnitude obtained for the P50 ($d = 1.55$) corresponds to an idealized patient-control distribution overlap of about 28%. Put another way, perhaps 72% of schizophrenia patients have abnormal P50 evoked potential responses. Accordingly, this seemingly arcane neurobehavioral mechanism wins the neuroscience sweepstakes. It is the single most sensitive indicator of schizophrenic illness in the published literature surveyed in this book.

The P50 effect is followed immediately by the finding that post-mortem schizophrenic brain tissue has elevated densities of the dopamine D4 receptor ($d = 1.48$). However, this body of evidence has been severely questioned. Many researchers in the field no longer regard the evidence for dopamine D4 abnormalities as convincing, because alternate ways of estimating the receptor yield negligible results (see chapter 6). It may be best to pass this finding by or at least to view it with extreme skepticism. In any case, it is followed very closely in overall strength by the deficit in verbal learning and memory. Effect sizes in this range ($d = 1.41$) mean that perhaps two-thirds of schizophrenia patients and healthy people can be distinguished from each other on the basis of verbal memory performance. On the other hand, perhaps a third of the patients have memory scores that are in normal ranges. This finding reflects the total number of words recalled over repeated trials rather than specific aspects of performance like retention over time or number of recall errors. Memory impairment is one of the most common consequences of any kind of brain insult, and general deficits like this one imply a correspondingly general kind of brain dysfunction, albeit one focused on the left, or language-dominant, cerebral hemisphere. The next largest effect is another dopamine-related abnormality, this time reflecting elevated dopamine D2 receptors in post-mortem patient tissue ($d = 1.37$). However, once again, the validity of the finding is questionable. These post-mortem findings all reflect results obtained from patient brain tissue that was exposed to dopamine-blocking medication. It is very likely that the brain adapts to dopamine blockade by growing more receptors (see chapter 6). Hence the average effect size probably reflects this adaptation to drug exposure as much as it reflects the biological basis of schizophrenia.

The general verbal memory finding is complemented by several large effects (i.e., $d \geq 1$) for deficits in other aspects of cognition. These aspects include deficient attention and perception (vulnerability to backward visual masking, dichotic listening, eye tracking) and impaired word generation and executive ability (Tower problem-solving tests). Similarly, lower general intellectual ability, as measured by IQ tests, language comprehension (Token Test), and the Stroop effect, also yield average effects that are close to $d = 1.0$. Just below this level of evidence is the literature on cognitive tasks used to "activate" the brain during positron emission tomography studies ($d = .80$). Many cognitive functions seem to be affected to some degree by schizophrenia, and the underlying brain disorder of the illness must be correspondingly widespread and extensive in nature.

It is natural to expect that cellular, neurochemical, and neuroanatomical features of schizophrenia should yield large effect sizes when compared with normal values. But the only other biological finding in this top group of large effects is the tendency for upper layers of the frontal cortex to show decreased numbers of neurons when compared with normal tissue ($d = 1.12$). This kind of result is consistent with prenatal origins for schizophrenia, perhaps during the second trimester of pregnancy. The finding may reflect arrested cell migration that failed to populate fully the upper layers of the cortex with neurons. The companion finding, increased densities in lower layers, has a slightly smaller effect size ($d = .87$) and is found further down the list. In addition, there are literatures in this range ($d = .86 - .92$) that relate to the hippocampus, a major substrate for memory formation, and these literatures are also based on post-mortem brain studies. The difference between normal and "drug-free" schizophrenic dopamine D2 densities is also found here ($d = .93$). Recall from chapter 6 that the term "drug-free" refers to tissue obtained from patients who were not receiving antipsychotic medication for days or weeks before death. In most cases the patients received dopamine-blocking drugs at some time in their lives.

Up to this point the reported abnormalities probably occur in 50–70% of the schizophrenia patient population. Below a benchmark of around $d = .8$, the findings increasingly represent large degrees of overlap and therefore poor discrimination between patients and healthy people. It is here where most of the brain-imaging studies are found. Many studies based on magnetic resonance and positron emission techniques yield effect sizes between $d = .7$ and $d = .1$. In other words, abnormal volume, metabolism, and blood flow in the temporal and frontal lobes occur in relatively small proportions of people with schizophrenia. Generally speaking, these imaging techniques yield smaller findings than techniques based on post-mortem tissue analysis. Indeed, it is possible to test the relative strength of evidence in different domains. Fourteen of the collected research literatures use post-mortem tissue analysis, and 18 use neuroimaging techniques like positron emission and magnetic resonance of living people. The average effect for all post-mortem literatures is $d = .78$, and for all neuroimaging literatures it is $d = .42$. The confidence intervals associated with each average effect (.21, .08) indicate that the post-mortem literatures yield significantly more powerful findings than the imaging literatures. This differential sensitivity applies even when the same brain structures are measured. For example, average effects for hippocampal volume reduction are larger when measured post mortem ($d = .92$) than when measured with magnetic resonance scans of living patients ($d = .41$). On the other hand, brain imaging can often escape the contaminating influence of antipsychotic medication exposure. This is made possible by the recruitment of drug-naive patients who are experiencing their first psychotic episode.

Also in this range of moderate and weak effects are more findings relevant to the developmental hypothesis of schizophrenia. Small proportions of patients sustained pregnancy and birth complications ($d = .32$) and endured aversive life experiences prior to illness ($d = .33$). In addition, findings relating to glutamate deficits in schizophrenia ($d = .57, .40, .38$), an alternative or complement to dopamine-based accounts, are found in this region of small effects. Thereafter the findings diminish rapidly into theoretical and statistical insignificance.

On balance, accordingly, this extensive, if not exhaustive, review of neuroscience and schizophrenia reveals a series of findings that range from moderately powerful effects to trivial ones. But the average size of an effect, the extent to which patients and healthy people differ, is only one aspect of evidence. The other key aspect is consistency and replication. If the same aspect of brain biology or function is measured in new groups of patients and control participants, does the same finding emerge? To be sure, findings may be consistently small as well as consistently large. However, in either case, if the confidence interval, a kind of margin of error within which the average can be expected to fall, includes zero, a researcher cannot be sure that the finding will be reproduced. Most people are aware of confidence intervals in the form of opinion polls and their ubiquitous rider that results are considered accurate but only within a number of percentage points 19 times out of 20. The same caution must be applied to the averaged statistics that represent each neuroscience literature. It turns out that in some cases, confidence intervals around the averages come perilously close to zero and in some cases they embrace it, indicating a very unreliable body of findings. This too is an aspect of evidence, and it constrains the security of knowledge about schizophrenia.

To index the consistency of neuroscience findings, I ranked the 54 average effects on the basis of their 95% confidence intervals. The smaller the interval the better. I kept track of every time this margin of error included zero when placed around the average effect. Considering the effects in this way shows that it is quite possible for negligible findings to be highly consistent. This applies to the evidence that people with schizophrenia are born more frequently in winter months. The average effect is so small ($d = .05$) that the patient−control overlap in birth months must be close to 96%. Yet the 17 studies that contribute to this average are very consistent in their findings, and this is indexed by the tiny confidence interval (.03). Therefore, the winter births average is an accurate and stable but trivial value. In contrast, the findings for abnormally low levels of homovanillic acid in cerebrospinal fluid, an index of dopamine activity, are both small in average size ($d = .11$) and so inconsistent that the bounds on accuracy include zero (i.e., $d = -.13$ to $d = .35$). And this is not to mention that the effect size reflects a deficiency of the metabolite in patients when an excess was predicted. Overall, out of the 54 neuroscience research literatures 14, or 26%, have margins of error that include zero. For the most part these unstable bodies of evidence are weak findings where the average effect is small and already close to zero. However, there are a few cases where the average d is moderate or even fairly large and still the interval includes zero. For example, the average finding for reduced numbers of serotonin receptors in the prefrontal cortex of schizophrenic brain samples is $d = .72$. However, the findings are extremely variable, and this variability yields a large margin of error. The true average effect for this literature may be as low as $d = -.02$ or as high as $d = 1.46$. In other words, a researcher may find excesses *or* deficits in serotonin receptors in the frontal brain tissue of people who had schizophrenia during life. The extreme instability of the cytoarchitectural literature is even more striking. Post-mortem tissue analysis reveals that on average at least half of the schizophrenia samples show cellular disorganization and disarray in the hippocampus ($d = .90$). Yet the findings are so variable that the true average d may be anywhere between zero and 1.8. Even when the expected values for the average effect do not actually include zero, the sheer size of the interval may still indicate a great deal of inconsistency in the findings. This certainly applies to the increased density of dopamine D4 (confidence interval = .94) and D2 receptors (confidence interval = .65) in schizophrenia and to the decrease in cells in the upper layers of frontal cortex (confidence interval = .87).

Therefore, both the average strength and the consistency of findings in a research literature are useful ways of evaluating evidence in schizophrenia science. And with both considerations in mind, it is possible to generate tables like table

Table 9.1 The most powerful and reliable neuroscience findings in schizophrenia research

Finding	Mean d	Confidence Interval	N
1. P50 evoked potential "gating" defect	1.55	1.21–1.89	20
2. Impaired general verbal memory	1.41	1.20–1.62	31
3. Vulnerability to backward visual masking	1.27	.78–1.76	18
4. Impaired attention in dichotic listening	1.16	.82–1.50	11
5. Impaired general intellectual ability	1.10	.86–1.34	35
6. Reduced ability to generate words	1.09	.92–1.26	27
7. Continuous Performance Test	1.04	.90–1.18	29
8. Saccadic frequency in eye tracking	1.03	.56–1.50	14

Note: The table shows average effect sizes (Cohen's *d*) in absolute values, corrected for sample size for each research literature as well as the 95% confidence interval for the average *d* and the number of studies (N) contributing to each meta-analysis. Average effects greater than or equal to *d* = 1.0 imply that more than 50% of schizophrenia patients demonstrate the reported abnormality. All eight research literatures have confidence intervals for the mean that are less than 50 decimal points.

9.1 and table 9.2, which represent the most powerful *and* most consistent as well as the weakest bodies of evidence in the neuroscience of schizophrenia. The research literatures in table 9.1 all obtained average *d* values greater than or equal to one and hence represent abnormalities that probably occur in a substantial majority of patients with the illness. But in addition, their margins of error do not exceed half of an effect size on either side of the average. Hence moderate to fairly large findings will almost always occur in these research fields. Consideration of table 9.1 shows that only eight bodies of evidence make the grade in terms of both strength and consistency. And further consideration reveals that there is a remarkable commonality among these literatures. They all involve cognitive and perceptual differences between schizophrenia patients and healthy people. Six of the eight are purely cognitive findings, obtained with tasks that require learning, reasoning, selective attention, visual or auditory perception, and expressive language. The other two, the P50 evoked potential and the saccadic frequency score from eye-tracking tests, use a physiological measurement to index a cognitive or mental event.

The complementary table of weakest literatures also has a commonality in that each entry is exclusively biological in nature. Six of the eight literatures have confidence intervals that include zero, the hallmark of questionable evidence. Part of this instability may be due to the small number of studies comprising literatures like maternal exposure to influenza or post-mortem glutamate assays. Margins of error are directly influenced by the number of contributing studies as well as by the variability of the findings themselves. Still, four unstable literatures in table 9.2 are based on at least 10 studies. Moreover, even when stability or the number of contributing studies is not a problem, the weakness of the average effect is striking.

The apparent strength and consistency of cognitive abnormalities in schizo-

Table 9.2 The weakest neuroscience findings in schizophrenia research

Finding	Mean d	Confidence Interval	N
1. Maternal exposure to influenza	.02	0–.04	4
2. Excess winter births and later illness	.05	.02–.08	17
3. Excess presynaptic glutamate sites	.08	−.14–.30	5
4. Deficient homovanillic acid levels	.11	−.13–.35	11
5. Left temporal lobe resting metabolism	.13	−.29–.55	11
6. Low hippocampal metabolism/blood flow	.25	−.23–.73	10
7. Low left temporal lobe resting blood flow	.25	−.02–.52	10
8. Reduced left temporal lobe volume	.25	.15–.35	25

Note: The table shows average effect sizes (Cohen's d) in absolute values, corrected for samples size for research literatures with a mean d less than .30. Confidence Interval is the 95% confidence interval for the mean d, and N is the number of studies contributing to the meta-analysis. Confidence intervals that include zero indicate highly unstable research literatures. The glutamate literature is based on post-mortem studies, the metabolism and blood flow literatures are based on positron emission tomography, and the temporal lobe volume literature is based on magnetic resonance imaging.

phrenia contrasts with the apparent weakness and inconsistency of many biological findings, and this prompts a question. Is there a systematic relationship between how strong the evidence is on the one hand and whether the evidence is cognitive or biological on the other hand? To answer this question I divided the 54 evidence summaries into the three groups mentioned at the outset. Recall that the largest group comprises 33 research literatures that are exclusively biological in nature. This includes all of the structural brain-imaging research, all of the post-mortem receptor assays, most possible developmental insults, and all of the positron tomography carried out with patients in a "resting" state. The next largest group consists of the 13 literatures that reflect exclusively cognitive and perceptual differences between patients and healthy people. These differences always involve test scores or performance indices that are based directly on behavior. Finally, there are the eight effect sizes that are psychophysiological in nature. They all require participants to engage in mental activity of some kind but also use a biological response to the activity as the measurement of interest. This group of eight literatures comprises studies where participants had to, say, attend to a moving stimulus and undergo concurrent measurement of their smooth pursuit eye movements. It also includes the evoked potential literatures using the P300 paradigm, where participants listen for novel events and produce positive electrical brain voltages in response to these events.

I have cast the results of this division of evidence into three graphs in figure 9.1. The top pair of distributions is based on the cognitive effect sizes. The average cognitive effect is $d = .99$, and it yields the degree of hypothetical overlap between patients and healthy people, about 45%, shown in the figure. The next best separation of schizophrenia patients and healthy people is achieved by the psychophysiological findings, with an average d of .78. Roughly half of pa-

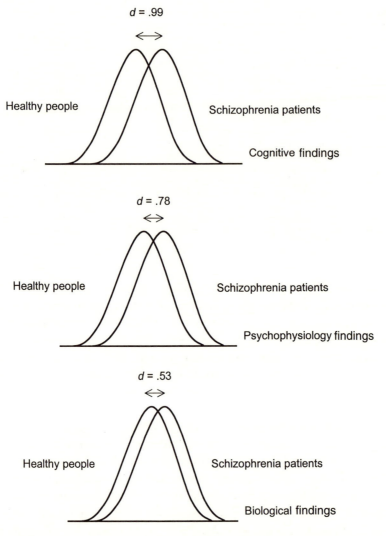

Figure 9.1. Cognitive, psychophysiological, and biological differences between schizophrenia patients and healthy people. The top pair of idealized distributions shows the averaged meta-analytic results for comparisons of cognitive processes like memory, perception, language, and attention. The effect size corresponds to a distribution overlap of about 45%. The second pair of distributions reflects average patient–control differences in eye tracking, evoked potential, and cognitive activation brain-scan studies. These distributions overlap by about 54%. The last pair reflects meta-analytic findings on biological differences, including brain structure, physiology, and neurochemistry. The estimated distribution overlap is about 65%. The cognitive differences are significantly greater than the biological differences between schizophrenia patients and healthy people.

tients could be considered indistinguishable from healthy people in eye tracking or evoked potential recordings or other psychophysiological measurements. The poorest discrimination is achieved by the neurobiological findings,
with an average effect of $d = .53$. In this case roughly 65% of the patients and
healthy people show similar kinds of cellular, neurochemical, or neuroanatomical characteristics.

If statistical tests are applied to the results in figure 9.1, they reveal that the
cognitive findings are significantly larger than the neurobiological results. The
psychophysiological literatures occupy a kind of middle ground. However, if
the same tests are applied to the stability findings and confidence intervals discussed previously, the differences are not significant. Hence cognitive and psychophysiological evidence is more powerful but not necessarily more consistent
than the biological evidence. Still, when the prevailing consistency level is combined with the small effect sizes of many findings in neurobiology, there is another pattern that emerges in the results. Out of 14 confidence intervals that include zero when they are placed around the average effect, 13 are found in the
neurobiological evidence. Only one occurs in the psychophysiological results,
and none occur in the cognitive findings. Thus, almost 40% of the neurobiological evidence on schizophrenia is so weak and unstable that the interval
within which differences between patients and healthy people are likely to fall
includes zero.

Within the domain of the neurobiological literatures the neuroimaging and
post-mortem studies contribute differentially to weakness and instability. Thus
evidence from post-mortem literatures (average $d = .78$) is significantly more
powerful than evidence from neuroimaging literatures (average $d = .42$). The
magnetic resonance literatures seem especially weak in their average effects ($d =$
.37). Yet the opposite holds for the stability of evidence. The average confidence interval for neuroimaging evidence (.30) is significantly smaller than the
average confidence interval for post-mortem evidence (.60). Part of this is because there are fewer studies in the post-mortem literatures. Thus, neuroimaging evidence is based on an average of about 15 studies for each average effect,
whereas post-mortem literatures draw on an average of only 6.5 studies for
each effect. Psychophysiological evidence has the strongest study base, with almost 23 studies for each average d, but the cognitive literatures are also well supported and stable (average confidence interval = .32), with 18 studies for each
average effect. All in all, biological literatures that are stable tend to be weak in
the magnitude of their findings, while those that have larger effect sizes tend to
be unstable. In comparison, most cognitive literatures are both fairly powerful
and fairly stable.

Accordingly, figure 9.1 does illustrate a systematic relationship between evidential strength and the extent to which findings are psychological or biological in nature. Regardless of the specific research question under study, the stronger

the psychological content, the greater the difference between schizophrenia patients and healthy research participants. Hence it is fair to say that schizophrenia manifests itself to a greater extent in defective cognition than in defective biology.

This apparent superiority of cognitive over biological evidence is puzzling. What does it really mean? After all, if schizophrenia is a brain disease, direct measurement of brain biology should yield the strongest differences between people with and without the disease. Perhaps the sensitivity of psychological measures to the illness lies in the fact that the diagnosis of schizophrenia itself incorporates psychological information. In other words, a person will not receive the diagnosis unless they differ psychologically from the general population. So it is not surprising if the accumulated research shows that thought and perception differentiate schizophrenia patients from healthy people. In a sense, cognitive findings simply recapitulate the diagnosis of the illness. In contrast, biological measures are not used in diagnostic decision-making, except to rule out medical disorders. They do not in any sense recapitulate the information used in the diagnosis of schizophrenia. Therefore, biological measures do not discriminate patients and controls as well as psychological measures do.

An analogous situation exists for cognitive and neurobiological findings in Alzheimer's disease (Zakzanis, 1998). Memory tests distinguish dementia patients from healthy old people much more efficiently than brain scans do. But then memory impairment figures in the dementia diagnosis in the first place. And even the best magnetic resonance machines cannot detect the microscopic cellular changes that underlie the disease. So it makes sense that cognitive measurement is more sensitive than biological measurement in at least some kinds of illness.

Yet it is not so easy to do away with the implications of figure 9.1. These cognitive and psychophysiological literatures use measures that do not actually figure in diagnostic decisions about schizophrenia any more than the biological measures do. Diagnosis is based on the presence of positive and negative symptoms and on the absence of alternative disorders. Tests of cognitive ability are not part of the *DSM-IV* (1994) criteria for schizophrenia. Indeed, cognitive tests generally fare poorly as predictors of the most powerful diagnostic symptoms—delusions and hallucinations (see chapter 2). Therefore, the argument that all psychological findings in schizophrenia research simply recapitulate the diagnosis is not true.

Another argument for dismissing the relative strength of psychological findings is to say that cognition is inherently more vulnerable than biology to a variety of general illness-related influences that have nothing to do with the specific nature of schizophrenia. These influences might include patient fatigue, stress, disinterest, poor general health, other psychiatric disorders, inadequate motivation, and the side effects of medication. Such influences may reduce patient scores on cognitive tests relative to healthy people and exaggerate the degree of separation between groups in the research findings. However, this argument assumes that biological aspects of patients are not under similar kinds of extraneous influence. And such an assumption is not justified in light of the compelling evidence that exposure to antipsychotic medication increases dopamine receptor densities. In comparison, medication has only slight and inconsistent influences on some cognitive tasks (Spohn & Strauss, 1989). In fact, it is hard to find anything that contaminates basic aspects of cognition in the way that medication exposure contaminates neurobiology (see chapter 6). Moreover, general health and nutritional status probably influences brain physiology and structure at least as much as it influences cognition. For example, the rate of tobacco smoking in schizophrenia patients is at least double the rate found in the general population (Hughes, Hatsukami, Mitchell, & Dahlgren, 1986). The active ingredients of tobacco, like nicotine, have widespread and significant physiological effects on a person, and these effects may amplify patient–control differences in biology independently of the schizophrenic disease process (see Fowler et al., 1996). In other words, a case could be made that biology is extremely vulnerable to influences that have nothing to do with the nature of schizophrenia. To be sure, there is evidence that cognitive and psychophysiological performance can also be effected by general clinical factors that are unrelated to schizophrenia (e.g., see chapter 3). But there is little reason to assume that such factors only influence psychology or that they only act to amplify and not reduce differences between schizophrenia patients and healthy people. Finally, if psychological processes are somehow inherently vulnerable to the presence or absence of extraneous factors, psychology should yield correspondingly variable and unstable findings. But this is simply not the case. The cognitive and psychophysiological findings underlying figure 9.1 are as stable and consistent as the biological findings based on brain imaging and more stable than findings based on post-mortem analysis. Hence it is difficult to dismiss in a facile way the relatively powerful validity of cognitive brain function in distinguishing schizophrenia patients and healthy people.

In summary, this extensive appraisal across many areas of neuroscience research reveals no common abnormality in all cases of schizophrenic illness. The strongest, most consistent evidence suggests that 50–70% of schizophrenia patients are deficient in sensory gating, perception, attention, eye tracking, memory, and other aspects of cognitive brain function. In comparison, most of the neurobiological abnormalities in the illness probably occur in a minority of patients. Moreover, close to 40% of the biological findings are so weak and variable that they may represent minor, unimportant, or chance abnormalities with no intrinsic link to schizophrenia. Clearly, the cognitive evidence wins the neuroscience sweepstakes. Yet even the cognitive findings do not characterize *all* patients with the illness. So now the imaginative challenge looms. What kind of

neurological illness manifests itself so incompletely in any aspect of brain structure and function? What kind of disease is more distinguished by its psychology
than by its biology?

The Promissory Note

One way of understanding the neuroscience evidence on the schizophrenia
puzzle is to say that it just reflects an illness that has received inadequate study,
with inadequate instruments, over an inadequate period of time. Researchers
are chasing a subtle neurological aberration, possibly like the one suggested by
Meehl (1990b), in the way individual neurons work. And they are chasing this
subtle defect with imaging techniques that cannot provide the detailed level of
observation needed to find what is wrong with the schizophrenic brain. At the
same time, the fine-grained analysis offered by post-mortem techniques is con-
founded by the fact that patient brain tissue was exposed to antipsychotic medication. However, in the near future, better receptor-binding ligands will become available, and the current generation of brain scanners will be replaced by
instruments that provide much more anatomical detail about the brain in living people with the illness. Bodies of evidence will accrue based on functional
magnetic resonance imaging and spectroscopy techniques. These techniques
index brain activity as well as brain structure but with higher spatial resolution
than positron emission scanning can achieve (see McCarley, Hsiao, Freedman,
Pfefferbaum, & Donchin, 1996). This century will see the extension of such
techniques to children at high risk for schizophrenia. The completion of the
human genome project and the development of neurogenetics will reveal the
genes that are linked to the illness. The gene products that turn the normal
nervous system into the schizophrenic nervous system will be identified and
understood. In other words, more research will yield the strong and consistent
evidence that is still lacking. Perhaps the prophecies of breakthrough by the end
of the old millenium were wrong, but neuroscience can promise the answers
early in the new millennium.

There are indeed some reasons for accepting this scientific promissory note,
especially in terms of technical advances in observation and measurement and
how such advances may furnish more powerful evidence. For example, if the
biological evidence summaries from the previous chapters are divided into
those based on brain scans of living patients and those based on microscopic
post-mortem analysis, a discrepancy emerges. The average effect size for brain
imaging studies is $d = .42$ (95% confidence interval = .08), compared with an
average $d = .78$ (95% confidence interval = .21) for post-mortem studies.
Across specific research topics, post-mortem levels of observation yield significantly more powerful findings than do observations based on brain scans of liv-

ing patients. To be sure, even the post-mortem level of observation produces, on average, findings where barely half of the schizophrenia patients are completely distinguishable from healthy people. But still, the discrepancy in evidence supports the idea that the brain will yield its secrets in relation to serious mental illness once adequately sensitive instruments are available. Perhaps breakthroughs are around the corner in fields like single nerve cell recording that are relevant to schizophrenia (Goldman-Rakic, 1999). And the history of science can supply many examples, from the telescope to the microscope, to further support the principle that technical advances and the march of time and effort will propel breakthroughs and discoveries. Thus the basic light microscope increased tremendously the resolving power and level of observation available to the naked eye, yet the advent of electron microscopes opened a world of minute natural detail far beyond the magnifying power of even the best light-based instruments. Perhaps neuroscience awaits an equivalent advance in technical capacity, with schizophrenia science as one of the first beneficiaries of the improvements.

On the other hand, better, more accurate instruments do not always produce stronger findings. For example, it was the older brain-scanning techniques like computerized axial tomography that found substantial abnormalities in the frontal brain of schizophrenia patients. In comparison, newer, more accurate techniques like magnetic resonance imaging show very small differences between patients and healthy people (Zakzanis & Heinrichs, 1999). Moreover, these differences may decline further as the resolving power of both magnetic resonance and positron emission scanning increases (Davidson, 1999). Similarly, the history of psychiatry shows that more refined genetic methods have sometimes reduced rather than enhanced the estimated heritability of schizophrenia (Gottesman, 1991, pp. 107–108). And the recent work on the neurochemistry of the illness has produced new and more complex issues and questions rather than a simple confirmation for the role of dopamine in schizophrenia (see chapter 6). It is not always the case that better instruments and increased quantity of research lead to discoveries that transform understanding in science.

In extreme form the promissory note argument holds that the relentless accretion of research findings will eventually yield the answer to the root problems of schizophrenia science. There are historical examples that support and refute this argument, and philosophers of science disagree about the ingredients of scientific discovery and progress (Kuhn, 1962; Meehl, 1990b; Popper, 1959). This argument represents one way, but not the only way, of looking at the evidential record on schizophrenia.

Multiple Disease States

There is another possibility that can account for the apparent modesty and the instability of many findings in the neuroscience sweepstakes. Perhaps the truth about schizophrenia is already there, but unrecognized. In 1984 Seeman and his associates (Seeman et al., 1984) reported post-mortem data on dopamine D2 densities in the basal ganglia of schizophrenia and control brain tissue. The distribution of dopamine receptor densities in the study was irregular, with two peaks in the schizophrenia patient sample instead of just one. The lower mode reflected an increase of 25% in the number of dopamine D2 binding sites, and the upper mode reflected an increase of 130% relative to control samples. The schizophrenia cases in each peak were similar in terms of medication history and in terms of technical aspects of tissue preparation after death. The data seemed to demonstrate that perhaps half of the patient brains were markedly abnormal in terms of receptor densities while the remaining half showed only slight elevations. Could it be that a proportion of patients has clear abnormalities in receptor densities, while the rest have small elevations, perhaps due to antipsychotic medication rather than to the disease process? In a more general sense as well, it is possible that moderate and even large effect sizes hide the existence of subpopulations of patients with different kinds of schizophrenic illness. Although few investigators report data distributions, there are other reports that also imply the existence of more than one schizophrenic disease state (e.g., Clementz et al., 1992; Iacono et al., 1992).

Thus another way of looking at the yield of neuroscience research, especially its failure to find abnormalities in all people with the illness, involves the possibility that several illnesses underlie the summarized findings reported in this book. Suppose there are different kinds of schizophrenia. One kind may involve an abnormal elevation in dopamine receptors; another kind may involve failed neuronal migration during early development; still another kind might stem from abnormal stress biology; and even more schizophrenias may exist. Each of these pathologies arises from independent genetic or environmental influences. If this scenario is true, and patients with different diseases are lumped together and given the same diagnosis, the scientific picture that emerges is bound to be one of modest and inconsistent findings, especially in terms of neurobiology. No wonder biological effect sizes seldom show that even a majority of patients actually have a suspected defect or abnormality. No wonder neurobiology findings are often hard to replicate. If there is more than one form of schizophrenic illness, more than one neurogenesis and etiology, and patients are combined into generic samples, effect sizes approximating $d = 3.0$ will never occur. Even if key aspects of one illness are detected, the presence of patients with other forms of schizophrenia in the research sample will reduce the effect size. Accordingly, the idea that schizophrenia is more than one illness and that heterogeneity of results reflects heterogeneity at every level, from genetics to cognition, is a second way of looking at the inconclusive research legacy of the last two decades. This idea may be helpful in understanding the evidence in figure 9.1 and where science should head in the future.

There is nothing new about the observation that schizophrenia is heterogeneous. Articles on schizophrenia often begin and end with cautionary statements to this effect. Increasingly, researchers and clinicians refer to the condition in plural form: the "schizophrenic disorders" (Bellak, 1979) or even the "schizophrenias" (Carson & Sanislow, 1993). Both Kraepelin (1919) and Bleuler (1950) were aware of the great clinical diversity of schizophrenia, and both pioneers thought it was an important issue in understanding the illness. Kraepelin described what he called "forms" of schizophrenia. Thus paranoid schizophrenia was considered a distinctive form of illness and contrasted with hebephrenic and catatonic forms of schizophrenia. In addition, Kraepelin was aware of the great variability in course and outcome for these patients, despite earlier impressions (Kraepelin, 1896) that they all ended in a demented "terminal state." Nonetheless, he equivocated on the implications of heterogeneity, asserting: "Whether dementia praecox in the extent here delimited represents *one uniform disease*, cannot be decided at present with certainty" (1919, p. 252).

Bleuler (1950) was more willing to consider the possibility that "dementia praecox" represented several diseases. He repeatedly referred to schizophrenia as a "group" of disorders rather than a single illness. He also divided the illness into paranoid, catatonic, hebephrenic, and simple subgroups on the basis of symptom profiles. Yet he did not believe that these separate symptom groupings were necessarily separate disease entities. Like Kraepelin, he hedged and argued that "at the present time, we cannot solve the problem of dissecting schizophrenia into its natural subdivisions"(p. 227).

Symptomatic and Alternative Subtypes of Schizophrenia

The symptom subgroups described by the early psychiatrists have persisted as diagnostic variants of schizophrenia to this day. Thus the *DSM-IV* (1994) includes criteria for paranoid, catatonic, hebephrenic (disorganized), and "residual" subtypes. However, persistence and longevity in diagnostic schemes do not automatically confer validity. Are these subtypes really different kinds of schizophrenia? Two basic kinds of evidence are helpful in evaluating subtypes: evidence of validity and evidence of stability. In other words, to what extent are patients who fall into different subtypes really different, not just in symptoms but in their biology and in the nature of their illness? If groups of paranoid, catatonic, and hebephrenic patients also differ in, for example, their family histories of schizophrenia, their cognitive deficits, and in their responsiveness to medication, these subtypes may actually correspond to different kinds of disease. Furthermore, if a patient with paranoid schizophrenia still meets criteria for this subtype 2 years after the initial diagnosis, the subtype is stable and perhaps distinct from other variations of the illness. In contrast, if a patient initially meets criteria for the paranoid subtype and then meets criteria for the catatonic subtype a year later, the subtype is unstable and perhaps not a truly distinct illness. In unstable situations the different subtypes probably represent changing phases of a single illness—transitions from paranoid to catatonic, to undifferentiated, and so forth—rather than multiple illnesses.

McGlashan and Fenton (1991) found five studies and one review that examined various validity and stability-related aspects of the classical subtypes. Most studies were concerned with the paranoid-nonparanoid distinction. No consistent pattern of greater or lesser heritability of the paranoid subtype of schizophrenia was found. However, three studies appeared to show better clinical outcome for the paranoid subtype relative to the other subtypes. There were also biological differences. One study reported lower monoamine oxydase (the enzyme that breaks down dopamine) activity in paranoid patients, and two studies found mild differences in blood chemistry that were not statistically significant. Three studies that compared subtypes with neurological and neuropsychological tests found no consistent differences. One study found evidence suggesting better cognitive functioning in paranoid patients than in other patients. There were also single studies implying later development of illness in paranoid than in hebephrenic or undifferentiated patients. There was little support for subtype differences in perinatal insults, season of birth, or social competence. On the question of stability, four studies reviewed by McGlashan and Fenton indicate that the paranoid subtype is the most stable of all the symptomatic distinctions. One study (Parnas, Jorgensen, Teasdale, Schulsinger, & Mednick, 1988) found that of 51 patients diagnosed initially as paranoid, 48 were still paranoid 6 years later. However, other studies reported much more modest stability for the paranoid subtype and generally found weak stability and considerable evidence of intersubtype progression in the case of the remaining symptomatic subtypes.

Distinctions like paranoid versus nonparanoid derive from clinical lore and observation. What if the distinction is more in the eye of the beholder than in the patient population? In other words, perhaps symptoms do not really cluster patients together in the way that the subtype criteria suggest. Perhaps subtypes are arbitrary groupings imposed on the patient population. For example, Carpenter and Strauss (1979) cluster-analyzed 600 patients with schizophrenia and found four clusters, or subtypes. However, they bore no resemblance to the classical distinctions. More recently, Helmes (1991) cluster-analyzed symptom data from a large sample and found little evidence of subtypes at all, and the clusters that were extracted did not correspond to the classical subtypes.

Hence, the "forms" of schizophrenia identified by Kraepelin (1919) and

Bleuler (1950) have endured, with modifications, to the present time, and they appear to be meaningful distinctions to clinicians. But the validity and stability of the old distinctions have not been demonstrated. The paranoid subtype has the most empirical support, although even this grouping does not emerge as a coherent symptom cluster in research studies. There are certainly insufficient grounds for concluding that the paranoid subtype represents an illness that is distinct from the rest of schizophrenia. In fact, the findings with respect to the validity and stability of symptomatic subtypes are themselves heterogeneous. There is little reason to believe that symptoms on their own offer a sound scientific way of organizing the diverse findings on the biology and psychology of schizophrenia. Yet efforts in this area have continued to the present day.

Consider some more recent and sophisticated attempts to parse schizophrenia on the basis of its symptoms. The promise of subtyping is that it may provide a means of organizing apparently disparate and incoherent research findings into a comprehensible set of homogeneous disorders. A useful schizophrenia typology should aggregate neurobiological and behavioral findings in such a way that heterogeneity is reduced and new ideas about underlying pathophysiology are brought to light. With this in mind, a distinction between positive and negative symptoms suggested by Strauss, Carpenter, and Bartko (1974) was elaborated by Crow (1980) into the concept of Type I and Type II schizophrenia. Type I schizophrenia was characterized by positive symptoms like delusions and hallucinations. Crow argued that these symptoms were the result of a hyperactive dopamine system in the brain. Therefore, Type I patients should respond well to antipsychotic medication and show marked reduction in their symptoms. In contrast, Type II schizophrenia comprised patients with negative symptoms like slowness, poverty of thought and action, withdrawal, and loss of motivation. It was argued that these patients would have enlarged cerebral ventricles, reflecting brain tissue losses more in keeping with traditional neurology. Hence Type II patients should be cognitively impaired and respond less well to dopamine-blocking drugs.

The Type I/Type II formulation attracted considerable interest and enthusiasm on the part of both clinicians and researchers. It had several of the ingredients of a useful typology. First, it made use of a readily observed symptomatic distinction. Second, it organized the apparent heterogeneity of two common findings in schizophrenia research: the fact that some, but not all, patients have enlarged ventricles on the basis of brain-scan studies and the fact that most, but not all, patients benefit from dopamine-blocking drugs. Third, it not only reduced the incoherence of research and clinical findings; it went on to pose distinct pathophysiologies to explain them. Finally, the Type I and Type II theory lent itself to empirical testing in a straightforward way.

It is unfortunate that the attractiveness of Crow's (1980) distinction was not backed up by consistent empirical support. Instead it was found that most patients had mixed positive and negative symptom profiles and few fell exclusively into one subtype. Initially supportive evidence was contradicted by later attempts to link ventricular enlargement or medication responsiveness with the subtypes. It was also found that negative as well as positive symptoms responded to antipsychotic drugs, which eliminated drug response as part and parcel of the illness distinction. Finally, positive and negative symptoms were found to be unstable so that patients moved between subtypes over time (see Zuckerman, 1999, pp. 325–331).

In recent years, symptom-based subtyping of schizophrenia has turned increasingly to empirically grounded divisions of the illness that derive from statistical clustering techniques like factor analysis. Three subtypes have been repeatedly identified. One involves primarily negative symptoms; another comprises thought disorder, bizarre, and inappropriate behavior; and a third consists of positive symptoms like delusions and hallucination (see Andreasen, Arndt, Alliger, Miller, & Flaum, 1995; Liddle, 1987). Stability over time and the fluctuating nature of many symptoms remains a problem, so that some patients evolve out of their initial subtype. However, Liddle argues that the syndromes of schizophrenia are best conceived of as dimensions of illness that can coexist in a single patient. These illness dimensions have distinct pathophysiologies, at least in theory, but they are not distinct diseases. Unlike many schizophrenia typologies, Liddle's scheme makes no claim to stability over time and no claim to exclusive illness categories. Each patient may fall into each of the three syndromes, and this may change over time. Liddle (1994,1996) points to evidence that the syndromes associate with different patterns of brain activity and with different cognitive tasks as validation for his illness dimensions.

Yet is this kind of approach really a solution to the heterogeneity problem in schizophrenia research? A three-way division may be the best way of organizing the symptoms of schizophrenia. But symptoms are a very insecure basis for organizing the illness itself. They are subjective states, and researchers and clinicians can only estimate the presence and severity of these states in another person (see chapter 2). Moreover, there are other, more objective features of schizophrenia that do not wax and wane over time as greatly as symptoms do. This applies to eye-tracking deficits and perhaps to the P300 evoked potential (see chapter 3). In other words, there may be better ways of parsing the illness. It is premature to give up on coexclusive illness subtypes until all the possibilities have been considered.

In view of the widespread evidence of neurobiological heterogeneity in schizophrenia, a corresponding proliferation of biologically based subtypes might be expected. However, there is no such proliferation. Researchers make use of symptomatic subtypes on occasion or ignore the issue altogether and treat schizophrenia as a single disease. A few exceptions do exist. For example, Kishimoto et al. (1987) reported three brain metabolism subtypes on the basis of positron emission tomography scans of 20 patients. One subtype comprised six patients with reduced glucose metabolism in the frontal area (hypofrontal subtype); another involved eight patients with reduced parietal lobe metabolism (hypoparietal subtype); and six patients had no reductions in metabolism (normal subtype). More recently, Clark, Kopala, James, Hurwitz, and Li (1993) also found evidence for a prefrontal metabolic subtype and suggested the existence of another patient subgroup with diffusely lowered brain metabolism.

An additional approach to subtyping involves the use of neurocognitive tasks rather than brain imaging or symptoms. Neurocognitive tasks provide behavioral information that is not available with conventional brain scanning and also furnish some information about local brain function, albeit with modest accuracy. In addition, neurocognitive tasks are more objective than symptom ratings, more valid as neurological indicators, and not reducible in any simple way to medication effects. Symptom-based typologies are always problematic to generate because of the confounding effect of antipsychotic medication, which modifies symptoms in most patients. Finally, there is an extensive knowledge base in neuropsychology stretching back to the last century. This knowledge base not only underpins the validity of individual cognitive tasks, it underpins hypotheses and conjectures about brain–behavior relationships. Major limitations of the approach include the fact that little is known about the stability of neurocognitive functioning over time in schizophrenia patients. In addition, selecting the most informative measures from dozens of tests can be a challenge.

As an example of the neurocognitive approach to the parsing of schizophrenia, consider a typology from my own research (Heinrichs & Awad, 1993; Heinrichs, Ruttan, Zakzanis, & Case, 1997). We used four tasks drawn from the research literature in neuropsychology and schizophrenia to subdivide a sample of schizophrenia patients. The tasks included the Wechsler Adult Intelligence Scale, (WAIS-R; Wechsler, 1981), the number of categories achieved on the Wisconsin Card Sorting Test (Heaton, 1981), the number of intrusion errors on recall trials from the California Verbal Learning Test (Delis et al., 1987) and the Purdue Pegboard (Purdue Research Foundation, n. d.). The card-sorting test was used as an index of executive function and mental flexibility, and the WAIS-R IQ was an estimate of general cognitive ability. The recall intrusion errors reflected verbal memory and medial-temporal lobe function, while the pegboard indexed manual dexterity and the motor system, including the basal ganglia.

Unlike symptom typologies that rely on placing patients into preconceived categories based on clinical ratings of behavior, our approach was empirically justified by the use of cluster analysis to find, not presume, subgroups of patients. We studied 104 chronic patients affiliated with a large psychiatric hospital in Toronto. The four task scores were recorded for each patient and submitted to cluster-analytic procedures that grouped patients on the basis of test score similarity. The procedure yielded a five-cluster solution as the most efficient way of organizing the patients' cognitive data. One subtype was distinguished primarily by low performance on the Wisconsin Card Sorting Test. These patients also had low to average intelligence and memory and motor function scores that were close to normal levels. We termed this the "executive" subtype. A second cluster comprised patients who were within average ranges on each of the four tasks ("normative") subtype. A third cluster consisted of patients with impaired card-sorting *and* impaired dexterity scores ("executive-motor") but with low to average intelligence and intact recall. The fourth cluster was termed "dementia" because the patients were impaired on all four tasks. The fifth subtype was termed "motor" because only the Purdue dexterity task was impaired.

These neurocognitive subtypes were similar in the number of patients per group, and they did not differ in medication or in years of education. However, because of the cross-sectional design, where patients are studied at only one point in time, there was no information on subtype stability. Hence, we obtained data on 55 of the original participants 3 years after the first study (see Heinrichs et al., 1997). In addition to stability and reliability concerns, it was possible to address the cognitive and clinical validity of the putative subtypes. The results indicated that the cognitive tests had fair to excellent reliability over 3 years. However, the subtypes themselves ranged from unstable at worst (executive) to moderately stable at best (executive-motor). The overall stability of the typology was similar to what is obtained with symptomatic subtypes. Also like symptom-based classifications, there was subtype progression, in that some patients moved from one subtype to another over the 3-year followup period. In terms of validity, independent cognitive tests supported the distinctiveness of the subtypes, and there was also evidence of subtype differences in quality of life and social functioning. The dementia subtype patients, in particular, were consistently disadvantaged relative to the other subtypes in terms of social and daily living skills. Hence the results were encouraging in that they showed the feasibility of parsing schizophrenia along neurocognitive rather than symptomatic lines. However, the new typology did not offer improved stability, and patients seemed to evolve from one subtype to another over the course of illness. Accordingly, compelling evidence that neurocognitive subtypes represent different illnesses is still lacking.

There are numerous alternative ways of parsing schizophrenia into more homogenous groups of patients. Yet this field of research has not attracted extensive interest. By and large, researchers continue to study schizophrenia as if it was a single illness, and they prefer to ignore the most radical implications of heterogeneity. In principle, any of the cognitive, neurobiological, or symptomatic features of the illness could be used to break schizophrenia down into component disorders. The main problem is to try and decide which neuroscience findings reflect the "natural subdivisions" of the illness and which find-ings are peripheral and represent dead ends. Is it possible, for example, to use the neuroscience effects reported in this book to assist the search for multiple ill-nesses in schizophrenia?

As a general rule, biological findings should be the preferred means of pars-ing schizophrenia because they lie closer than behavior to the neurogenesis of the illness. Hence there may be subsets of patients with abnormalities in differ-ent aspects of neurobiology, and these patients may represent distinct forms of illness. These subsets could include a group of patients with elevated dopamine D2 densities in the basal ganglia. Perhaps another group has deficient resting frontal brain metabolism and blood flow, and still other patients are distin-guished by temporal lobe defects. All of these subgroups can be identified with brain-imaging techniques that are applied to living patients. In contrast, any use of brain tissue analysis to subdivide schizophrenia must be post mortem. How-ever, psychophysiological evidence may also serve subtyping purposes, even though such evidence is only vaguely related to the neural systems implicated in schizophrenia. Indeed, efforts are under way in the field of eye tracking to see whether subgroups of impaired and normal patients differ in ways that hold promise for the heterogeneity problem (e.g. Ross, Buchanan, Medoff, Lahti, & Thaker, 1998).

It is also possible to use the meta-analytic findings of the previous chapters to speculate about disease variants, even when the findings are not practical as guides for subtyping research. For example, there may be a neurodevelopmen-tal form of schizophrenia caused by maturational failure and arrested cell mi-gration, perhaps focused on the prefrontal region of the brain. There may be a form of illness that arises from a damaged hippocampus interacting with in-creased stress hormone release during adolescence. There may even be a schizo-phrenia that springs from deficiencies in glutamate. Investigating any of these possibilities will require both major technical advances and acceptance of mul-tiple illness models as working hypotheses in schizophrenia research. But perhaps the greatest challenge facing attempts to parse the illness involves obtaining suf-ficiently large numbers of patients for study (see Bellak, 1994). At present, a clinical sample of 100 patients is considered a large study, but if several diseases exist within the *DSM-IV* (1994) schizophrenia umbrella, then many hundreds of patients will be required for subtyping studies. In a way, the challenge of het-erogeneity amounts to nothing less than a multiplication of the all the chal-lenges involved in the single disease model of schizophrenia. As if one puzzling disease is not enough, now researchers face an unknown number. This daunting prospect may continue to slow attempts at parsing schizophrenia despite the po-tential that such attempts have for major discoveries and insights (Heinrichs, 1993).

The Anomaly at the Frontier of Mind and Brain

Consider one more possibility. Perhaps the kind of illness that produces the findings reviewed in this book is an illness that cannot be accommodated within current views of brain function, behavior, and neurological disease. What if the findings that have accumulated with respect to schizophrenia violate or contradict in a basic kind of way the current neuroscience approach to mental illness? The synthesis of evidence shows that no abnormality in brain or behavior can be found in all people with a schizophrenia diagnosis. Yet within the spectrum of evidence, cognitive abnormalities occur with substantially greater prevalence than do biological abnormalities. Indeed, more than a third of the biological research literatures are not only very modest in strength but unstable and unreliable as well. Perhaps this situation means something important about the adequacy of neuroscience thought in relation to the schizophrenia puzzle. Perhaps it also means something important about the adequacy of attempts to understand the mind in neurological terms.

The ideas developed by Kuhn (1962, 1977) on the nature of change in science provide a way of articulating this third possibility. Central to these ideas is the concept of a paradigm, or a set of achievements that models problems and solutions to problems for the community of scientists working in a given field. The diligent application of beliefs, methods, and knowledge inspired by an accepted paradigm constitutes the activity of "normal" science. As a collective enterprise, normal science focuses on solving puzzles and on unexplained phenomena in the field of investigation. Thus the dominant paradigm is gradually extended and elaborated as its usefulness is demonstrated in relation to an increasing number of scientific questions. Yet in Kuhn's (1962) framework, the enterprise of normal science periodically encounters anomalies—problems and puzzles that resist solution. The expectations inspired by the paradigm do not materialize, and the puzzle remains unsolved. When this happens, scientists sometimes redouble their efforts and succeed in solving the puzzle within the existing paradigm. Anomalous problems or findings may also be set aside for later attention and sometimes they are just ignored. But anomalies occasionally lead to a scientific crisis because of the sheer inability of the dominant paradigm to explain and solve them. The paradigm becomes overextended and is itself drawn into question. During such crises, alternative paradigms are first generated and then adopted. Previously potent but less effective models and explanations recede into history. In this way Copernicus replaced geocentric with heliocentric views to explain anomalies of planetary motion. Lavoisier replaced phlogiston theory with oxygen theory to explain combustion. And Darwin proposed natural selection to account for nagging anomalies that bedeviled Victorian views of natural history. And all of this offers another way of looking at the past and present neuroscience evidence on schizophrenia.

First, the past.

During the mid- to late nineteenth century, medical science provided repeated demonstrations that disturbances of mind and behavior were caused by focal brain pathology. Initially, the associated paradigm rested on fairly "coarse" types of brain damage, large infarctions and brain abscesses. It also rested on fairly coarse or obvious behavioral disturbances—paralysis, arrested speech, severely impaired comprehension. With the advent of more powerful microscopes and tissue-staining techniques, more subtle kinds of pathology were detected. For example, microscopic cellular changes were discovered in diseases like senile dementia. The application of these increasingly refined tools to mental illness brought about the "first" biological psychiatry at the beginning of the twentieth century (Shorter, 1997, pp. 69–112). But the application of the brain disorder–behavior disorder paradigm to schizophrenia was stillborn. The brains of patients with the illness did not reveal the expected pathology. Hence the madness puzzle was set aside, almost abandoned, for several decades. Schizophrenia remained outside the domain of neurology. Psychoanalysis beckoned psychiatry away from neuroscience; indeed, it beckoned psychiatry away from science altogether.

One way of looking at the failure of the first biological psychiatry to solve schizophrenia is to say that the medical paradigm was too primitive in its conceptual foundations to deal with something as complex as madness. The paradigm created the expectation that a clinical state, defined by symptoms, would associate with observable brain pathology. And this worked for many disorders, from stroke to tumor to infection. It even worked for clinical states that were primarily psychological, like aphasia, amnesia, and dementia—disorders of language, memory, and intellect, respectively. The paradigm worked despite the fact that the physicians and scientists who employed it knew little about the nature of language, memory, or intelligence. Most of the sophistication in the medical paradigm was biological. Common-sense notions of mind and behavior along with careful clinical observation were sufficient. The paradigm only required the demonstration of *dependencies* between mind and brain. Neurology and psychiatry lacked a theory or a model of how mind was *reducible* to brain, but it didn't matter because the paradigm still worked for most disorders. It worked for most disorders, but not apparently for schizophrenia.

It is important to note that a theory of mind and brain is not the same as saying, for example, that the left cerebral hemisphere governs language and the right hemisphere governs spatial perception. A theory of mind and brain is not the same as a hypothesis that the hippocampus is essential for the formation of new memories or that the amygdala mediates the learning of fear. It is not enough to argue that there is no memory function without a hippocampus and no fear without an amygdala. These are simply assertions about the dependency between mind and brain. A real theory begins where dependencies end. A real theory addresses basic problems like: How are memories and fears translated into the language of neurobiology? A theory of mind and brain specifies how mental events like thoughts, ideas, wishes, fears, memories, and pleasures can be understood in terms of neurological events like transmitter release, receptor binding, neuronal firing, and postsynaptic inhibition and excitation. There was no theory of mind and brain at the turn of the century. Instead, some fairly crude facts about brain—behavior dependencies had been gathered, and it was hoped that a similar dependency would be found for schizophrenia. But it wasn't.

Yet that was long ago, and a much more refined and sophisticated neuroscience with a long track record of success was applied to schizophrenia in the 1980s. This fueled the "second," or resurgent, biological psychiatry (see Andreasen, 1984; Shorter, 1997, pp. 239–287). With the addition of advanced neuroimaging technology, the principle that mental states, including mental illnesses, are linked to events in the brain was again applied to schizophrenia. Most recently, traditional and neurochemical concepts of pathology have been complemented by ideas of altered brain circuitry, failed brain maturation, and cellular disorganization. And the subsequent growth of research and ideas has produced the evidence reviewed and summarized in this book and presented in tables 9.1 and 9.2 and in figure 9.1.

The problem is that neuroscience still uses the old medical paradigm and lacks a theory and a model of how biological events become mental events that become schizophrenia. The explosion of knowledge concerning the nervous system has been mostly a biological explosion. Many conditions still involve observable pathologies, and mental events can still be relegated to diagnostic criteria and otherwise ignored. But the evidence suggests that schizophrenia is in a class of disorders that cannot be understood without a workable theory of mind and brain. Why do schizophrenia patients differ more from healthy people in their cognition than in their neurobiology? Why are there no abnormalities that are shared by all patients? Why is the knowledge base in support of schizophrenia as a disturbance in neurobiology so insecure? It must be that schizophrenia is a disorder of the working brain as a psychological system, a disorder of the brain in action. Yet without a model of how to understand this action and how to relate mental to neurological activity, neuroscience cannot take the next step and solve the schizophrenia puzzle—the anomaly of madness.

What would such a model or theory of mind and brain look like? Now there's a question. For a flavor of the possibilities, consider what has happened in cognitive science over the last decade within the framework of parallel distributed processing theory and connectionism (McClelland & Rumelhart, 1986; Rumelhart & McClelland, 1986). Connectionist theory proposes that mental activity emerges from large numbers of basic information-processing units that have weighted connections with each other and form pathways. Information inheres in the pattern of activation that exists between the connected units. In other words, information exists within the network as a whole but not at any one location. In reality these units could be individual neurons or groups of related neurons. Like neurons, the units are subject to influence from other units, and this influence may be excitatory or inhibitory. The combination of influences creates the unit's activation level—the neuron's firing rate or probability of firing. Once activation occurs, it is spread to other units through output connections. In addition to being excitatory or inhibitory, these connections may vary from weak to strong, and this is embodied in the idea of connection weights. Accordingly, the aggregate of incoming influences on a neuron or group of neurons depends on the number and weight of different connections. Highly connected units that serve a specific cognitive function, say, perceiving the meaning of a shape, are grouped as a module. There may be input modules dedicated to sensory analysis and perception and output modules dedicated to particular responses, and there may be mediating or intermediate modules as well. Mental work or processing involves the spread of activation among units within a module and between different modules. Knowledge in an everyday sense is the ability to supply a correct or at least useful and appropriate answer or response to a question or problem. But in terms of connectionist theory and this kind of neural network, knowledge inheres in the connection weights between units. It follows that if knowledge comprises a set of connection weights, then learning comprises the alteration and adjustment of these weights in response to corrective feedback.

One of the advantages of thinking about mind and brain puzzles in connectionist terms is that network models make biological sense. Previously, researchers relied on weak analogies between brains and computers. Like neurons in the brain, the simulated networks of connectionist theory work simultaneously or "in parallel" to a great extent. Simultaneous processing that is distributed across a network is much more "brainlike" than the extremely rapid but stepwise processing carried out by a computer. Moreover, connectionist theory holds that learning and memory reside in the connection weights between the units in the distributed network. This is also feasible for the brain. Information in the brain is not stored at particular locations or retrieved for use the way it is in a computer. Finally, connectionist models not only make biological sense, they can be designed to carry out activities like reading printed text out loud or recognizing objects from shading and shape. In other words, they can simulate mental work. And these models can be refined and tested for accuracy and efficiency by using—ironically—a computer (see Churchland, 1995; Crick, 1994).

But what does any of this have to do with schizophrenia? For one thing, it is possible to think of the neurogenesis of the illness in connectionist terms. In simulated neural networks, connection weights between neurons are often randomized initially. However, in the real brain, neural networks are probably predisposed by genes to carry out certain activities. A good example of this is language learning, which seems to occur in young brains that are genetically "primed" to develop communication skills (see Pinker, 1994). If there are network modules for language, there may be modules for social cognition and for representations of the body and personal history. Well-worn pathways used to interpret external and internal events may exist in cerebral space. Perhaps schizophrenia involves a pathological redistribution of connection weights, an alteration of synaptic strength in several high-level neural networks. This alteration may be primed to occur by faulty genetics and then precipitated by hormonal changes in adolescence. It may be a transitory redistribution that is subject to internal correction or to drugs. The pathology inheres in the synaptic strengths between thousands of neurons that form the basis for the interpretation of external events and personal history. It seems unlikely that this pathology is reducible to cell numbers or densities in a straightforward way. It also seems unlikely that simply measuring neurotransmitter receptors or looking at shifts in brain metabolism will reveal the pathology of the working mind and brain in detail.

Remember Ruth, the woman with tactile and olfactory hallucinations, and her experience of smelling and feeling a sluglike creature around her neck. Suppose that the brain contains a network that could be termed a self-representation or self-schema module. It includes the brain's "picture" of the body. It also comprises a diverse web of connections among memories, sights and sounds, smells and sensations that form the basis of personal knowledge. Usually, units in this network have strong connection weights with each other, and most incoming sensory events do not activate the self-representation system. However, a subset of sensory events that stem from the body is capable of activating the system. In this way a person recognizes his or her own physical sensations and is aware of the body. The self-representation module can spread activation into expressive or output modules so that a person acts and interacts with the environment. But suppose further that connection strengths are altered, the system is perturbed, so that sensory events from the body no longer activate self-representations, they activate modules that represent environmental schemas or events. The body smell, touch of clothing, and skin sensations that Ruth previously recognized as her own no longer activate self-representations. She experiences her own body as something alien.

Now consider William and his delusions of divine powers and relationship to Christ. Cognitive networks and modules incorporating cultural beliefs and religious concepts might ordinarily have weak connection weights or little synaptic strength with self-representation networks. However, if the system of neural networks that comprises the mind is perturbed and weights are altered pathologically, activation may spread between modules that are usually barely linked. Personal knowledge and religious knowledge networks are joined, creating delusions of divinity. Finally, even James, the man convinced of a parasite in his brain, can be understood this way. Part of the self-representation network loses integrity with the rest of the network and is subject to activation by modules that represent external events or ways of organizing external events. James's own thoughts are no longer a part of him; they are due to external forces, and a parasite that speaks through his brain is the product of this decoupling of mental modules.

Of course these imaginative sketches are gross oversimplifications and do not do justice to the complexity and detail of connectionist models or to the simulation of cognitive processes. And it is one thing to simulate cognitive brain activity and another to determine if neural networks really exist and function in the ways proposed. But a few researchers have already applied parallel-distributed processing principles to the study of symptoms (Hoffman & McGlashan, 1993; Hoffman & Rapaport, 1994, pp. 255–267; McGlashan & Hoffman, 2000) and to cognitive deficits (Cohen & Servan-Schreiber, 1992, 1993) in schizophrenia. While such efforts have focused on very limited aspects of the illness, they may represent the beginnings of much more complex views about the neurological basis of schizophrenia. If pathology inheres in perturbed or altered activity patterns that are distributed across wide areas of the brain, more than new instruments will be needed to track down these patterns. New ways of thinking about neurotransmitter systems, receptor characteristics, regional brain architecture, and neurophysiology will be needed. New ways of thinking about thinking will be needed. And the answers to schizophrenia may completely upset the apple cart of traditional medical science and biological psychiatry. Solving the schizophrenia puzzle may carry neuroscience to new conceptions of mind and behavior and in the process cause a revolution.

Conclusion

It is tempting to end a book like this with happy forecasts, to prophesy imminent relief from suffering and scientific ignorance. Instead I have offered only a cautious appraisal and three uncertain possibilities. There is no way of knowing, at present, which view of schizophrenia science will turn out to be correct. Most researchers accept the first or promissory note view of the evidence. This acceptance is a conservative, "normal science" response to some perplexing facts. Normal science insists that continued application of prevailing assumptions and the steady improvement of technology will show the way to the biological truth about schizophrenia. The multiple illnesses view takes a less conservative position by arguing that the weakness and inconsistency of the evidence are due to the existence of different kinds of illness. Studying diverse conditions as a single disease state is guaranteed to produce inconsistent findings that apply to some patients and not to others. Everyone pays lip service to the heterogeneity problem, but only a small number of researchers do more and actually study multiple illness models of schizophrenia. No doubt the third hypothesis, the notion of anomaly, a revolution in waiting, has a radical kind of appeal. It may even be true. But I worry that diehards who still blame schizophrenia on the cruelty of mothers or on society's intolerance for eccentricity will seize and distort the meaning of this possibility. Perhaps misconceived notions and exaggerations are inevitable in relation to this, the most human and the most psychological of illnesses. But I will not add to them. So at the very end I offer only a description and no prophecy about the end of madness.

Schizophrenia is the flaw that is woven into the fabric of a child's life. It is the sudden wound in the mind's secret body, the hemorrhage of meaning disguised as wisdom. It is the clever voice, singing lies. It is the illness of the imagination, beyond imagination; beyond the comfort of memory, beyond the reach of human tenderness and the hope of safety. It is the illness that conspires against love. It is the illness that forces what is intimate and what is alien into strange unions. It is the illness that comes and goes on a tide of chemistry and in its wake leaves a violent sorrow and a longing for the pleasures of darkness. Tomorrow may bring the answers that escaped in the past, the answers that lead to cause and cure. In the meantime, madness is among us and diminishes to the extent that we care for those who endure it.

REFERENCES

Studies included in meta-analyses are indicated with an asterisk.

Ackerly, S. S., & Benton, A. L. (1948). Report of a case of bilateral frontal lobe defect. *Research and Publications of the Association for the Research of Nervous and Mental Disease, 27,* 479–504.

Addington, J., & Addington, D. (1991). Positive and negative symptoms of schizophrenia: Their course and relationship over time. *Schizophrenia Research, 5,* 51–59.

★Adler, L. E., Hoffer, L. D., Wiser, A., & Freedman, R. (1993). Normalization of auditory physiology by cigarette smoking in schizophrenic patients. *American Journal of Psychiatry, 150,* 1856–1861.

Adler, L. E., Olincy, A., Waldo, M., Harris, J. G., Griffith, J., Stevens, K., Flach, K., Nagamoto, H., Bickford, P., Leonard, S., & Freedman, R. (1998). Schizophrenia, sensory gating, and nicotinic receptors. *Schizophrenia Bulletin, 24,* 189–202.

★Adler, L. E., Pachtman, E., Franks, R. D., Pecevich, M., Waldo, M. C., & Freedman, R. (1982). Neurophysiological evidence for a defect in neuronal mechanisms involved in sensory gating in schizophrenia. *Biological Psychiatry, 17,* 639–654.

★Adler, L. E., Waldo, M. C., Tatcher, A., Cawthra, E., Baker, N., & Freedman, R. (1990). Lack of relationship of auditory gating defects to negative symptoms in schizophrenia. *Schizophrenia Research, 3,* 131–138.

★Akbarian, S., Bunney, W. E., Jr., Potkin, S. G., Wigal, S. B., Hagman, J. O., Sandman, C. A., & Jones, E. G. (1993). Altered distribution of nicotinamide-adenine dinucleotide phosphate-diaphorase cells in frontal lobe of schizophrenics implies disturbances of cortical development. *Archives of General Psychiatry, 50,* 169–177.

*Akbarian, S., Kim, J. J., Potkin, S. G., Hagman, J. O., Tafazzoli, A., Bunney, W. E., Jr., & Jones, E. G. (1995). Gene expression for glutamic acid decarboxylase is reduced without loss of neurons in prefrontal cortex of schizophrenics. *Archives of General Psychiatry, 52,* 258–266.

*Akbarian, S., Kim, J. J., Potkin, S. G., Hetrick, W. P, Bunney, W. E., Jr., & Jones, E. G. (1996). Maldistribution of interstitial neurons in prefrontal white matter of the brains of schizophrenic patients. *Archives of General Psychiatry, 53,* 425–436.

Alanen, Y. O., Hagglund, V., Harkonen, P., & Kunnunen, P. (1968). On psychodynamics and conjoint psychotherapy of schizophrenic men and their wives. *Psychotherapy and Psychosomatics, 16,* 299–300.

Aleman, A., Hijman, R., de Haan, E. H., & Kahn, R. S. (1999). Memory impairment in schizophrenia: A meta-analysis. *American Journal of Psychiatry, 156,* 1358–1366.

*Al-Khani, M. A., Bebbington, P. E., Watson, J. P., & House, F. (1986). Life events and schizophrenia: A Saudi Arabian study. *British Journal of Psychiatry, 148,* 12–22.

*Allen, H. A. (1982). Dichotic monitoring and focused versus divided attention in schizophrenia. *British Journal of Psychiatry, 21,* 205–212.

*Allen, J. S., Matsunaga, K., Harisalihazade, S., & Stark, L. (1990). Smooth pursuit eye movements of normal and schizophrenic subjects tracking an unpredictable target. *Biological Psychiatry, 28,* 705–720.

*Al-Mousawi, A. H., Evans, N., Ebmeier, K. P., Roeda, D., Chaloner, F., & Ashcroft, G. W. (1996). Limbic dysfunction in schizophrenia and mania: A study using 18F-labelled fluorodeoxyglucose and positron emission tomography. *British Journal of Psychiatry, 169,* 509–516.

*Aloia, M. S., Gourovitch, M. L., Missar, D., Pickar, D., Weinberger, D. R., & Goldberg, T. E. (1998). Cognitive substrates of thought disorder: II. specifying a candidate cognitive mechanism. *American Journal of Psychiatry, 155,* 1677–1684.

*Altshuler, L. L., Bartzokis, G., Grieder, T., Curran, J., & Mintz, J. (1998). Amygdala enlargement in bipolar disorder and hippocampal reduction in schizophrenia: An MRI study demonstrating neuroanatomic specificity. *Archives of General Psychiatry, 55,* 663–664.

*Altshuler, L. L., Casanova, M. F., Goldberg, T. E., & Kleinman, J. E. (1990). The hippocampus and parahippocampus in schizophrenia, suicide and control brains. *Archives of General Psychiatry, 47,* 1029–1034.

*Altshuler, L. L., Conrad, A., Kovelman, J. A., & Scheibel, A. (1987). Hippocampal pyramidal cell orientation in schizophrenia: A controlled neurohistologic study of the Yakovlev collection. *Archives of General Psychiatry, 44,* 1094–1098.

*Amador, X. F., Flaum, M., Andreasen, N. C., Strauss, D. H., Yale, S. A., Clark, S. C., & Gorman, J. M. (1994). Awareness of illness in schizophrenia and schizoaffective and mood disorders. *Archives of General Psychiatry, 51,* 826–836.

Amador, X. F., Sackheim, H. A., Mukherjee, S., Halperin, R., Neeley, P., Maclin, E., & Schnur, D. (1991). Specificity of smooth pursuit eye movement and visual fixation abnormalities in schizophrenia: Comparison to mania and normal controls. *Schizophrenia Research, 5,* 135–144.

American Psychiatric Association. (1980). *Diagnostic and statistical manual of mental disorders* (3rd ed.). Washington, DC: Author.

American Psychiatric Association. (1994). *Diagnostic and statistical manual of mental disorders* (4th ed.). Washington, DC: Author.

Amin, F., Davidson, M., Kahn, R. S., Schmeidler, J., Stern, R., Knott, P. J., & Apter, S. (1995). Assessment of the central dopaminergic index of plasma HVA in schizophrenia. *Schizophrenia Bulletin, 21,* 53–66.

★Amminger, G. P., Pape, S., Rock, D., Roberts, S. A., Ott, S. L., Squires-Wheeler, E., Kestenbaum, C., & Erlenmeyer-Kimling, L. (1999). Relationship between childhood behavioral disturbance and later schizophrenia in the New York High-Risk project. *American Journal of Psychiatry, 156,* 525–530.

★Anderson, J., Gordon, E., Barry, R. J., Rennie, C., Beumont, P. J. V., & Meares, R. (1995). Maximum vaiance of late component event related potentials (190–240ms) in unmedicated schizophrenic patients. *Psychiatry Research, 56,* 229–236.

★Anderson, J., Gordon, E., Barry, R. J., Rennie, C. J., Gonsalvez, C., Pettigrew, G., Beumont, P. J. V., & Meares, R. (1995). Event related response variability in schizophrenia: Effect of intratrial target subsets. *Psychiatry Research, 56,* 237–243.

★Anderson, S. A., Volk, D. W., & Lewis, D. A. (1996). Increased density of microtubule associated protein 2–immunoreactive neurons in the prefrontal white matter of schizophrenic subjects. *Schizophrenia Research, 19,* 111–119.

Anderson, S. W., Damasio, H., Jones, R. D., & Tranel, D. (1991). Wisconsin Card Sorting Test performance as a measure of frontal lobe damage. *Journal of Clinical and Experimental Neuropsychology, 13,* 909–922.

★Anderson, S. W., & Tranel, D. (1989). Awareness of disease states following cerebral infarction, dementia and head trauma: Standardized assessment. *Clinical Neuropsychologist, 3,* 327–339.

Andreasen, N. C. (1982). Negative symptoms in schizophrenia: Definition and reliability. *Archives of General Psychiatry, 39,* 784–788.

Andreasen, N. C. (1984). *The Scale for Assessment of Positive Symptoms (SAPS).* Iowa City: University of Iowa Press.

Andreasen, N. C. (1985). *The broken brain: The biological revolution in psychiatry.* New York: Harper & Row.

Andreasen, N. C. (1989). The American concept of schizophrenia. *Schizophrenia Bulletin, 15,* 519–531.

Andreasen, N. C. (1991). Assessment issues and the cost of schizophrenia. *Schizophrenia Bulletin, 17,* 475–481.

Andreasen, N. C., Arndt, S., Alliger, R., Miller, D., & Flaum, M. (1995). Symptoms of schizophrenia: Methods, meanings, and mechanisms. *Archives of General Psychiatry, 52,* 341–351.

★Andreasen, N. C. Arndt, S., Swayze, V., Cizadlo, T., Flaum, M., O'Leary, D., Ehrhardt, J. C., & Yuh, W. T. (1994). Thalamic abnormalities in schizophrenia visualized through magnetic resonance image averaging. *Science, 266,* 294–298.

★Andreasen, N. C., Ehrhardt, J. C., Swayze, V. W., II, Alliger, R. J., Yuh, W. T., Cohen, G., & Ziebell, S. (1990). Magnetic resonance imaging of the brain in schizophrenia: The pathophysiologic significance of structural abnormalities. *Archives of General Psychiatry, 47,* 35–44.

Andreasen, N. C., & Flaum, M. (1991). Schizophrenia: The characteristic symptoms. *Schizophrenia Bulletin, 17,* 27–49.

Andreasen, N. C., & Grove, W. (1979). The relationship between schizophrenic language, manic language and aphasia. In J. Gruzelier & P. Flor-Henry (Eds.), *Developments in psychiatry: Vol. 3. Hemisphere asymmetries of function in psychopathology* (pp. 373–390). Amsterdam: Elsevier.

★Andreasen, N. C., Hurtig, R. R., Kesler, M. L., & O'Leary, D. S. (1996). Auditory attentional deficits in patients with schizophrenia: A positron emission tomography study. *Archives of General Psychiatry, 53,* 633–641.

★Andreasen, N. C., Nasrallah, H. A., Dunn, V., Olson, S. C., Grove, W. M., Ehrhardt, J. C., Coffman, J. A., & Crossett, J. H. (1986). Structural abnormalities in the frontal system in schizophrenia. A magnetic resonance imaging study. *Archives of General Psychiatry, 43,* 136–144.

★Andreasen, N. C., O'Leary, D. S., Flaum, M., Nopoulos, P., Watkins, G. L., Boles Ponto, L. L., & Hichwa, R. D. (1997). Hypofrontality in schizophrenia: Distributed dysfunctional circuits in neuroleptic-naive patients. *Lancet, 349,* 1730–1734.

★Aparicio-Legarza, M. I., Cutts, A. J., Davis, B., & Reynolds, G. P. (1997). Deficits of [3H]D-aspartate binding to glutamate uptake sites in striatal and accumbens tissue in patients with schizophrenia. *Neuroscience Letters, 232,* 13–16.

★Aparicio-Legarza, M. I., Davis, B., Hutson, P. H., & Reynolds, G. P. (1998). Increased density of glutamate/N-methyl-D-aspartate receptors in putamen from schizophrenic patients. *Neuroscience Letters, 241,* 143–146.

★Arango, C., Bartko, J. J., Gold, J. M., & Buchanan, R. W. (1999). Prediction of neuropsychological performance by neurological signs in schizophrenia. *American Journal of Psychiatry, 156,* 1349–1357.

★Ariel, R. N., Golden, C. J., Berg, R. A., Quaife, M. A., Dirksen, J. W., Forsell, T., Wilson, J., & Graber, B. (1983). Regional cerebral blood flow in schizophrenics: Tests using the xenon Xe 133 inhalation method. *Archives of General Psychiatry, 40,* 258–263.

Arndt, S., Alliger, R. J., & Andreasen, N. C. (1991). The distinction of positive and negative symptoms: The failure of a two-dimensional model. *British Journal of Psychiatry, 158,* 317–322.

★Arnold, S. E., Franz, B. R., Gur, R. C., Gur, R. E., Shapiro, R. M., Moberg, P. J., & Trojanowki, J. Q. (1995). Smaller neuron size in schizophrenia in hippocampal subfields that mediate cortical-hippocampal interactions. *American Journal of Psychiatry, 152,* 738–748.

Arnold, S. E., & Trojanowski, J. Q. (1996). Recent advances in defining the neuropathology of schizophrenia. *Acta Neuropathologie, 92,* 217–231.

★Arora, R. C., & Meltzer, H. Y. (1991). Serotonin2 (5–HT2) receptor binding in the frontal cortex of schizophrenic patients. *Journal of Neural Transmission, 85,* 19–29.

★Aschauer, H. N., Meszaros, K., Willinger, U., Reiter, E., Heiden, A. M., Lenzinger, E., Beran, H., & Resinger, E. (1994). The season of birth of schizophrenics and schizoaffectives. *Psychopathology, 27,* 298–302.

Axelrod, B. N., & Millis, S. R. (1994). Preliminary standardization of the Cognitive Estimation Test. *Assessment, 1,* 269–274.

*Baare, W. F., Pol, H. E., Hijman, R., Mali, W. P., Viergever, M. A., & Kahn, R. S. (1999). Volumetric analysis of frontal lobe regions in schizophrenia: Relation to cognitive function and symptomatology. *Biological Psychiatry, 45,* 1597–1605.

Baddeley, A. D., & Hitch, G. J. (1994). Developments in the concept of working memory. *Neurospychology, 8,* 485–493.

Bagdy, G., Perenyi, A., Frecska, E., Revai, K., Papp, Z., Fekete, M. I., & Arato, M. (1985). Decrease in dopamine, its metabolites and noradrenaline in cerebrospinal fluid of schizophrenic patients after withdrawal of long-term neuroleptic treatment. *Psychopharmacology, 85,* 62–64.

*Bagedahl-Strindlund, M., Rosencrantz-Larsson, L., & Wilkner-Svanfeldt, P. (1989). Children of mentally ill mothers: Social situation and psychometric testing of mental development. *Scandinavian Journal of Social Medicine, 17,* 171–179.

Bakan, D. (1966). The test of significance in psychological research. *Psychological Bulletin, 66,* 423–437.

*Baker, C. A., & Morrison, A. P. (1998). Cognitive processes in auditory hallucinations: Attributional biases and metacognition. *Psychological Medicine, 28,* 1199–1208.

*Baker, N., Adler, L. E., Franks, R. D., Waldo, M., Berry, S., Nagamoto, H., Muckle, A., & Freedman, R. (1987). Neurophysiological assessment of sensory gating in psychiatric inpatients: Comparison between schizophrenia and other diagnoses. *Biological Psychiatry, 22,* 603–617.

Ball, M. J. (1983). Granulovacuolar degeneration. In B. Reisberg (Ed.), *Alzheimer's disease: The standard reference* (pp. 52–68). New York: Free Press.

Ball, M. J., & Lo, P. (1977). Granulovacuolar degeneration in the aging brain and in dementia. *Journal of Neuropathology and Experimental Neurology, 36,* 474–487.

Balogh, D. W., & Merritt, R. D. (1987). Visual masking and the schizophrenia spectrum: Interfacing clinical and experimental methods. *Schizophrenia Bulletin, 13,* 679–698.

*Barch, D. M., Carter, C. S., Perlstein, W., Baird, J., Cohen, J. D., & Schooler, N. (1999). Increased Stroop facilitation effects are not due to increased automatic spreading activation. *Schizophrenia Research, 39,* 51–64.

Barchas, J. D., Faull, K. F., Quinn, B., & Elliot, G. R. (1994). Biochemical aspects of the psychotic disorders. In G. J. Siegel, B. W. Agranoff, W. R. Albers, & P. B. Molinoff (Eds.), *Basic neurochemistry: Molecular, cellular and medical aspects* (5th ed., pp. 959–977). New York: Raven Press.

*Baribeau-Baun, J., Picton, T. W., & Gosselin, J. Y. (1983). Schizophrenia: a neurophysiological evaluation of abnormal information processing. *Science, 219,* 874–876.

*Barr, W. B., Ashtari, M., Bilder, R. M., Degreef, G., & Lieberman, J. A. (1997). Brain morphometric comparison of first-episode schizophrenia and temporal lobe epilepsy. *British Journal of Psychiatry, 170,* 515–519.

*Barrett, K., McCallum, W. C., & Pocock, P. V. (1986). Brain indicators of altered attention and information processing in schizophrenic patients. *British Journal of Psychiatry, 148,* 414–420.

*Barta, P. E., Pearlson, G. D., Powers, R. E., Richards, S. S., & Tune, L. E. (1990). Auditory hallucinations and smaller superior temporal gyral volume in schizophrenia. *American Journal of Psychiatry, 147,* 1457–1462.

*Bartha, R., al-Semaan, Y. M., Williamson, P. C., Drost, D. J., Malla, A. K., Carr, T. J.,

Densmore, M., Canaran, G., & Neufeld, R. W. (1999). A short echo proton magnetic resonance spectroscopy study of the left mesial-temporal lobe in first-onset schizophrenic patients. *Biological Psychiatry, 45*, 1403–1411.

Bateson, G., Jackson, D. D., Haley, J., & Weakland, J. (1956). Toward a theory of schizophrenia. *Behavioral Science, 1*, 251–264.

Bauer, R. M. (1993). Agnosia. In K. M. Heilman & E. Valenstein (Eds.), *Clinical neuropsychology* (3rd ed., pp. 215–278). New York: Oxford University Press.

Bauer, R. M., Tobias, B., & Valenstein, E. (1993). Amnesic disorders. In K. M. Heilman & E. Valenstein (Eds.), *Clinical neuropsychology* (3rd ed., pp. 523–602). New York: Oxford University Press.

Bear, D. M., & Fedio, P. (1977). Quantitative analysis of interictal behavior in temporal lobe epilepsy. *Archives of Neurology, 34*, 454–467.

*Beatty, W. W., Jocic, Z., Monson, N., & Staton, D. (1993). Memory and frontal lobe dysfunction in schizophrenia and schizoaffective disorder. *Journal of Nervous and Mental Disease, 181*, 448–453.

*Bebbington, P. Wilkins, S., Jones, P., Foerster, A., Murray, R., Toone, B., & Lewis, S. (1993). Life events and psychosis: Initial results from the Camberwell Collaborative Psychosis Study. *British Journal of Psychiatry, 162*, 72–79.

*Becker, T., Elmer, K., Schneider, F., Schneider, M., Grodd, W., Bartels, M., Heckers, S., & Beckmann, H. (1996). Confirmation of reduced temporal limbic structure volume on magnetic resonance imaging in male patients with schizophrenia. *Psychiatry Research, 67*, 135–143.

Begleiter, H., Porjesz, B., Bihari, & Kissin, B. (1984). Event-related brain potentials in boys at risk for alcoholism, *Science, 225*, 1493–1496.

Bekhterev, V. M. (1900). Demonstration eines Gehirns mit Zerstörung der vorderen und inneren Theile der Hirnrinde beider Schlafenlappen. *Neurologisches Zeitblatt, 19*, 990–991.

Bellak, L. (1979). A "mini-max:" A research strategy for establishing subgroups of the schizophrenic syndrome. *Schizophrenia Bulletin, 5*, 443–446.

Bellak, L. (1994). The schizophrenic syndrome and attention deficit disorder. Thesis, anti-thesis, and synthesis? *American Psychologist, 49*, 25–29.

*Benes, F. M., Davidson, J., & Bird, E. D. (1986). Quantitative cytoarchitectural studies of the cerebral cortex of schizophrenics. *Archives of General Psychiatry, 43*, 31–35.

*Benes, F. M., McSparren, J., Bird, E. D., SanGiovanni, J. P., & Vincent, S. L. (1991). Deficits in small interneurons in prefrontal and cingulate cortices of schizophrenic and schizoaffective patients. *Archives of General Psychiatry, 48*, 996–1001.

*Benes, F. M., Sorensen, I., & Bird, E. D. (1991). Reduced neuronal size in posterior hippocampus of schizophrenic patients. *Schizophrenia Bulletin, 17*, 597–608.

*Benes, F. M., Vincent, S. L., Marie, A., & Khan, Y. (1996). Up-regulation of GABAA receptor binding on neurons of the prefrontal cortex in schizophrenic subjects. *Neuroscience, 75*, 1021–1031.

Benson, D. F. (1993). Aphasia. In K. M. Heilman & E. Valenstein (Eds.), *Clinical neuropsychology* (3rd ed.). New York: Oxford University Press.

Benson, D. F., & Stuss, D. T. (1990). Frontal lobe influences on delusions: A clinical perspective. *Schizophrenia Bulletin, 16*, 403–411.

Bentall, R. P. (1990). The illusion of reality: A review and integration of psychological research on hallucinations. *Psychological Bulletin, 107*, 82–95.

Bentall, R. P. (1994). Cognitive biases and abnormal beliefs. Towards a model of persecutory delusions. In A. S. David & J. C. Cutting (Eds.), *The neuropsychology of schizophrenia* (pp. 337–360). Brain damage, behaviour and cognition series. London: Lawrence Erlbaum.

*Bentall, R. P., Baker, G. A., & Havers, S. (1991). Reality monitoring and psychotic hallucinations. *British Journal of Clinical Psychology, 30*, 213–222.

*Bentall, R. P., & Kaney, S. (1996). Abnormalities of self-representation and persecutory delusions: A test of a cognitive model of paranoia. *Psychological Medicine, 26*, 1231–1237.

*Bentall, R. P., Kaney, S., & Bowen-Jones, K. (1995). Persecutory delusions and recall of threat-related, depression-related and neutral words. *Cognitive Therapy and Research, 19*, 445–457.

*Bentall, R. P., Kaney, S., & Dewey, M. E. (1991). Paranoia and social reasoning: An attribution theory analysis. *British Journal of Clinical Psychology, 30*, 13–23.

*Bentall, R. P., & Slade, P. D. (1985). Reality testing and auditory hallucinations: A signal detection analysis. *British Journal of Clinical Psychology, 24*, 159–169.

Benton, A. L. (1968). Differential behavioral effects in frontal lobe disease. *Neuropsychologia, 6*, 53–60.

*Bergman, A. J., & Walker, E. (1995). The relationship between cognitive functions and behavioral deviance in children at risk for psychopathology. *Journal of Child Psychology and Psychiatry and Allied Disciplines, 36*, 265–278.

*Bergman, A. J., Wolfson, M. A., & Walker, E. F. (1997). Neuromotor functioning and behavior problems in children at risk for psychopathology. *Journal of Abnormal Child Psychology, 25*, 229–237.

*Berk, M., Terre-Blanche, M. J., Maude, C., Lucas, M. D., Mendelsohn, M., & O'Neill-Kerr, A. J. (1996). Season of birth and schizophrenia: Southern Hemisphere data. *Australian and New Zealand Journal of Psychiatry, 30*, 220–222.

*Berman, K. F., Doran, A. R., Pickar, D., & Weinberger, D. R. (1993). Is the mechanism of prefrontal hypofunction in depression the same as in schizophrenia? Regional cerebral blood flow during cognitive activation. *British Journal of Psychiatry, 162*, 183–192.

*Berman, K. F., Zec, R. F., & Weinberger, D. R. (1986). Physiologic dysfunction of dorsolateral prefrontal cortex in schizophrenia: II. Role of neuroleptic treatement, attention and mental effort. *Archives of General Psychiatry, 43*, 126–135.

*Besche, C., Passerieux, C., Segui, J., Sarfati, Y., Laurent, J. P., & Hardy-Bayle, M. C. (1997). Syntactic and semantic processing in schizophrenic patients evaluated by lexical-decision tasks. *Neuropsychology, 11*, 498–505.

*Bilder, R. M., Lipschutz-Broch, L., Reiter, G., Geisler, S. H., Mayerhoff, D. I., & Lieberman, J. A. (1992). Intellectual deficits in first-episode schizophrenia: Evidence for progressive deterioration. *Schizophrenia Bulletin, 18*, 437–448.

Bilder, R. M., Mukherjee, S. M., Rieder, R. O., & Pandurangi, A. K. (1985). Symptomatic and neuropsychological components of defect states. *Schizophrenia Bulletin, 11*, 409–419.

*Bilder, R. M., Wu, H., Bogerts, B., Degreef, G., Ashtari, M., Alvir, J. M., Snyder, P. J., & Lieberman, J. A. (1994). Absence of regional hemispheric volume assymmetries in first-episode schizophrenia. *American Journal of Psychiatry, 151*, 1437–1447.

*Biver, F., Goldman, S., Luxen, A., Delvenne, V., De Maertelaer, V., De La Fuente, J., Mendlewicz, J., & Lotstra, F. (1995). Altered frontostriatal relationship in unmedicated schizophrenic patients. *Psychiatry Research, 61*, 161–171.

*Blackwood, D. H., Ebmeier, K. D., Muir, W. J., Sharp, C. W., Glabus, M., Walker, M., Souza, V., Duncan, J. R., & Goodwin, G. M. (1994). Correlation of regional cerebral blood flow equivalents measured by single photon emission computerized tomography with P300 latency and eye movement abnormality in schizophrenia. *Acta Psychiatrica Scandinavica, 90*, 157–166.

*Blackwood, D. H., & Muir, W. J. (1990). Cognitive brain potentials and their application. *British Journal of Psychiatry, 157*, 96–101.

*Blackwood, D. H., St. Clair, D. M., Muir, W. J., & Duffy, J. C. (1991). Auditory P300 and eye tracking dysfunction in schizophrenic pedigrees. *Archives of General Psychiatry, 48*, 899–909.

*Blackwood, D. H., Whalley, L. J., Christie, J. E., Blackburn, I. M., St. Clair, D. M., & McInnes, A. (1987). Changes in auditory P300 event-related potential in schizophrenia and depression. *British Journal of Psychiatry, 150*, 154–160.

Blackwood, D. H., Young, A. H., McQueen, J. K., Martin, M. J., Roxborough, H. M., Muir, W. J., St. Clair, D. M., & Kean, D. M. (1991). Magnetic resonance imaging in schizophrenia: Altered brain morphology associated with P300 abnormalities and eye tracking dysfunction. *Biological Psychiatry, 30*, 753–769.

Bleuler, E. (1950). *Dementia praecox, or the group of schizophrenias* (J. Zinkin, Trans.). New York: International Universities Press. (Original work published 1911).

*Blum, N. A., & Freides, D. (1995). Investigating thought disorder in schizophrenia with the lexical decision task. *Schizophrenia Research, 16*, 217–224.

*Bobes, M. A., Lei, Z. X., Ibanez, S., Yi, H., & Valdes-Sosa, M. (1996). Semantic matching of pictures in schizophrenia: A cross-cultural ERP study. *Biological Psychiatry, 40*, 189–202.

*Bogerts, B., Falkai, P., Haupts, M., Greve, B., Ernst, S., Tapernon-Franz, U., & Heinzmann, U. (1990). Post-mortem volume measurements of limbic system and basal ganglia structures in chronic schizophrenics: Initial results from a new brain collection. *Schizophrenia Research, 3*, 295–301.

*Bogerts, B., Lieberman, J. A., Ashtari, M., Bilder, R. M., Degreef, G., Lerner, G., Johns, C., & Masiar, S. (1993). Hippocampus-amygdala volumes and psychopathology in chronic schizophrenia. *Biological Psychiatry, 33*, 236–246.

*Bogerts, B., Meertz, E., & Schonfeldt-Bausch, R. (1985). Basal ganglia and limbic system pathology in schizophrenia: A morphometric study of brain volume and shrinkage. *Archives of General Psychiatry, 42*, 784–791.

*Boutros, N., Nasrallah, H., Leighty, R., Torello, M., Tueting, P., & Olson, S. (1997). Auditory evoked potentials: Clinical versus research applications. *Psychiatry Research, 69*, 183–195.

*Boutros, N. N., Belger, A., Campbell, D., D'Souza, C., & Krystal, J. (1999). Comparison of four components of sensory gating in schizophrenia and normal subjects: a preliminary report. *Psychiatry Research, 88*, 119–130.

Boutros, N. N., Overall, J., & Zouridakis, G. (1991). Test-retest reliability of the P50 mid-latency auditory evoked response. *Psychiatry Research, 39*, 181–192.

Braff, D. L. (1993). Information processing and attention dysfunctions in schizophrenia. *Schizophrenia Bulletin, 19*, 233–259.

Braff, D. L., & Saccuzzo, D. P. (1982). Effect of antipsychotic medication on speed of information processing in schizophrenic patients. *American Journal of Psychiatry, 139*, 1127–1130.

Braff, D. L., & Saccuzzo, D. P. (1985). The time course of information-processing deficits in schizophrenia. *American Journal of Psychiatry, 142*, 170–174.

*Brecher, M., & Begleiter, H. (1983). Event-related potentials to high-incentive stimuli in unmedicated schizophrenic patients. *Biological Psychiatry*, 18, 661–674.

*Breese, C. R., Freedman, R., & Leonard, S. S. (1995). Glutamate receptor subtype expression in human postmortem brain tissue from schizophrenics and alcohol abusers. *Brain Research, 674*, 82–90.

*Breier, A., Buchanan, R. W., Elkashef, A., Munson, R. C., Kirkpatrick, B., & Gellad, F. (1992). Brain morphology and schizophrenia: A magnetic resonance imaging study of limbic, prefrontal cortex and caudate structures. *Archives of General Psychiatry, 49*, 921–926.

Breslin, N. A., & Weinberger, D. R. (1991). Neurodevelopmental implications of findings from brain imaging studies of schizophrenia. In S. A. Mednick & T. D. Cannon (Eds.), *Fetal neural development and adult schizophrenia* (pp. 199–215). New York: Cambridge University Press.

Brickner, R. M. (1934). An interpretation of frontal lobe function based upon the study of a case of partial bilateral frontal lobectomy. *Research and Publications of the Association for the Research of Nervous and Mental Disease, 13*, 259–351.

Brickner, R. M. (1936). *The intellectual functions of the frontal lobes*. New York: Macmillan.

Broca, P. (1861). Remarques sur le siège de la faculté du langage articulé suivies d'une observation d'aphémie. *Bulletin de la Societe d'Anatomie Paris, 2*, 330–357.

Brodmann, K. (1909). *Vergleichende Lokalisationslehre der Grosshirnrinde in ihren Prinzipien dargestellt auf Grund des Zellenbaues*. Leipzig: Barth.

*Brown, K. W., White, T., & Palmer, D. (1992). Movement disorders and psychological tests of frontal lobe function in schizophrenic patients. *Psychological Medicine, 22*, 69–77.

Brown, R. G., & Marsden, C. D. (1988). Internal versus external cues and the control of attention in Parkinson's disease. *Brain, 111*, 323–345.

Brown, S., & Schaefer, E. A. (1888). An investigation into the functions of the occipital and temporal lobe of the monkey's brain. *Philosophical Transactions of the Royal Society, 179* (part B), 303–327.

*Bryant, N. L., Buchanan, R. W., Vladar, K., Breier, A., & Rothman, M. (1999). Gender differences in temporal lobe structures of patients with schizophrenia: a volumetric MRI study. *American Journal of Psychiatry, 156*, 603–609.

Buchanan, R. W. (1995). Clozapine: Efficacy and safety. *Schizophrenia Bulletin, 21*, 579–591.

Buchanan, R. W., & Carpenter, W. T. (2000). Schizophrenia: Introduction and overview. In B. J. Sadock & V. A. Sadock (Eds.), *Kaplan and Sadock's comprehensive textbook of psychiatry* (Vol. 1). (7th ed., pp. 1096–1110). Philadelphia: Lippincott Williams & Wilkins.

★Buchanan, R. W., Breier, A., Kirkpatrick, B., Elkashef, A., Munson, R. C., Gellad, F., & Carpenter, W. T., Jr. (1993). Structural abnormalities in deficit and non-deficit schizophrenia. *American Journal of Psychiatry, 150,* 59–65.

★Buchanan, R. W., Strauss, M. E., Breier, A., Kirkpatrick, B., & Carpenter, W. T., Jr. (1997). Attentional impairments in deficit and nondeficit forms of schizophrenia. *American Journal of Psychiatry, 154,* 363–370.

★Buchanan, R. W., Vladar, K., Barta, P. E., & Pearlson, G. D. (1998). Structural evaluation of the prefrontal cortex in schizophrenia. *American Journal of Psychiatry, 155,* 1049–1055.

★Buchsbaum, M. S., DeLisi, L. E., Holcomb, H. H., Cappelletti, J., King, A. C., Johnson, J., Hazlett, E., Dowling-Zimmerman, S., Post, R. M., Morihisa, J., Carpenter, W., Cohen, R., Pickar, D., Weinberger, D. R., Margolin, R., & Kessler, R. (1984). Anteroposterior gradients in cerebral glucose use in schizophrenia and affective disorders. *Archives of General Psychiatry, 41,* 1159–1166.

Buchsbaum, M. S., & Haier, R. J. (1983). Psychopathology: Biological approaches. *Annual Review of Psychology, 34,* 401–430.

★Buchsbaum, M. S., Haier, R. J., Potkin, S. G., Nuechterlein, K., Bracha, H. S., Katz, M., Lohr, J., Wu, J., Lottenberg, S., & Jerabek, P. A. (1992). Frontostriatal disorder of cerebral metabolism in never-medicated schizophrenics. *Archives of General Psychiatry, 49,* 935–942.

★Buchsbaum, M. S., Nuechterlein, K. H., Haier, R. J., Wu, J., Sicotte, N., Hazlett, E., Asarnow, R., Potkin, S., & Guich, S. (1990). Glucose metabolic rate in normals and schizophrenics during the Continuous Performance Test assessed by positron emission tomography. *British Journal of Psychiatry, 156,* 216–227.

Buckley, P. F., Moore, C., Long, H., Larkin, C., Thompson, P., Mulvany, F., Redmond, O., Stack, J. P., Ennis, J. T., & Waddington, J. L. (1994). 1H-magnetic resonance spectroscopy of the left temporal and frontal lobes in schizophrenia: Clinical, neurodevelopmental and cognitive correlates. *Biological Psychiatry, 36,* 792–800.

Bunney, B. G., Potkin, S. G., & Bunney, W. E. (1997). Neuropathological studies of brain tissue in schizophrenia. *Journal of Psychiatric Research, 31,* 159–173.

★Burnet, P. W., Eastwood, S. L., & Harrison, P. J. (1996). 5-HT1A and 5-HT2A receptor mRNAs and binding site densities are differentially altered in schizophrenia. *Neuropsychopharmacology, 15,* 442–455.

★Bustini, M., Stratta, P., Daneluzzo, E., Pollice, R., Prosperini, P., & Rossi, A. (1999). Tower of Hanoi and WCST performance in schizophrenia: problem-solving capacity and clinical correlates. *Psychiatry Research, 33,* 285–290.

Butler, R. W., & Braff, D. L. (1991). Delusions: A review and integration. *Schizophrenia Bulletin, 17,* 633–647.

Butler, R. W., Roisman, I., Hill, J. M., & Tuma, R. (1993). The effects of frontal brain impairment on fluency: Simple and complex paradigms. *Neuropsychology, 7,* 519–529.

Butzlaff, R. L., & Hooley, J. M. (1998). Expressed emotion and psychiatric relapse: A meta-analysis. *Archives of General Psychiatry, 55,* 547–552.

*Cadenhead, K. S., Geyer, M. A., Butler, R. W., Perry, W., Sprock, J., & Braff, D. L. (1997). Information processing deficits of schizophrenia patients: Relationship to clinical ratings, gender, and medication status. *Schizophrenia Research, 28*, 51–62.

Cadenhead, K. S., Light, G. A., Geyer, M. A., & Braff, D. L. (2000). Sensory gating deficits assessed by the P50 event-related potential in subjects with schizotypal personality disorder. *American Journal of Psychiatry, 157*, 55–59.

*Cadenhead, K. S., Serper, Y., & Braff, D. L. (1998). Transient versus sustained visual channels in the visual backward masking deficits of schizophrenia patients. *Biological Psychiatry, 43*, 132–138.

Cahill, L., Haier, R. J., Fallon, J., Alkire, M. T., Tang, C., Keator, D., Wu, J., & McGaugh, J. L. (1996). Amygdala activity at encoding correlated with long-term, free recall of emotional information. *Proceedings of the National Academy of Science USA, 93*, 8016–8021.

*Campana, A., Duci, A., Gambini, O., & Scarone, S. (1999). An artificial neural network that uses eye-tracking performance to identify patients with schizophrenia. *Schizophrenia Bulletin, 25*, 789–799.

*Campion, D., Thibaut, F., Denise, P., Courtin, P., Pottier, M., & Levillain, D. (1992). SPEM impairment in drug-naive schizophrenic patients: Evidence for a trait marker. *Biological Psychiatry, 32*, 891–902.

Canavan, A. G., Passingham, R. E., Marsden, C. D., Quinn, N., Wyke, M, & Polkey, C. E. (1989). The performance on learning tasks of patients in the early stages of Parkinson's disease. *Neuropsychologia, 27*, 141–156.

Cannon, M., Cotter, D., Coffey, V. P., Sham, P. C., Takei, N., Larkin, C., Murray, R. M., & O'Callaghan, E. (1996). Prenatal exposure to the 1957 influenza epidemic and adult schizophrenia: A follow-up study. *British Journal of Psychiatry, 168*, 368–371.

*Cannon, M., Jones, P., Gilvarry, C., Rifkin, L., McKenzie, K., Foerster, A., & Murray, R. M. (1997). Premorbid social functioning in schizophrenia and bipolar disorder: Similarities and differences. *American Journal of Psychiatry, 154*, 1544–1550.

Cannon, T. D. (1996). Abnormalities of brain structure and function in schizophrenia: Implications for aetiology and pathophysiology. *Annals of Medicine, 28*, 533–539.

*Cantor-Graae, E., McNeil, T. F., Sjöstrom, K., Nordstrom, L. G., & Rosenlund, T. (1997). Maternal demographic correlates of increased history of obstetric complications in schizophreina. *Journal of Psychiatric Research, 31*, 347–357.

Cardno, A. G., & Gottesman, I. I. (2000). Twin studies of schizophrenia: From bow-and-arrow concordances to Star Wars Mx and functional genomics. *American Journal of Medical Genetics, 97*, 12–17.

Carlsson, M., & Carlsson, A. (1990). Interactions between glutamatergic and mono-aminergic systems within the basal ganglia: Implications for schizophrenia and Parkinson's disease. *Trends in Neuroscience, 13*, 272–276.

Carlsson, A., Hansson, L. O., Waters, N., & Carlsson, M. L. (1997). Neurotransmitter aberrations in schizophrenia: New perspectives and therapeutic implications. *Life Sciences, 61*, 75–94.

Carpenter, M. D. (1976). Sensitivity to syntactic structure: Good versus poor premorbid schizophrenics. *Journal of Abnormal Psychology, 85*, 41–50.

Carpenter, W. T., Heinrichs, D. W., & Wagman, A. M. (1988). Deficit and non-deficit forms of schizophrenia: The concept. *American Journal of Psychiatry, 145,* 578–583.

Carpenter, W. T., & Strauss, J. S. (1979). Diagnostic issues in schizophrenia. In L. Bellak (Ed.), *Disorders of the schizophrenic syndrome* (pp. 291–319). New York: Basic Books.

Carson, R. C., & Sanislow, C. A., III. (1993). The schizophrenias. In P. B. Sutker & H. E. Adams (Eds.), *Comprehensive handbook of psychopathology* (2nd ed., pp. 295–333). New York: Plenum Press.

Case, R. (1985). *Intellectual development: Birth to adulthood.* Orlando, FL: Academic Press.

Catts, S. V., Ward, P. B., Lloyd, A., Huang, X. F., Dixon, G., Chahl, L., Harper, C., & Wakefield, D. (1997). Molecular biological investigations into the role of the NMDA receptor in the pathophysiology of schizophrenia. *Australian and New Zealand Journal of Psychiatry, 31*(1), 17–26.

Chapman, L. J., & Chapman, J. P. (1973). Problems in the measurement of cognitive deficits. *Psychological Bulletin, 79,* 380–385.

Chen, E. Y., Wilkins, A. J., & McKenna, P. J. (1994). Semantic memory is both impaired and anomalous in schizophrenia. *Psychological Medicine, 24,* 193–202.

★Chen, Y., Levy, D. L., Nakayama, K., Matthysse, S., Palafox, G., & Holzman, P. S. (1999). Dependence of impaired eye tracking on deficient velocity discrimination in schizophrenia. *Archives of General Psychiatry, 56,* 155–161.

Chiulli, S., Yeo, R. A., Haaland, K. Y., & Garry, P. (1989). Complex Figure copy and recall in the elderly. *Journal of Clinical and Experimental Neuropsychology, 11,* 95.

★Christison, G. W., Casanova, M. F., Weinberger, D. R., Rawlings, R., & Kleinman, J. E. (1989). A quantitative investigation of hippocampal pyramidal cell size, shape, and variability of orientation in schizophrenia. *Archives of General Psychiatry, 46,* 1027–1032.

Christison, G. W., Kirch, D. G., & Wyatt, R. J. (1991). When symptoms persist: Choosing among alternative somatic treatments for schizophrenia. *Schizophrenia Bulletin, 17,* 217–245.

Chua, S. E., & Murray, R. M. (1996). The neurodevelopmental theory of schizophrenia: Evidence concerning structure and neuropsychology. *Annals of Medicine, 28,* 547–555.

★Chung, R. K., Langeluddecke, P., & Tennant, C. (1986). Threatening life events in the onset of schizophrenia, schizophreniform psychosis and hypomania. *British Journal of Psychiatry, 148,* 680–685.

Churchland, P. M. (1995). *The engine of reason, the seat of the soul.* Cambridge: MIT Press.

★Clark, C., Kopala, L., Hurwitz, T., Li, D. (1991). Regional metabolism in microsmic patients with schizophrenia. *Canadian Journal of Psychiatry, 36,* 645–650.

Clark, C. M., Kopala, L., James, G., Hurwitz, T., & Li, D. (1993). Metabolic subtypes in patients with schizophrenia. *Biological Psychiatry, 33,* 86–92.

Cleghorn, J. M., Garnett, E. S., Nahmias, C., Brown, G. M. Kaplan, R .D., Szechtman, H., Szechtman, B., Franco, S., Dermer, S. W., & Cook, P. (1990). Regional brain metabolism during auditory hallucinations in chronic schizophrenia. *British Journal of Psychiatry, 157,* 562–570.

★Cleghorn, J. M., Garnett, E. S., Nahmias, C., Firnau, G., Brown, G. M., Kaplan, R. D., Szechtman, H., & Szechtman, B. (1989). Increased frontal and reduced parietal glucose metabolism in acute untreated schizophrenia. *Psychiatry Research, 28,* 119–133.

Cleghorn, J. M., Kaplan, R. D., Szechtman, B., Szechtman, H., & Brown, G. M. (1990). Neuroleptic drug effects on cognitive function in schizophrenia. *Schizophrenia Research, 3,* 211–219.

★Clementz, B. A., Geyer, M. A., & Braff, D. L. (1998). Poor P50 suppression among schizophrenia patients and their first-degree biological relatives. *American Journal of Psychiatry, 155,* 1691–1694.

★Clementz, B. A., Grove, W. M., Iacono, W. G., & Sweeney, J. A. (1992). Smooth-pursuit eye movement dysfunction and liability for schizophrenia: Implications for genetic modelling. *Journal of Abnormal Psychology, 101,* 117–129.

★Clementz, B. A., McDowell, J. E., & Zisook, S. (1994). Saccadic system functioning among schizophrenia patients and their first-degree biological relatives. *Journal of Abnormal Psychology, 103,* 277–287.

Clementz, B. A., & Sweeney, J. A. (1990). Is eye movement dysfunction a biological marker for schizophrenia? A methodological review. *Psychological Bulletin, 108,* 77–92.

★Coburn, K. L., Shillcutt, S. D., Tucker, K. A., Estes, K. M., Brin, F. B., Merai, P. & Moore, N. C. (1998). P300 delay and attenuation in schizophrenia: Reversal by neuroleptic medication. *Biological Psychiatry, 44,* 466–474.

★Coffman, J. A., Schwarzkopf, S. B., Olson, S. C., & Nasrallah, H. A. (1989). Midsagittal cerebral anatomy by magnetic resonance imaging: The importance of slice position and thickness. *Schizophrenia Research, 2,* 287–294.

Cohen, B. D. (1978). Referent communication disturbances in schizophrenia. In S. Schwartz (Ed.), *Language and cognition in schizophrenia* (pp. 1–34). Hillsdale, NJ: Erlbaum.

Cohen, H. (1981). The evolution of the concept of disease. In A. L. Caplan, H. Engelhardt Jr., & J. J. McCartney (Eds.), *Concepts of health and disease* (pp. 209–220). London: Addison-Wesley.

Cohen, J. (1988). *Statistical power analysis for the behavioral sciences* (2nd ed.). New York: Academic Press.

Cohen, J. (1994). The earth is round (p < .05). *American Psychologist, 49,* 997–1003.

★Cohen, J. D., Barch, D. M., Carter, C., & Servan-Schreiber, D. (1999). Context-processing deficits in schizophrenia: Converging evidence from three theoretically motivated cognitive tasks. *Journal of Abnormal Psychology, 108,* 120–133.

Cohen, J. D., & Servan-Schreiber, D. (1992). Context, cortex and dopamine: A connectionist approach to behavior and biology in schizophrenia. *Psychological Review, 99,* 45–77.

Cohen, J. D., & Servan-Schreiber, D. (1993). A theory of dopamine function and its role in cognitive deficits in schizophrenia. *Schizophrenia Bulletin, 19,* 85–104.

★Cohen, R. M., Nordahl, T. E., Semple, W. E., Andreason, P., Litman, R. E., & Pickar, D. (1997). The brain metabolic patterns of clozapine- and fluphenazine-treated patients with schizophrenia during a continuous performance task. *Archives of General Psychiatry, 54,* 481–486.

★Cohen, R. M., Nordahl, T. E., Semple, W. E., Andreason, P., & Pickar, D. (1998). Abnormalities in the distributed network of sustained attention predict neuroleptic treatment response in schizophrenia. *Neuropsychopharmacology, 19,* 36−47.

*Cohen, R. M., Semple, W. E., Gross, M., Nordahl, T. E., DeLisi, L. E., Holcomb, H. H., King, A. C., Morihisa, J. M., & Pickar, D. (1987). Dysfunction in a prefrontal substrate of sustained attention in schizophrenia. *Life Science, 40,* 2031−2039.

Cohen, R. Z., Seeman, M. V., Gotowiec, A., & Kopala, L. (1999). Earlier puberty as a predictor of later onset of schizophrenia in women. *American Journal of Psychiatry, 156,* 1059−1064.

Cohen, S. (1964). Drugs for the troubled mind. *Medical World News,* 92−109.

Collicutt, J. R., & Hemsley, D. R. (1981). A psychophysical investigation of auditory functioning in schizophrenia. *British Journal of Clinical Psychology, 20,* 199−204.

*Condray, R., Steinhauer, S. R., van Kammen, D. P., & Kasparek, A. (1996). Working memory capacity predicts language comprehension in schizophrenic patients. *Schizophrenia Research, 20,* 1−13.

*Conrad, A. J., Abebe, T., Austin, R., Forsythe, S., & Scheibel, A. B. (1991). Hippocampal pyramidal cell disarray in schizophrenia as a bilateral phenomenon. *Archives of General Psychiatry, 48,* 413−317.

Conrad, A. J., & Scheibel, A. B. (1987). Schizophrenia and the hippocampus: The embryological hypothesis extended. *Schizophrenia Bulletin, 13,* 577−587.

Coon, H., Byerley, W., Holik, J., Hoff, M., Myles-Worsley, M., Lannfelt, L., Sokoloff, P., Schwartz, J-C., Waldo, M., Freedman, R., & Plaetke, R. (1993). Linkage analysis of schizophrenia with five dopamine receptor genes in nine pedigrees. *American Journal of Human Genetics, 52,* 327−334.

Cooper, J. R., Bloom, F. E., & Roth, R. H. (1996). *The biochemical basis of neuropharmacology* (7th ed.). New York: Oxford University Press.

Corcoran, R., Cahill, C., & Frith, C. D. (1997). The appreciation of visual jokes in people with schizophrenia: A study of "mentalizing" ability. *Schizophrenia Research, 24,* 319−327.

*Corey-Bloom, J., Jernigan, T., Archibald, S., Harris, M. J., & Jeste, D. V. (1995). Quantitative magnetic resonance imaging of the brain in late-life schizophrenia. *American Journal of Psychiatry, 152,* 447−449.

Corkin, S. (1984). Lasting consequences of bilateral medial temporal lobectomy: Clinical course and experimental findings in H.M. *Seminars in Neurology, 4,* 249−259.

*Cornblatt, B. A., & Erlenmeyer-Kimling, L. (1985). Global attentional deviance as a marker of risk for schizophrenia: Specificity and predictive validity. *Journal of Abnormal Psychology, 94,* 470−486.

Cornblatt, B. A., & Keilp, J. G. (1994). Impaired attention, genetics and the pathophysiology of schizophrenia. *Schizophrenia Bulletin, 20,* 31−46.

*Cornblatt, B. A., Lenzenweger, M. F., Dworkin, R. H., & Erlenmeyer-Kimling, L. (1992). Childhood attentional dysfunctions predict social deficits in unaffected adults at risk for schizophrenia. *British Journal of Psychiatry, 161,* 59−64.

*Cornblatt, B. A., Lenzenweger, M. F., & Erlenmeyer-Kimling, L. (1989). The Continuous Performance Test, Identical Pairs version: II. Contrasting attentional profiles in schizophrenic and depressed patients. *Psychiatry Research, 29,* 65−86.

*Cowell, P. E., Kostianovsky, D. J., Gur, R. C., Turetsky, B. I., & Gur, R. E. (1996). Sex differences in neuroanatomical and clinical correlations in schizophrenia. *American Journal of Psychiatry, 153*, 799–805.

Creese, I., Burt, D. R., & Snyder, S. H. (1976). Dopamine receptor binding predicts clinical and pharmacological potencies of anti-schizophrenic drugs. *Science, 192*, 481–483.

Crick, F. (1994). *The astonishing hypothesis*. London: Touchstone Books.

★Cross, A. J., Crow, T. J., & Owen, F. (1981). 3H-Flupenthixol binding in post-mortem brains of schizophrenics: Evidence for a selective increase in dopamine D2 receptors. *Psychopharmacology, 74*, 122–124.

Crosson, B., Sartork, J., Jenny, A .B., & Nabors, N. A. (1993). Increased intrusions during verbal recall in traumatic and non-traumatic lesions of the temporal lobe. *Neuropsychology, 7*, 193–208.

Crow, T. J. (1980). Positive and negative schizophrenic symptoms and the role of dopamine: II. *British Journal of Psychiatry, 137*, 383–386.

Crowe, S. F., & Kuttner, M. (1991). Differences between schizophrenia and the schizophrenia-like psychosis of temporal lobe epilepsy: Support for the two-process view of schizophrenia. *Neuropsychiatry, Neuropsychology, and Behavioral Neurology, 4*, 127–135.

★Csernansky, J. G., Joshi, S., Wang, L., Haller, J. W., Gado, M., Miller, J. P., Grenander, U., & Miller, M. I. (1998). Hippocampal morphometry in schizophrenia by high dimensional brain mapping. *Proceedings of the National Academy of Science USA, 95*, 11406–11411.

★Cullum, C. M., Harris, J. G., Waldo, M. C., Smernoff, E., Madison, A., Nagamoto, H. T., Griffith, J., Adler, L. E., & Freedman, R. (1993). Neurophysiological and neuropsychological evidence for attentional dysfunction in schizophrenia. *Schizophrenia Research, 10*, 131–141.

Curtis, V. A., Bullmore, E. T., Morris, R. G., Brammer, M. J., Williams, S. C., Simmons, A., Sharma, T., Murray, R. M., & McGuire, P. K. (1999). Attenuated frontal activation in schizophrenia may be task dependent. *Schizophrenia Research, 37*, 35–44.

Cutting, J. (1985). *The psychology of schizophrenia*. Edinburgh: Churchill Livingstone.

Damasio, A. R., & Anderson, S. W. (1993). The frontal lobes. In K. M. Heilman & E. Valenstein (Eds.), *Clinical neuropsychology* (3rd ed., pp. 409–460). New York: Oxford University Press.

★d'Amato, T., Guillaud-Bataille, J.M., Rochet, T., Jay, M., Mercier, C., Terra, J.L., & Dalery, J. (1996). No season-of-birth effect in schizophrenic patients from a tropical island in the Southern Hemisphere. *Psychiatry Research, 60*, 205–210.

Daniel, D. G., Goldberg, T. E., Gibbons, R. D., & Weinberger, D. R. (1991). Lack of a bimodal distribution of ventricular size in schizophrenia: A Gaussian mixture analysis of 1056 cases and controls. *Biological Psychiatry, 30*, 887–903.

Darwin, C. (1958). *The origin of species*. New York: New Library of World Literature. (Originally published 1859).

★Dassa, D., Azorin, J. M., Ledoray, V., Sambuc, R., & Giudicelli, S. (1996). Season of birth and schizophrenia: Sex difference. *Progress in Neuropsychopharmacology and Biological Psychiatry, 20*, 243–251.

David, A. S. (1994). The neuropsychological origin of auditory hallucinations. In A. S.

David & J. C. Cutting (Eds.), *The neuropsychology of schizophrenia* (pp. 269–313). Brain damage, behaviour and cognition series. Hove, UK: Erlbaum.

David, A. S., & Cutting, J. C. (1993). Visual imagery and visual semantics in the cerebral hemispheres in schizophrenia. *Schizophrenia Research, 8*, 263–271.

David, A. S., & Cutting, J. C. (1994). The neuropsychology of schizophrenia: Introduction and overview. In A. S. David & J. C. Cutting (Eds.), *The neuropsychology of schizophrenia.* (pp. 1–14). Brain damage, behaviour and cognition series. Hove, UK: Erlbaum.

*Davidson, L. (1999). Neurobiology of the frontal and temporal lobes in schizophrenia: A meta-analytic review of neuroimaging and neuropathological findings. Unpublished master's thesis, Department of Psychology, York University, Toronto, Canada.

*Davidson, M., Reichenberg, A., Rabinowitz, J., Weiser, M., Kaplan, Z., & Mark, M. (1999). Behavioral and intellectual markers for schizophrenia in apparently healthy male adolescents. *American Journal of Psychiatry, 156*, 1328–1335.

Davies, L. M., & Drummond, M. F. (1990). The economic burden of schizophrenia. *Psychiatric Bulletin, 14*, 522–525.

Dawson, M. E., Nuechterlein, K. H., Schell, A. M., Gitlin, M., & Ventura, J. (1994). Autonomic abnormalities in schizophrenia. State or trait indicators? *Archives of General Psychiatry, 51*, 813–824.

Deakin, J. F., & Simpson, M. D. (1997). A two-process theory of schizophrenia: Evidence from studies in post-mortem brain. *Journal of Psychiatry Research, 31*, 277–295.

*Deakin, J. F., Slater, P., Simpson, M. D., Gilchrist, A. C., Skan, W. J., Royston, M. C., Reynolds, G. P., & Cross, A. J. (1989). Frontal cortical and left temporal glutamatergic dysfunction in schizophrenia. *Journal of Neurochemistry, 52*, 1781–1786.

*Dean, B., & Hayes, W. (1996). Decreased frontal cortical serotonin2A receptors in schizophrenia. *Schizophrenia Research, 21*, 133–139.

*Dean, B., Hayes, W., Opeskin, K., Naylor, L., Pavey, G., Hill, C., Keks, N., & Copolov, D. L. (1996). Serotonin2 receptors and the serotonin transporter in the schizophrenic brain. *Behavioral Brain Research, 73*, 169–175.

*Dean, B., Hussain, T., Hayes, W., Scarr, E., Kitsoulis, S., Hill, C., Opeskin, K., & Copolov, D. L. (1999). Changes in serotonin2A and GABA(A) receptors in schizophrenia: Studies on the human dorsolateral prefrontal cortex. *Journal of Neurochemistry, 72*, 1593–1599.

*Dean, B., Scarr, E., Bradbury, R., & Copolov, D. (1999). Decreased hippocampal (CA3) NMDA receptors in schizophrenia. *Synapse, 32*, 67–69.

*Dean, R. S., Gray, J. W., & Seretny, M. L. (1987). Cognitive aspects of schizophrenia and primary affective depression. *International Journal of Clinical Neuropsychology, 9*, 33–36.

*Deicken, R. F., Pegues, M., & Amend, D. (1999). Reduced hippocampal N-acetylaspartate without volume loss in schizophrenia. *Schizophrenia Research, 37*, 217–223.

Delay, J., Deniker, P., & Harl, J. M. (1952). Utilisation en thérapeutique psychiatrique d'une phenothiazine d'action centrale élective. *Annales Medico-Psychologiques, 110*, 112–117.

Delis, D., Kramer, J. H., Kaplan, E., & Ober, B. A. (1987). *California Verbal Learning Test Manual—Adult Version.* San Antonio, TX: Psychological Corporation.

*Delisi, L. E., Buchsbaum, M. S., Holcomb, H. H., Langston, K. C., King, A. C., Kessler, R., Pickar, D., Carpenter, W. T., Morihisa, J. M., Margolin, R., & Weinberger, D.R. (1989). Increased temporal lobe glucose use in chronic schizophrenic patients. *Biological Psychiatry, 25,* 835–851.

*Delisi, L. E., Hoff, A. L., Neale, C., & Kushner, M. (1994). Asymmetries in the superior temporal lobe in male and female first-episode schizophenic patients: Measures of the planum temporale and superior temporal gyrus by MRI. *Schizophrenia Research, 12,* 19–28.

*DeLisi, L. E., Hoff, A. L., Schwartz, J. E., Shields, G. W., Halthore, S. N., Gupta, S. M., Henn, F. A., & Anand, A. K. (1991). Brain morphology in first episode schizophrenic-like psychotic patients: A quantitative magnetic resonance imaging study. *Biological Psychiatry, 29,* 159–175.

Delisi, L. E., Sakuma, M., Kushner, M., Finer, D. L., Hoff, A. L., & Crow, T. J. (1997). Anomalous cerebral asymmetry and language processing in schizophrenia. *Schizophrenia Bulletin, 23,* 255–271.

*Delisi, L. E., Stritzke, P., Riordan, H., Holan, V., Boccio, A., Kushner, M., McClelland, J., Van Eyl, O., & Anand, A. (1992). The timing of brain morphological changes in schizophrenia and their relationship to clinical outcome. *Biological Psychiatry, 31,* 241–254.

*DeMyer, M. K., Gilmor, R. L., Hendrie, H. C., DeMyer, W. E., Augustyn, G. T., & Jackson, R. K. (1988). Magnetic resonance brain images in schizophrenic and normal subjects: Influence of diagnosis and education. *Schizophrenia Bulletin, 14,* 21–37.

De Renzi, E. & Faglioni, P. (1978). Normative data and screening power of a shortened version of the Token Test. *Cortex, 14,* 41–49.

Diamond, D. B. (1997). The fate of the ego in contemporary psychiatry with particular reference to etiologic theories of schizophrenia. *Psychiatry: Interpersonal and Biological Processes, 60,* 67–88.

Diefendorf, A. R., & Dodge, R. (1908). An experimental study of the ocular reactions of the insane from photographic records. *Brain, 31,* 451–489.

Dingledine, R., & McBain, C. J. (1994). Excitatory amino acid transmitters. In G. J. Siegel, B. W. Agranoff, W. R. Albers, & P. B. Molinoff (Eds.), *Basic neurochemistry: Molecular, cellular and medical aspects* (5th ed., pp. 367–399). New York: Raven Press.

Docherty, N., Schnur, M., & Harvey, P. D. (1988). Reference performance and positive and negative thought disorder: A follow-up study of manics and schizophrenics. *Journal of Abnormal Psychology, 97,* 437–442.

Docherty, N. M., Evans, I. M., Sledge, W. H., Seibyl, J. P., & Krystal, J. H. (1994). Affective reactivity of language in schizophrenia. *Journal of Nervous and Mental Disease, 182,* 98–102.

*Done, D. J., Crow, T. J., Johnstone, E. C., & Sacker, A. (1994). Childhood antecedents of schizophrenia and affective illness: Social adjustment at ages 7 and 11. *British Medical Journal, 309,* 699–703.

Done, D. J., & Frith, C. D. (1984). The effect of context during word perception in schizophrenic patients. *Brain and Language, 23,* 318–336.

*Dudley, R. E., John, C. H., Young, A. W., & Over, D. E. (1997). The effect of self-referent material on the reasoning of people with delusions. *British Journal of Clinical Psychology, 36,* 575–584.

*Dworkin, R. H., Cornblatt, B. A., Friedmann, R., Kaplansky, L. M., Lewis, J. A., Rinaldi, A., Shilliday, C., & Erlenmeyer-Kimling, L. (1993). Childhood precursors of affective versus social deficits in adolescents at risk for schizophrenia. *Schizophrenia Bulletin, 19,* 563–577.

*Dworkin, R. H., Lewis, J. A., Cornblatt, B. A., & Erlenmeyer-Kimling, L. (1994). Social competence deficits in adolescents at risk for schizophrenia. *Journal of Nervous and Mental Disease, 182,* 103–108.

Dykstra, L. (1992). Drug action. In J. Grabowski & G. R. Van den Bos (Eds.), *Psychopharmacology: Basic mechanisms and applied interventions* (pp. 63–96). Master lectures in psychology series. Washington, DC: American Psychological Association.

*Earle-Boyer, E. A., Serper, M. R., Davidson, M., & Harvey, P. D. (1991). Continuous performance tests in schizophrenic patients: Stimulus and medication effects on performance. *Psychiatry Research, 37,* 47–56.

*Eastwood, S. L., Kerwin, R. W., & Harrison, P. J. (1997). Immunoautoradiographic evidence for a loss of alpha-amino-3–hydroxy-5–methyl-4–isoxazole propionate-preferring non-N-methyl-D-aspartate glutamate receptors within the medial temporal lobe in schizophrenia. *Biological Psychiatry, 41,* 636–643.

*Ebert, D., Feistel, H., Barocka, A., Kaschka, W., & Mokrusch, T. (1993). A test-retest study of cerebral blood flow during somatosensory stimulation in depressed patients with schizophrenia and major depression. *European Archives of Psychiatry and Clinical Neuroscience, 242,* 250–254.

Ebert, J. D., Loewy, A. G., Miller, R. S., & Schneiderman, H. A. (1973). *Biology.* New York: Holt Rinehart & Winston.

*Ebmeier, K. P., Glabus, M., Potter, D. D., & Salzen, E. A. (1992). The effect of different high-pass filter settings on peak latencies in the event-related potentials of schizophrenics, patients with Parkinson's disease and controls. *Electroencephalography and Clinical Neurophysiology, 84,* 280–287.

Edwards, C. R. (1983). The analysis of symptoms and signs. In J. Macleod (Ed.), *Clinical examination* (6th ed., pp. 30–55). Edinburgh, UK: Churchill Livingstone.

*Egan, M. F, Duncan, C. C. Suddath, R. L. Kirch, D. G., Mirsky, A. F., & Wyatt, R. J. (1994). Event-related potential abnormalities correlate with structural brain alterations and clinical features in patients with chronic schizophrenia. *Schizophrenia Research, 11,* 259–271.

Eikmeier, G., Lodemann, E., Zerbin, D., & Gastpar, M. (1992). P300, clinical symptoms, and neuropsychological parameters in acute and remitted schizophrenia: A preliminary report. *Biological Psychiatry, 31,* 1065–1069.

*Elkins, I. J., Cromwell, R. L., & Asarnow, R. F. (1992). Span of apprehension in schizophrenic patients as a function of distractor masking and laterality. *Journal of Abnormal Psychology, 101,* 53–60.

Ellenberger, H. F. (1970). *The discovery of the unconscious: The history and evolution of dynamic psychiatry.* New York: Basic Books.

Erlenmeyer-Kimling, L. (1987). Biological markers for the liability to schizophrenia. In H. Helmchen & F. Henn (Eds.), *Biological perspectives of schizophrenia* (pp. 33–56). New York: Wiley.

★Erlenmeyer-Kimling, L., Roberts, S. A., Rock, D., Adamo, U. H., Shapiro, B. M., & Pape, S. (1998). Prediction from longitudinal assessments of high-risk children. In M. F. Lenzenweger and R. H. Dworkin (Eds.), *Origins and development of schizophrenia: Advances in experimental psychopathology* (pp. 427–445). Washington, DC: American Psychiatric Association.

★Falkai, P., & Bogerts, B. (1986). Cell loss in the hippocampus of schizophrenics. *European Archives of Psychiatry and Neurological Science, 236*, 154–161.

★Falkai, P., Bogerts, B., Schneider, T., Greve, B., Pfeiffer, U., Pilz, K., Gonsiorzcyk, C., Majtenyi, C., & Ovary, I. (1995). Disturbed planum temporale asymmetry in schizophrenia: A quantitative post-mortem study. *Schizophrenia Research, 14*, 161–176.

Falkai, P., Honer, W. G., David, S., Bogerts, B., Majtenyi, C., & Bayer, T. A. (1999). No evidence for astrogliosis in brains of schizophrenic patients: A post-mortem study. *Neuropathology and Applied Neurobiology, 25*, 48–53.

Fancher, R. E. (1996). *Pioneers of psychology* (3rd ed.). New York: Norton.

Faraone, S. V., Tsuang, M. T., & Tsuang, D. W. (1999). *Genetics of mental disorders.* New York: Guilford.

★Farde, L., Wiesel, F. A. Hall, H., Halldin, C., Stone-Elander, S., & Sedvall, G. (1987). No D2 receptor increase in PET study of schizophrenia. *Archives of General Psychiatry, 44*, 671–672.

★Farde, L., Wiesel, F. A., Stone-Elander, S., Halldin, C., Nordstrom, A. L., Hall, H., & Sedvall, G. (1990). D2 dopamine receptors in neuroleptic-naive schizophrenic patients: A positron emission tomography study with [11C] raclopride. *Archives of General Psychiatry, 47*, 213–219.

★Farkas, T., Wolf, A. P., Jaeger, J., Brodie, J. D., Christman, D. R., & Fowler, J. S. (1984). Regional brain glucose metabolism in chronic schizophrenia: A positron emission transaxial tomographic study. *Archives of General Psychiatry, 41*, 293–300.

Fedio, P. & Martin, A. (1983). Ideative-emotive behavioral characteristics of patients following left or right temporal lobectomy. *Epilepsia, 24*, S117–S130.

Fein, G. G., Jacobson, J. L., Jacobson, S. W., Schwartz, P. M., & Dowler, J. K (1984). Prenatal exposure to polychlorinated biphenyls: Effects on birth size and gestational age. *Journal of Pediatrics, 105*, 315–320.

Feinberg, T. E., & Shapiro, R. M. (1989). Misidentification-reduplication and the right hemisphere. *Neuropsychiatry, Neuropsychology and Behavioral Neurology, 2*, 39–48.

Fenichel, O. (1945). *The psychoanalytic theory of neurosis.* New York: Norton.

Ferracuti, S., Accornero, N., & Manfredi, M. (1991). Atypical psychosis associated with left temporal arachnoid cyst: Report of four cases. *Integrative Psychiatry, 7*, 132–139.

Fish, B. (1975). Biologic antecedents of psychosis in children. In D. X. Freedman (Ed.), *The biology of the major psychoses: A comparative analysis* (pp. 49–80). New York: Raven Press.

Fish, B. (1977). Neurobiologic antecedents of schizophrenia in children: Evidence for an inherited, congenital neurointegrative defect. *Archives of General Psychiatry, 34*, 1297–1313.

Fish, B., Marcus, J., Hans, S. L., Auerbach, J. G., & Perdue, S. (1992). Infants at risk for schizophrenia: Sequalae of a genetic neurointegrative defect. A review and replication analysis of pandysmaturation in the Jerusalem Development Study. *Archives of General Psychiatry, 49*, 221–235.

Fisher, R. A. (1947). *The design of experiments.* Edinburgh, UK: Oliver & Boyd.

*Flaum, M., Swayze, V. W., II, O'Leary, D. S., Yuh, W. T., Ehrhardt, J. C., Arndt, S. V., & Andreasen, N. C. (1995). Effects of diagnosis, laterality, and gender on brain morphology in schizophrenia. *American Journal of Psychiatry, 152,* 704–714.

Ford, J. M. (1999). Schizophrenia: The broken P300 and beyond. *Psychophysiology, 36,* 667–682.

*Ford, J. M., Mathalon, D. H., Marsh, L. Faustman, W. O., Harris, D. Hoff, A. L. Beal, M. Pfefferbaum, A. (1999). P300 is related to clinical state in severely and moderately ill patients with schizophrenia. *Biological Psychiatry, 46,* 94–101.

*Ford, J. M., White, P. M., Csernansky, J. G., Faustman, W. O., Roth, W. T., & Pfefferbaum, A. (1994). ERPs in schizophrenia: Effects of antipsychotic medication. *Biological Psychiatry, 31,* 1065–1068.

*Ford, J. M., White, P. M., Lim, K. O., & Pfefferbaum, A. (1994). Schizophrenics have fewer and smaller P300s: A single-trial analysis. *Biological Psychiatry, 35,* 96–103.

Fowler, J. S., Volkow, N. D., Wang, G. -J., Pappas, N., Logan, J., MacGregor, R., Alexoff, D., Shea, C., Schlyer, D., Wolf, A. P., Warner, D., Zezulkova, I., & Cilento, R. (1996). Inhibition of monoamine oxidase B in the brains of smokers. *Nature, 379,* 733–736.

Fowles, D. C. (1992). Schizophrenia: Diathesis-stress revisited. *Annual Review of Psychology, 43,* 303–336.

Frame, C. L., & Oltmanns, T. F. (1982). Serial recall by schizophrenic and affective patients during and after psychotic episodes. *Journal of Abnormal Psychology, 91,* 311–318.

*Frangou, S., Sharma, T., Alarcon, G., Sigmudsson, T., Takei, N., Binnie, C., & Murray, R. M. (1997). The Maudsley Family Study: II. Endogenous event-related potentials in familial schizophrenia. *Schizophrenia Research, 23,* 45–53.

Franke, P., Maier, W., Hain, C., & Klingler, T. (1992). Wisconsin Card Sorting Test: An indicator of vulnerability to schizophrenia? *Schizophrenia Research, 6,* 243–249.

*Franke, P., Maier, W., Hardt, J., & Hain, C. (1993). Cognitive functioning and anhedonia in subjects at risk for schizophrenia. *Schizophrenia Research, 10,* 77–84.

*Franke, P., Maier, W., Hardt, J., Hain, C., & Cornblatt, B. A. (1994). Attentional abilities and measures of schizotypy: Their variation and covariation in schizophrenic patients, their siblings, and normal control subjects. *Psychiatry Research, 54,* 259–272.

*Franzek, E., & Beckmann, H. (1992). Season-of-birth effect reveals the existence of etiologically different groups of schizophrenia. *Biological Psychiatry, 32,* 375–378.

*Freedman, R., Adler, L. E., Waldo, M. C., Pachtman, E., & Franks, R. D. (1983). Neurophysiological evidence for a defect in inhibitory pathways in schizophrenia: Comparison of medicated and drug-free patients. *Biological Psychiatry, 18, 537–551.*

*Freedman, R., Hall, M., Adler, L. E., & Leonard, S. (1995). Evidence in postmortem brain tissue for decreased numbers of hippocampal nicotinic receptors in schizophrenia. *Biological Psychiatry, 38,* 22–33.

Freud, S. (1900). *Die Traumdeutung.* Vienna: Deuticke.

*Friedman, D., Cornblatt B., Vaughn, H., Jr., & Erlenmeyer-Kimling, L. (1986). Event-related potentials in children at risk for schizophrenia during two versions of the Continuous Performance Test. *Psychiatry Research, 18,* 161–177.

Friedman, L., & Squires-Wheeler, E. (1994). Event-related potentials (ERPs) as indicators of risk for schizophrenia. *Schizophrenia Bulletin, 20*, 63–74.

Frith, C. D. (1979). Consciousness, information processing and schizophrenia. *British Journal of Psychiatry, 134*, 225–235.

Frith, C. D. (1987). The positive and negative symptoms of schizophrenia reflect impairments in the perception and initiation of action. *Psychological Medicine, 17*, 631–648.

Frith, C .D. (1992). *The cognitive neuropsychology of schizophrenia.* Hillsdale, NJ: Erlbaum.

Frith, C. D. (1994). Theory of mind in schizophrenia. In A. S. David & J. C. Cutting (Eds.), *The neuropsychology of schizophrenia.* Brain damage, behaviour and cognition series (pp. 147–161). Hove, UK: Erlbaum.

Frith, C. D., & Corcoran, R. (1996). Exploring "theory of mind" in people with schizophrenia. *Psychological Medicine, 26*, 521–530.

Frith, C. D., & Done, D. J. (1988). Towards a neuropsychology of schizophrenia. *British Journal of Psychiatry, 153*, 437–443.

Frith, C. D., & Done, D. J. (1989). Experiences of alien control in schizophrenia reflect a disorder in the central monitoring of action. *Psychological Medicine, 19*, 359–363.

★Frodl, T., Meisenzahl, E. M., Gallinat, J., Hegerl, U., & Moller, H. J. (1998). Markers from event-related potential subcomponents and reaction time for information processing dysfunction in schizophrenia. *European Archives of Psychiatry and Clinical Neuroscience, 248*, 307–313.

★Frodl-Bauch, T., Gallinat, J., Meisenzahl, E. M., Moller, H. J., & Hegerl, U. (1999). P300 subcomponents reflect different aspects of psychopathology in schizophrenia. *Biological Psychiatry, 45*, 116–126.

Fromm-Reichmann, F. (1948). Notes on the development of treatments of schizophrenics by psychoanalytic psychotherapy. *Psychiatry, 2*, 263–273.

Fromm-Reichmann, F. (1959). *Psychoanalysis and psychotherapy, selected papers.* Chicago: University of Chicago Press.

Frost, J. J. (1990). Imaging the serotonergic system by positron emission tomography. *Annals of the New York Academy of Science, 600*, 273–280.

★Fukuzako, H., Fukuzako, T., Hashiguchi, T., Hokazono, Y., Takeuchi, K., Hirakawa, K., Ueyama, K., Takigawa, M., Kajiya, Y., Nakajo, M., & Fujimoto, T. (1996). Reduction in hippocampal formation volume is caused mainly by its shortening in chronic schizophrenia: Assessment by MRI. *Biological Psychiatry, 39*, 938–945.

★Fukuzako, H., Yamada, K., Kodama, S., Yonezawa, T., Fukuzako, T., Takenouchi, K., Kajiya, Y., Nakajo, M., & Takigawa, M. (1997). Hippocampal volume asymmetry and age at illness onset in males with schizophrenia. *European Archives of Psychiatry and Clinical Neuroscience, 247*, 248–251.

Gardner, H. (1975). *The shattered mind.* New York: Knopf.

Garety, P. A., & Freeman, D. (1999). Cognitive approaches to delusions: a critical review of theories and evidence. *British Journal of Clinical Psychology, 38*, 113–154.

Garety, P. A., & Hemsley, D. R. (1994). *Delusions: Investigations into the psychology of delusional reasoning.* New York: Oxford University Press.

★Garety, P. A., Hemsley, D. R., & Wessely, S. (1991). Reasoning in deluded schizophrenic and paranoid patients: Biases in performance on a probabilistic inference task. *Journal of Nervous and Mental Disease, 179*, 194–201.

Gathercole, S. E. (1994). Neuropsychology and working memory: A review. *Neuropsychology, 8*, 494–505.

*Gattaz, W. F., Waldmeier, P., & Beckmann, H. (1982). CSF monoamine metabolites in schizophrenic patients. *Acta Psychiatrica Scandinavica, 66*, 350–360.

Gazzaniga, M. S. (1985). *The social brain: Discovering the networks of the mind.* New York: Basic Books.

*Geraud, G., Arne-Bes, M. C., Guell, A., & Bes, A. (1987). Reversibility of hemodynamic hypofrontality in schizophrenia. *Journal of Cerebral Blood Flow and Metabolism, 7*, 9–12.

Gilbert, S. F. (1997). *Developmental biology.* Sunderland, MA: Sinauer.

*Gjedde, A., & Wong, D. F. (1987). Positron tomographic quantification of neuroreceptors in human brain in vivo—with special reference to the D2 dopamine receptors in caudate nucleus. *Neurosurgical Review, 10*, 9–18.

*Glabus, M. F., Blackwood, D. H. R., Ebmeier, K. P., Souza, V., Walker, M. T., Sharp, C. W., Dunan, J. T., & Muir, W. (1994). Methodological considerations in measurement of the P300 component of the auditory oddball ERP in schizophrenia. *Electroencephalography and Clinical Neurophysiology, 90*, 123–134.

Goel, V., & Grafman, J. (1995). Are the frontal lobes implicated in "planning" functions? Interpreting data from the Tower of Hanoi. *Neuropsychologia, 33*, 623–642.

Goldberg, E., Bilder, R. M., Hughes, J. E., Antin, S. P., & Matti, S. (1989). A reticulo-frontal disconnection syndrome. *Cortex, 25*, 687–695.

*Goldberg, T. E., Aloia, M. S., Gourovitch, M. L., Missar, D., Pickar, D. Weinberger, D. R. (1998). Cognitive substrates of thought disorder: I. The semantic system. *American Journal of Psychiatry, 155*, 1671–1676.

*Goldberg, T. E., Patterson, K. J., Taqqu, Y. & Wilder, K. (1998). Capacity limitations in short-term memory in schizophrenia: Tests of competing hypotheses. *Psychological Medicine, 28*, 665–673.

*Goldberg, T. E., Saint-Cyr, J. A., & Weinberger, D. R. (1990). Assessment of procedural learning and problem solving in schizophrenic patients by Tower of Hanoi type tasks. *Journal of Neuropsychiatry and Clinical Neuroscience, 2*, 165–173.

Goldberg, T. E., & Weinberger, D. R. (1995). A case against subtyping in schizophrenia. *Schizophrenia Research, 17*, 147–152.

Goldman-Rakic, P. S. (1992). Working memory and the mind. *Scientific American, 267*, 110–117.

Goldman-Rakic, P. S. (1996). The prefrontal landscape: Implications of functional architecture for understanding human mentation and the central executive. *Philosophical Transactions of the Royal Society, 351*, 1445–1453.

Goldman-Rakic, P. S. (1999). The physiological approach: Functional architecture of working memory and disordered cognition in schizophrenia. *Biological Psychiatry, 46*, 650–661.

*Goldstein, J. M., Goodman, J. M., Seidman, L. J., Kennedy, D. N., Makris, N., Lee, H., Tourville, J., Caviness, V. S. Jr., Faraone, S. V., & Tsuang, M. T. (1999). Cortical abnormalities in schizophrenia identified by structural magnetic resonance imaging. *Archives of General Psychiatry, 56*, 537–547.

★Goldstein, M. J. (1985). Family factors that antedate the onset of schizophrenia and related disorders: The results of a fifteen year prospective longitudinal study. *Acta Psychiatrica Scandinavica Suppl., 319*, 7–18.

★Gonsalvez, C. J., Gordon, E., Anderson, J., Pettigrew, G., Barry, R. J., Rennie, C., & Meares, R. (1995). Numbers of preceding nontargets differentially affect responses to targets in normal volunteers and patients with schizophrenia: A study of event-related potentials. *Psychiatry Research, 58*, 69–75.

★Gooding, D. C., Iacono, W. G., & Beiser, M. (1994). Temporal stability of smooth-pursuit eye tracking in first-episode psychosis. *Psychophysiology, 31*, 62–67.

Goodman, R. (1994). Brain development. In M. Rutter & D. F. Hay (Eds.), *Development through life: A handbook for clinicians* (pp. 49–78). Oxford: Blackwell Scientific.

★Goodman, S. H. (1987). Emory University Project on Children of Disturbed Parents. *Schizophrenia Bulletin, 13*, 411–423.

Gottesman, I. I. (1991). *Schizophrenia genesis: The origins of madness.* New York: Freeman.

Gottesman, I. I. (1994). Complications to the complex inheritance of schizophrenia. *Clinical Genetics, 46*, 116–123.

Gottesman, I. I., & Shields, J. (1972). *Schizophrenia and genetics: A twin study vantage point.* New York: Academic Press.

Gottesman, I. I., & Shields, J. (1982). *Schizophrenia. The epigenetic puzzle.* Cambridge, UK: Cambridge University Press.

Granholm, E., Morris, S. K., Sarkin, A. J., Asarnow, R. F. & Jeste, D. V. (1997). Pupillary responses index overload of working memory resources in schizophrenia. *Journal of Abnormal Psychology, 106*, 458–467.

Gray, J. A. (1998). Integrating schizophrenia. *Schizophrenia Bulletin, 24*, 249–266.

Gray, J. A., Feldon, J., Rawlins, J. N., Hemsley, D. R., & Smith, A. D. (1991). The neuropsychology of schizophrenia. *Behavioral and Brain Sciences, 14*, 1–84.

★Green, M., & Walker, E. (1986a). Attentional performance in positive- and negative-symptom schizophrenia. *Journal of Nervous and Mental Disease, 174*, 208–213.

★Green, M., & Walker, E. (1986b). Symptom correlates of vulnerability to backward masking in schizophrenia. *American Journal of Psychiatry, 143*, 181–186.

Green, M. F., & Kinsbourne, M. (1990). Subvocal activity and auditory hallucinations: Clues for behavioral treatments? *Schizophrenia Bulletin, 16*, 617–625.

★Green, M. F., Nuechterlein, K. H., Breitmeyer, B., & Mintz, J. (1999). Backward masking in unmedicated schizophrenia patients in psychotic remission: possible reflection of aberrant cortical oscillation. *American Journal of Psychiatry, 156*, 1367–1373.

★Griffith, J., Hoffer, L. D., Adler, L. E., Zerbe, G. O., & Freedman, R. (1995). Effects of sound intensity on a mid-latency evoked response to repeated auditory stimuli in schizophrenic and normal subjects. *Psychophysiology, 32*, 460–466.

★Griffith, J. J., Mednick, S. A., Schulsinger, F., & Diderichsen, B. (1980). Verbal associative disturbances in children at high risk for schizophrenia. *Journal of Abnormal Psychology, 89*, 125–131.

★Grillon, C., Ameli, R., Courchesne, E., & Braff, D. L. (1991). Effects of task relevance and attention on P3 in schizophrenic patients. *Schizophrenia Research, 4*, 11–21.

★Grillon, C., Courchesne, E., Ameli, R., Geyer, M. A., & Braff, D. L. (1990). Increased distractibility in schizophrenic patients: Electrophysiologic and behavioral evidence. *Archives of General Psychiatry, 47*, 171–179.

*Grimwood, S., Slater, P., Deakin, J. F., & Hutson, P. H. (1999). NR2B-containing NMDA receptors are up-regulated in temporal cortex in schizophrenia. *Neuroreport, 10,* 461–465.

*Grove, W. M., Clementz, B. A., Iacono, W.G., & Katsanis, J. (1992). Smooth pursuit ocular motor dysfunction in schizophrenia: Evidence for a major gene. *American Journal of Psychiatry, 149,* 1362–1368.

*Grove, W. M., Lebow, B. S., Clementz, B.A., Cerri, A., Medus, C., & Iacono, W.G. (1991). Familial prevalence and co-aggregation of schizotypy indicators: A multitrait family study. *Journal of Abnormal Psychology, 100,* 115–121.

*Guenther, W., Brodie, J. D., Bartlett, E. J., Dewey, S. L., Henn, F. A., Volkow, N. D., Alper, K., Wolkin, A., Cancro, R., & Wolf, A. P. (1994). Diminished cerebral metabolic response to motor stimulation in schizophrenics: A PET study. *European Archives of Psychiatry and Clinical Neuroscience, 244,* 115–125.

*Guich, S. M., Buchsbaum, M. S., Burgwald, L., Wu, J. C., Haier, R., Asarnow, R., Nuechterlein, K., & Potkin, S. (1989). Effect of attention on frontal distribution of delta activity and cerebral metabolic rate in schizophrenia. *Schizophrenia Research, 2,* 439–448.

*Gunduz, H., Woerner, M. G., Alvir, J. M., Degreef, G., Lieberman, J. A. (1999). Obsteric complications in schizophrenia, schizoaffective disorder and normal comparison subjects. *Schizophrenia Research, 40,* 237–243.

*Gunther-Genta, F., Bovet, P., & Hohlfeld, P. (1994). Obstetric complications and schizophrenia: A case-control study. *British Journal of Psychiatry, 164,* 165–170.

*Gur, R. E., Cowell, P., Turetsky, B. I., Gallacher, F., Cannon, T., Bilker, W., & Gur, R. C. (1998). A follow-up magnetic resonance imaging study of schizophrenia. Relationship of neuroanatomical changes to clinical and neurobehavioral measures. *Archives of General Psychiatry, 55,* 145–152.

*Gur, R. E., Mozley, D., Resnick, S. M., Mozley, L. H., Shtasel, D. L., Gallacher, F., Arnold, S. E., Karp, J. S., Alavi, A., Reivich, M., & Gur, R. C. (1995). Resting cerebral glucose metabolism in first-episode and previously treated patients with schizophrenia relates to clinical features. *Archives of General Psychiatry, 52,* 657–667.

*Gur, R. E., Resnick, S. M., Alavi, A., Gur, R. C., Caroff, S., Dann, R., Silver, F. L., Saykin, A. J., Chawluk, J. B., Kushner, M., & Reivich, M. (1987). Regional brain function in schizophrenia: I. A positron emission tomography study. *Archives of General Psychiatry, 44,* 119–125.

*Gureje, O., & Adewunmi, A. (1988). Life events and schizophrenia in Nigerians: A controlled investigation. *British Journal of Psychiatry, 153,* 367–375.

Gusella, J. F., Wexler, N. S., Connealy, P. M., Naylor, S. L., Anderson, M. A., Tanzi, R. E., Watkins, P. C., Ottina, K., Wallace, M. R., & Sakaguchi, A. Y. (1983). A polymorphic DNA marker genetically linked to Huntington's disease. *Nature, 306,* 234–238.

*Guterman, Y., & Josiassen, R. C. (1994). Sensory gating deviance in schizophrenia in the context of task related effects. *International Journal of Psychophysiology, 18,* 1–12.

*Haddock, G., Slade, P. D., & Bentall, R. P. (1995). Auditory hallucinations and the verbal transformation effect: The role of suggestions. *Personality and Individual Differences, 19,* 301–306.

*Haddock, G., Slade, P. D., Prasaad, R. & Bentall, R. P. (1996). Functioning of the phonological loop in auditory hallucinations. *Personality and Individual Differences, 20*, 753–760.

Haddock, G., Wolfenden, M., Lowens, I., Tarrier, N., & Bentall, R. P. (1995). Effect of emotional salience on thought disorder in patients with schizophrenia. *British Journal of Psychiatry, 167*, 618–620.

Hafner, H., & an der Heiden, W. (1999). The course of schizophrenia in the light of modern follow-up studies: The ABC and WHO studies. *European Archives of Psychiatry and Clinical Neurosciences, 249* (suppl. 4), 14–26.

*Hain, C., Maier, W., Klingler, T., & Franke, P. (1993). Positive/negative symptomatology and experimental measures of attention in schizophrenic patients. *Psychopathology, 26*, 62–68.

Halberstadt, A. L. (1995). The phencyclidine-glutamate model of schizophrenia. *Clinical Neuropharmacology, 18*, 237–249.

*Hallett, S., & Green, P. (1983). Possible defects of interhemispheric integration in children of schizophrenics. *Journal of Nervous and Mental Disease, 171*, 421–425.

*Hallett, S., Quinn, D., & Hewitt, J. (1986). Defective interhemispheric integration and anomalous language lateralization in children at risk for schizophrenia. *Journal of Nervous and Mental Disease, 174*, 418–427.

*Hans, S. L., Marcus, J., Henson, L., Auerbach, J. G., & Mirsky, A. F. (1992). Interpersonal behavior of children at risk for schizophrenia. *Psychiatry, 55*, 314–335.

Harlow, J. M. (1848). Passage of an iron rod through the head. *Boston Medical and Surgical Journal, 39*, 389–393.

Harlow, J. M. (1868). Recovery from the passage of an iron bar through the head. *Publications of the Massachusetts Medical Society, 2*, 327–347.

Harrison, P. J. (1999). The neuropathology of schizophrenia. A critical review of the data and their interpretation. *Brain, 122*, 593–624.

Harrow, M., Lanin-Kettering, L, & Miller, J. G., (1989). Impaired perspective and thought pathology in schizophrenic and psychotic disorders. *Schizophrenia Bulletin, 15*, 605–623.

Harvey, P., Winters, K. C., Weintraub, S., & Neale, J. M. (1981). Distractibility in children vulnerable to psychopathology. *Journal of Abnormal Psychology, 90*, 298–304.

Harvey, P. D. (1983). Speech competence in manic and schizophrenic psychoses: The association between clinically rated thought disorder and cohesion and reference performance. *Journal of Abrnormal Psychology, 92*, 368–377.

*Harvey, P. D. (1985). Reality monitoring in mania and schizophrenia: The association of thought disorder and performance. *Journal of Nervous and Mental Disease, 173*, 67–73.

Harvey, P. D., Docherty, N. M., Serper, M. R., & Rasmussen, M. (1990). Cognitive deficits and thought disorder: II. An eight month follow-up study. *Schizophrenia Bulletin, 16*, 147–156.

Harvey, P. D., Earle-Boyer, E. A., & Levinson, J. C. (1986). Distractibility and discourse failure: Their association in mania and schizophrenia. *Journal of Nervous and Mental Disease, 174*, 274–279.

Harvey, P. D., Earle-Boyer, E. A., & Levinson, J. C. (1988). Cognitive deficits and thought disorder: A retest study. *Schizophrenia Bulletin, 14*, 57–66.

Harvey, P. D., Earle-Boyer, E. A., Wielgus, M. S., & Levinson, J. C. (1986). Encoding, memory, and thought disorder in schizophrenia and mania. *Schizophrenia Bulletin, 12*, 252–261.

*Harvey, P. D., Keefe, R. S. E., Moskowitz, J., Putrram, K. M., Mohs, R. C., & Davis, K. L. (1990). Attentional markers of vulnerability to schizophrenia: Performance of medicated and unmedicated patients and normals. *Psychiatry Research, 33*, 179–188.

Harvey, P. D., & Pedley, M. (1989). Auditory and visual distractibility in schizophrenia: Clinical and medication status correlations. *Schizophrenia Research, 2*, 295–300.

Harvey, P. D., & Serper, M. R. (1990). Linguistic and cognitive failures in schizophrenia: A multivariate analysis. *Journal of Nervous and Mental Disease, 178*, 487–493.

*Harvey, P. D., Weintraub, S., & Neale, J. M. (1982). Speech competence of children vulnerable to psychopathology. *Journal of Abnormal Child Psychology, 10*, 373–387.

*Hatta, T., Ayetani, N., & Yoshizaki, K. (1984). Dichotic listening by chronic schizophrenic patients. *International Journal of Neuroscience, 23*, 75–80.

*Havermans, R., Honig, A., Vuurman, E. F., Krabbendam, L., Wilmink, J., Lamers, T., Verheecke, C. J., Jolles, J., Romme, M. A., & van Praag, H. M. (1999). A controlled study of temporal lobe structure volumes and P300 responses in schizophrenic patients with persistent auditory hallucinations. *Schizophrenia Research, 38*, 151–158.

*Hazlett, E. A., Buchsbaum, M. S., Haznedar, M. M., Singer, M. B., Germans, M. K., Schnur, D. B., Jimenez, E. A., Buchsbaum, B. R., & Troyer, B. T. (1998). Prefrontal cortex glucose metabolism and startle eyeblink modification abnormalities in unmedicated schizophrenia patients. *Psychophysiology, 35*, 186–198.

Heaton, R. K. (1981). *Wisconsin Card Sorting Test manual*. Odessa, FL: Psychological Assessment Resources.

Heaton, R. K., Chelune, G. J., Talley, J. L., Kay, G. G., & Curtiss, G. (1993). *Wisconsin Card Sorting Test manual: Revised and expanded*. Odessa, FL: Psychological Assessment Resources.

Hebb, D. O. (1945). Man's frontal lobes: A critical review. *Archives of Neurology and Psychiatry, 54*, 421–438.

Hebb, D. O., & Penfield, W. (1940). Human behavior after extensive bilateral removals from the frontal lobes. *Archives of Neurology and Psychiatry, 44*, 421–438.

*Heckers, S., Heinsen, H., Heinsen, Y. C., & Beckmann, H. (1990). Limbic structures and lateral ventricle in schizophrenia. A quantitative postmortem study. *Archives of General Psychiatry, 47*, 1016–1022.

Heckers, S., Rauch, S. L., Goff, D., Savage, C. R., Schacter, D. L., Fischman, A. J., & Alpert, N. M. (1998). Impaired recruitment of the hippocampus during conscious recollection in schizophrenia. *Nature Neuroscience, 1*, 318–323.

Hedges, L. V., & Olkin, I. (1985). *Statistical methods for meta-analysis*. New York: Academic Press.

*Hegerl, U., Gaebel, W., Gutzman, H., & Ulrich, G. (1988). Auditory evoked potentials as possible predictors of outcome in schizophrenic outpatients. *International Journal of Psychophysiology, 6*, 207–214.

Heilbrun, A. B., Jr. (1980). Impaired recognition of self-expressed thought in patients with auditory hallucinations. *Journal of Abnormal Psychology, 89*, 728–736.

Heilbrun, A. B., Jr., & Blum, N. A. (1984). Cognitive vulnerability to auditory hallucination: Impaired perception of meaning. *British Journal of Psychiatry, 144,* 508–512.

Heilbrun, A. B., Jr., Blum, N., & Haas, M. (1983). Cognitive vulnerability to auditory hallucination: Preferred imagery mode and spatial location of sounds. *British Journal of Psychiatry, 143,* 294–299.

Heilbrun, A. B., Jr., Diller, R., Fleming, R., & Slade, L. (1986). Strategies of disattention and auditory hallucinations in schizophrenics. *Journal of Nervous and Mental Disease, 174,* 265–273.

Heilman, K. M., Bowers, D., & Valenstein, E. (1993). Emotional disorders associated with neurological diseases. In K. M. Heilman & E. Valenstein (Eds.), *Clinical neuropsychology* (3rd ed., pp. 461–497). New York: Oxford University Press.

Heilman, K. M., & Valenstein, E. (1993). Introduction. In K. M. Heilman & E. Valenstein (Eds.), *Clinical neuropsychology* (3rd ed., pp. 1–16). New York: Oxford University Press.

Heilman, K. M., Watson, R. T., & Valenstein, E. (1993). Neglect and related disorders. In K. M. Heilman & E. Valenstein (Eds.), *Clinical neuropsychology* (3rd ed., pp. 279–336). New York: Oxford University Press.

Heinrichs, R. W. (1990). Variables associated with Wisconsin Card Sorting Test performance in neuropsychiatric patients referred for assessment. *Neuropsychiatry, Neuropsychology, and Behavioral Neurology, 3,* 107–112.

Heinrichs, R. W. (1993). Schizophrenia and the brain: Conditions for a neuropsychology of madness. *American Psychologist, 48,* 221–233.

Heinrichs, R. W., & Awad, A. G. (1993). Neurocognitive subtypes of chronic schizophrenia. *Schizophrenia Research, 9,* 49–58.

Heinrichs, R. W., Ruttan, L., Zakzanis, K. K., & Case, D. (1997). Parsing schizophrenia with neurocognitive tests: Evidence of stability and validity. *Brain and Cognition, 35,* 207–224.

★Heinrichs, R. W., & Zakzanis, K. K. (1998). Neurocognitive deficit in schizophrenia: A quantitative review of the evidence. *Neuropsychology, 12,* 426–445.

Helmes, E. (1991). Subtypes of schizophrenia: Real or apparent? Paper presented at the annual meeting of the Canadian Psychological Association, Calgary, Alberta, Canada.

★Helmeste, D. M., Tang, S. W., Bunney, W. E., Jr., Potkin, S. G., & Jones, E. G. (1996). Decrease in sigma but no increase in striatal dopamine D4 sites in schizophrenic brains. *European Journal of Pharmacology, 314,* R3–R5.

Hemsley, D. R. (1994). A cognitive model for schizophrenia and its possible neural basis. *Acta Psychiatrica Scandinavica Suppl. 384,* 80–86.

★Hemsley, D. R., & Richardson, P. H. (1980). Shadowing by context in schizophrenia. *Journal of Nervous and Mental Disease, 168,* 141–145.

Henik, A., Nissimov, E., Priel, B., & Umansky, R. (1995). Effects of cognitive load on semantic priming in patients with schizophrenia. *Journal of Abnormal Psychology, 104,* 576–584.

★Hess, E. J., Bracha, H. S., Kleinman, J. E., & Creese, I. (1987). Dopamine receptor subtype imbalance in schizophrenia. *Life Science, 40,* 1487–1497.

Heston, L. L. (1966). Psychiatric disorders in foster home reared children of schizophrenic mothers. *British Journal of Psychiatry, 112,* 819–825.

*Hietala, J., Syvalahti, E., Vuorio, K., Nagren, K., Lehikoinen, P., Ruotsalainen, U., Rakkolainen, V., Lehtinen, V., & Wegelius, U. (1994). Striatal D2 dopamine receptor characteristics in neuroleptic-naive schizophrenic patients studied with positron emission tomography. *Archives of General Psychiatry, 51*, 116–123.

*Highley, J. R., McDonald, B., Walker, M. A., Esiri, M. M., & Crow, T. J. (1999). Schizophrenia and temporal lobe asymmetry: A post-mortem stereological study of tissue volume. *British Journal of Psychiatry, 175*, 127–134.

Hillyard, S. A., & Kutas, M. (1983). Electrophysiology of cognitive processing. *Annual Review of Psychology, 34*, 33–61.

Hirsch, S. R., Das, I., Garey, L. J., & de Belleroche, J. (1997). A pivotal role for glutamate in the pathogenesis of schizophrenia and its cognitive dysfunction. *Pharmacology, Biochemistry and Behavior, 56*, 797–802.

*Hodges, A., Byrne, M., Grant, E., & Johnstone, E. (1999). People at risk of schizophrenia. Sample characteristics of the first 100 cases in the Edinburgh High-Risk Study. *British Journal of Psychiatry, 174*, 547–553.

Hoffman, R. E. (1986). Verbal hallucinations and language production processes in schizophrenia. *Behavioral and Brain Sciences, 9*, 503–517.

Hoffman, R. E. (1991). The Duphar Lecture: On the etiology of alien, nonself attributes of schizophrenic " voices." *Psychopathology, 24*, 347–355.

Hoffman, R. E. (1999). New methods for studying hallucinated "voices" in schizophrenia. *Acta Psychiatrica Scandinavica Suppl. 395*, 89–94.

Hoffman, R. E., & McGlashan, T. H. (1993). Parallel distributed processing and the emergence of schizophrenic symptoms. *Schizophrenia Bulletin, 19*, 119–140.

*Hoffman, R. E., & Rapaport, J. (1994). A psycholinguistic study of auditory/verbal hallucinations: Preliminary findings. In A. S. David & J. C. Cutting (Eds.), *The neuropsychology of schizophrenia* (pp. 255–267). Brain damage, behaviour, and cognition series. Hove, UK: Erlbaum.

*Hoffman, R. E., Rapaport, J., Mazure, C. M., & Quinlan, D. M. (1999). Selective speech perception alterations in schizophrenic patients reporting hallucinated "voices." *American Journal of Psychiatry, 156*, 393–399.

*Holinger, D. P., Faux, S. F., Shentan, M. E., Sokol, N. S., Seidman, L. J., Green, A. I., & McCarley, R. W. (1992). Reversed temporal region asymmetries of P300 topography in left and right handed schizophrenic subjects. *Electroencephalography and Clinical Neurophysiology, 84*, 532–537.

Holzman, P. S., Kringlen, E., Matthysse, S., Flanagan, S. D., Lipton, R. B., Cramer, S., Levin, S., Lange, K., & Levy, D. L. (1988). A single dominant gene can account for eye tracking dysfunctions and schizophrenia in offspring of discordant twins. *Archives of General Psychiatry, 45*, 641–647.

Holzman, P. S., & Matthysse, S. (1990). The genetics of schizophrenia: A review. *Psychological Science, 1*, 279–286.

Holzman, P. S., Proctor, L. R., & Hughes, D. W. (1973). Eye-tracking patterns in schizophrenia. *Science, 181*, 179–181.

Holzman, P. S., Solomon, C. M., Levin, S., & Waternaux, C. S. (1984). Pursuit eye movement dysfunctions in schizophrenia: Family evidence for specificity. *Archives of General Psychiatry, 41*, 136–139.

*Hook, S., Gordon, E., Lazzaro, I., Burke, C., Anderson, J., Zurynski, Y., Snars, J., & Meares, R. (1995). Regional differentiation of cortical activity in schizophrenia: A complementary approach to conventional analysis of regional cerebral blood flow. *Psychiatry Research, 61*, 85–93.

*Hsiao, J. K., Colison, J., Bartko, J. J., Doran, A. R., Konicki, P. E., Potter, W. Z., & Pickar, D. (1993). Monoamine neurotransmitter interactions in drug-free and neuroleptic-treated schizophrenics. *Archives of General Psychiatry, 50*, 606–614.

Hughes, J. R., Hatsukami, D. K., Mitchell, J. E., & Dahlgren, L. A. (1986). Prevalence of smoking among psychiatric outpatients. *American Journal of Psychiatry, 143*, 993–997.

*Hultman, C. M., Ohman, A., Cnattingius, S., Wieselgren, I. M., & Lindstrom, L. H. (1997). Prenatal and neonatal risk factors for schizophrenia. *British Journal of Psychiatry, 170*, 128–133.

*Hultman, C. M., Sparen, P., Takei, N., Murray, R. M., & Cnattingius, S. (1999). Prenatal and perinatal risk factors for schizophrenia, affective psychosis, and reactive psychosis of early onset: Case-control study. *British Medical Journal, 318*, 421–426.

Hunt, M. M. (1962). *Mental hospital.* New York: Pyramid Books.

Huntington, E. (1938). *Season of birth: Its relation to human abilities.* New York: Wiley.

*Huq, S. F., Garety, P. A., & Hemsley, D. R. (1988). Probabilistic judgments in deluded and non-deluded subjects. *Quarterly Journal of Experimental Psychology, 40*, 801–812.

Hustig, H. H., & Hafner, R. J. (1990). Persistent auditory hallucinations and their relationship to delusions and mood. *Journal of Nervous and Mental Disease, 178*, 264–267.

Iacono, W. G. (1985). Psychophysiologic markers of psychopathology: A review. *Canadian Psychology, 26*, 96–112.

Iacono, W. G. (1998). Identifying psychophysiological risk for psychopathology: Examples from subtsance abuse and schizophrenia research. *Psychophysiology, 35*, 621–637.

Iacono, W. G., & Lykken, D. T. (1979). Electro-oculographic recording and scoring of smooth pursuit and saccadic eye tracking: A parametric study using monozygotic twins. *Psychophysiology, 16*, 94–107.

Iacono, W. G., & Lykken, D. T. (1981). Two-year retest stability of eye tracking performance and a comparison of electro-oculographic and infrared recording techniques: Evidence of EEG in the electro-oculogram. *Psychophysiology, 18*, 49–55.

*Iacono, W. G., Moreau, M., Beiser, M., Fleming, J. A., & Lin, T. Y. (1992). Smooth-pursuit eye tracking in first-episode psychotic patients and their relatives. *Journal of Abnormal Psychology, 101*, 104–116.

Ingraham, L. J. & Kety, S. S. (2000). Adoption studies of schizophrenia. *American Journal of Medical Genetics, 97*, 18–22.

Iqbal, K., & Wisniewski, H. M. (1983). Neurofibrillary tangles. In B. Reisberg (Ed.), *Alzheimer's disease: The standard reference.* New York: Free Press.

Ishigaki, T., & Tanno, Y. (1999). The signal detection ability of patients with auditory hallucinations: Analysis using the continuous performance test. *Psychiatry and Clinical Neurosciences, 53*, 471–476.

*Ito, M., Kanno, M., Mori, Y., & Niwa, S. (1997). Attention deficits assessed by Continuous Performance Test and Span of Apprehension Test in Japanese schizophrenic patients. *Schizophrenia Research, 23*, 205–211.

Iversen, L. L. (1978). Inactivation of neurotransmitters. *Synapse, 18*, 137–153.

*Iwanami, A., Kanamori. R., Isono, H., Okajima, Y., & Kamijima, K. (1996). Impairment of inhibition of unattended stimuli in schizophrenia patients: Event-related potential correlates during selective attention. *Neuropsychobiology, 34*, 57–62.

*Iwanami, A., Suga, I., Kaneko, T., Sugiyama, A., & Nakatani, Y. (1994). P300 component of event-related potentials in methamphetamine psychosis and schizophrenia. *Progress in Neuropsychopharmacology and Biological Psychiatry, 18*, 465–475.

Jablensky, A. (1995). Schizophrenia: Recent epidemiologic issues. *Epidemiological Review, 17*, 10–20.

Jablensky, A., Sartorius, N., Ernberg, G., Anker, M., Korten, A., Cooper, J. E., Day, R., & Bertelsen, A. (1992). Schizophrenia: Manifestations, incidence and course in different cultures. A World Health Organization ten-country study. *Psychological Medicine Supplement, 20*, 1–97.

Jacob, T. (Ed.). (1986). *Family interaction and psychopathology: Theories, methods, and findings.* New York: Plenum Press.

Jacobs, P. A., & Sherman, S. L. (1985). The fragile (X): A marker for the Martin-Bell syndrome. *Disease Markers, 3*, 9–25.

*Jacobsen, B., & Kinney, D. K. (1980). Perinatal complications in adopted and non-adopted schizophrenics and their controls: Preliminary results. *Acta Psychiatrica Scandinavica, 62*, 337–342.

*James, A. C., Crow, T. J., Renowden, S., Wardell, A. M., Smith, D. M., & Anslow, P. (1999). Is the course of brain development in schizophrenia delayed? Evidence from onsets in adolescence. *Schizophrenia Research, 40*, 1–10.

Jansen, L. M., Gispen-de Wied, C. C., Gademan, P. J., De Jonge, R. C., van der Linden, J. A., & Kahn, R. S. (1998). Blunted cortisol response to a psychosocial stressor in schizophrenia. *Schizophrenia Research, 33*, 87–94.

*Javitt, D. C., Doneshka, P., Grochowski, S., & Ritter, W. (1995). Impaired mismatch negativity generation reflects widespread dysfunction of working memory in schizophrenia. *Archives of General Psychiatry, 52*, 550–558.

Jenkins, M. R., & Culbertson, J. L. (1996). Prenatal exposure to alcohol. In R. L. Adams & O. A. Parsons (Eds.), *Neuropsychology for clinical practice: Etiology, assessment, and treatment of common neurological disorders* (pp. 409–452). Washington, DC: American Psychological Association.

*Jernigan, T. L., Sargent, T. T., 3rd., Pfefferbaum, A., Kusubov, N., & Stahl, S. M. (1985). 18–fluorodeoxyglucose PET in schizophrenia. *Psychiatry Research, 16*, 317–329.

*Jeste, D. V., & Lohr, J. B. (1989). Hippocampal pathologic findings in schizopohrenia: A morphometric study. *Archives of General Psychiatry, 46*, 1019–1024.

Jibiki, I., Maeda, T., Kubota, T., & Yamaguchi, N. (1993). 1231–IMP SPECT brain imaging in epileptic psychosis: A study of two cases of temporal lobe epilepsy with schizophrenia-like syndrome. *Neuropsychobiology, 28*, 207–211.

*Jin, Y., Bunney, W. E., Jr., Sandman, C A., Patterson, J. V., Fleming, K., Moenter, J. R., Kalali, A. H., Hetrick, W. P., & Potkin, S. G. (1998). Is P50 supression a measure of sensory gating in schizophrenia? *Biological Psychiatry, 43*, 873–878.

⋆Jin, Y., Potkin, S. G., Patterson, J. V., Sandman, C. A., Hetrick, W. P., Bunney, W. E., Jr. (1997). Effects of P50 temporal variability on sensory gating in schizophrenia. *Psychiatry Research, 70,* 71−81.

Johanson, C.E. (1992). Biochemical mechanisms and pharmacological principles of drug action. In J. Grabowski & G. R. Van den Bos (Eds.), *Psychopharmacology: Basic mechanisms and applied interventions* (pp. 15−58). Washington, DC: American Psychological Association.

Johnson, M. K., & Raye, C. L. (1981). Reality monitoring. *Psychological Review, 88,* 67−85.

⋆Jones, I. H., Hay, D. A., Kirkby, K. C., Daniels, B. A., & Mowry, B. J. (1997). Season of birth and schizophrenia in Tasmania. *Australian and New Zealand Journal of Psychiatry, 31,* 57−61.

Jones-Gotman, M., & Milner, B. (1977). Design fluency: The invention of nonsense drawings after focal cortical lesions. *Neuropsychologia, 14,* 653−674.

⋆Jonsson, S. A., Luts, A., Guldberg-Kjaer, N., & Brun, A. (1997). Hippocampal pyramidal cell disarray correlates negatively to cell number: Implications for the pathogenesis of schizophrenia. *European Archives of Psychiatry and Clinical Neuroscience, 247,* 120−127.

⋆Joyce, J. N., Shane, A., Lexow, N., Winokur, A., Casanova, M. F., & Kleinman, J. E. (1993). Serotonin uptake sites and serotonin receptors are altered in the limbic system of schizophrenics. *Neuropsychopharmacology, 8,* 315−336.

⋆Judd, L. L., McAdams, L., Budnick, B., & Braff, D. L. (1992). Sensory gating deficits in schizophrenia: New results. *American Journal of Psychiatry, 149,* 488−493.

⋆Judd Finkelstein, J. R., Cannon, T. D., Gur, R. E., Gur, R. C., & Moberg, P. (1997). Attentional dysfunctions in neuroleptic-naïve and neuroleptic-withdrawn schizophrenic patients and their siblings. *Journal of Abnormal Psychology, 106,* 203−212.

Julien, R. M. (1995). *A primer of drug action: A concise, non-technical guide to the actions, uses and side effects of psychoactive drugs.* New York: Freeman.

Jung, C. G. (1939). On the psychogenesis of schizophrenia. In H. Read, M. Fordham, G. Adler, & W. McGuire (Eds.), *The collected works of C. G. Jung* (R. F. C. Hull, Trans., pp. 233−249). Princeton, NJ: Princeton University Press.

Jung, C. G. (1956). Recent thoughts on schizophrenia. In H. Read, M. Fordham, G. Adler, & W. McGuire (Eds.), *The collected works of C. G. Jung* (R. F. C. Hull, Trans., pp. 250−255). Princeton, NJ: Princeton University Press.

Jung, C. G. (1958). *The undiscovered self* (R. F. C. Hull, Trans.). Boston: Little Brown.

Jung, C. G. (1960). The psychology of dementia praecox (Original work published 1907). In H. Read, M. Fordham, G. Adler, & W. McGuire (Eds.), *The collected works of C. G. Jung* (R. F. C. Hull, Trans., pp. 1−4). Princeton, NJ: Princeton University Press.

⋆Jyoti Rao, K. M., Anathnarayanan, C. V., Gangadhar, B. N., & Janakiramaiah, N. (1995). Smaller P300 amplitude in schizophrenics in remission. *Neuropsychobiology, 32,* 171−174.

⋆Kalus, P., Senitz, D., & Beckmann, H. (1997). Cortical layer I changes in schizophrenia: A marker for impaired brain development? *Journal of Neural Transmission, 104,* 549−559.

Kane, J. M. (1989). The current status of neuroleptic therapy. *Journal of Clinical Psychiatry, 50,* 322–328.

*Kaney, S., & Bentall, R. P. (1992). Persecutory deulusions and the self-serving bias: Evidence from a contingency judgment task. *Journal of Nervous and Mental Disease, 180,* 773–780.

*Kaney, S., Bowen-Jones, K., Dewey, M. E. & Bentall, R. P. (1997). Two predictions about paranoid ideation: Deluded, depressed and normal participants' subjective frequency and consensus judgments for positive, neutral and negative events. *British Journal of Clinical Psychology, 36,* 349–364.

*Kaney, S., Wolfenden, M., Dewey, M. E., & Bentall, R. P. (1992). Persecutory delusions and recall of threatening propositions. *British Journal of Clinical Psychology, 31,* 85–87.

Karon, B. P., & Widener, A. J. (1994). Is there really a schizophrenogenic parent? *Psychoanalytic Psychology, 11,* 47–61.

*Kathmann, N., & Engel, R. R. (1990). Sensory gating in normals and schizophrenics: A failure to find strong P50 suppression in normals. *Biological Psychiatry, 27,* 1216–1226.

*Kawasaki, Y., Maeda, Y., Suzuki, M., Urata, K., Higashima, M., Kiba, K., Yamaguchi, N., Matsuda, H., & Hisada, K. (1993). SPECT analysis of regional cerebral blood flow changes in patients with schizophrenia during the Wisconsin Card Sorting Test. *Schizophrenia Research, 10,* 109–116.

Kay, S. R., Fiszbein A., & Opler, L. A. (1987). The positive and negative syndrome scale (PANSS) for schizophrenia. *Schizophrenia Bulletin, 13,* 261–276.

*Keefe, R. S. E., Lees Roitman, S. E., Harvey, P. D., Blum, C. S., DuPre, R. L., Prieto, P. M., Davidson, M., & Davis, K. L. (1995). A pen-and-paper human analogue of a monkey prefrontal cortex activation task: Spatial working memory in patients with schizophrenia. *Schizophrenia Research, 17,* 25–33.

*Kelsoe, J. R., Jr., Cadet, J. L., Pickar, D., & Weinberger, D. R. (1988). Quantitative neuroanatomy in schizophrenia: A controlled magnetic resonance imaging study. *Archives of General Psychiatry, 45,* 533–541.

*Kendell, R. E., Juszczak, E., & Cole, S. K. (1996). Obstetric complications and schizophrenia: A case control study based on standardised obstetric records. *British Journal of Psychiatry, 168,* 556–561.

*Kendell, R. E., & Kemp, I. W. (1989). Maternal influenza in the etiology of schizophrenia. *Archives of General Psychiatry, 46,* 878–882.

Kendler, K. S. (2000). Schizophrenia: genetics. In B. J. Sadock & V. A. Sadock (Eds.), *Kaplan and Sadock's comprehensive textbook of psychiatry* (Vol. 1). (7th ed., pp. 1147–1159). Philadelphia: Lippincott Williams & Wilkins.

Kendler, K. S., Gallagher, T. J., Abelson, J. M., & Kessler, R. C. (1996). Lifetime prevalence, demographic risk factors, and diagnostic validity of nonaffective psychosis as assessed in a U.S. community sample: The National Comorbidity Survey. *Archives of General Psychiatry, 53,* 1022–1031.

*Kendler, K. S., Gruenberg, A. M., & Strauss, J. S. (1982). An independent analysis of the Copenhagen sample of the Danish Adoption Study of Schizophrenia: V. The relationship between childhood social withdrawal and adult schizophrenia. *Archives of General Psychiatry, 39,* 1257–1261.

*Kerwin, R., Patel, S., & Meldrum, B. (1990). Quantitative autoradiographic analysis of glutamate binding sites in the hippocampal formation in normal and schizophrenic brain postmortem. *Neuroscience, 39*, 25–32.

Kety, S. S., Rosenthal, D., Wender, P. H., & Schulsinger, F. (1968). The types and prevalence of mental illness in the biological and adoptive families of adopted schizophrenics. *Journal of Psychiatric Research, 6(Suppl.)* 345–362.

*Kidogami, Y., Yoneda, H., Asaba, H., & Sakai, T. (1991). P300 in first degree relatives of schizophrenics. *Schizophrenia Research, 6*, 9–13.

*Kim, C. E., Lee, Y. S., Lim, Y. H., Noh, I. Y., & Park, S. H. (1994). Month of birth and schizophrenia in Korea: Sex, family history, and handedness. *British Journal of Psychiatry, 164*, 829–831.

Kim, J. S., Kornhuber, H. H., Schmid-Burgk, W., & Holzmuller, B. (1980). Low cerebrospinal fluid glutamate in schizophrenic patients and a new hypothesis on schizophrenia. *Neuroscience Letters, 20*, 379–382.

Kimura, D. (1961). Some effects of temporal-lobe damage on auditory perception. *Canadian Journal of Psychology, 15*, 156–165.

Kimura, D. (1964). Left–right differences in the perception of melodies. *Quarterly Journal of Experimental Psychology, 16*, 355–358.

Kimura, D. (1967). Functional asymmetry of the brain in dichotic listening. *Cortex, 3*, 163–178.

*Kinderman, P. (1994). Attentional bias, persecutory delusions and the self-concept. *British Journal of Medical Psychology, 67*, 53–66.

*Kinderman, P., & Bentall, R. P. (1996). Self-discrepancies and persecutory delusions: Evidence for a model of paranoid ideation. *Journal of Abnormal Psychology, 105*, 106–113.

*Kinderman, P., & Bentall, R. P. (1997). Causal attributions in paranoia and depression: Internal, personal, and situational attributions for negative events. *Journal of Abnormal Psychology, 106*, 341–345.

*Kinderman, P., Kaney, S., Morley, S., & Bentall, R. P. (1992). Paranoia and the defensive attributional style: Deluded and depressed patients' attributions about their own attributions. *British Journal of Medical Psychology, 65*, 371–383.

Kirch, D. G., Wagman, A. M., Goldman-Rakic, P. S. (1991). Commentary: The acquisition and use of human brain tissue in neuropsychiatric research. *Schizophrenia Bulletin, 17*, 593–596.

*Kishimoto, H., Kuwahara, H., Ohno, S., Takazu, O., Hama, Y., Sato, C., Ishii, T., Nomura, Y., Fujita, H., & Miyauchi, T. (1987). Three subtypes of chronic schizophrenia identified using 11C-glucose positron emission tomography. *Psychiatry Research, 21*, 285–292.

*Klein, C., & Andresen, B. (1991). On the influence of smoking upon smooth pursuit eye movements of schizophrenics and normal controls. *Journal of Psychophysiology, 5*, 361–369.

*Klein, R. H., & Salzman, L. F. (1981). Response-contingent learning in children at risk. *Journal of Nervous and Mental Disease, 169*, 249–252.

*Kleinschmidt, A., Falkai, P., Huang, Y., Schneider, T., Furst, G., & Steinmetz, H. (1994). In vivo morphometry of planum temporale asymmetry in first-episode schizophrenia. *Schizophrenia Research, 12*, 9–18.

Kleist, K. (1923). *Kriegsverletzungen des Gehirns in ihrer Bedeutung für die Hirnlokalisation* (Vol. 4). Leipzig: Barth.

★Kling, A. S., Metter, E. J., Riege, W. H., & Kuhl, D. E. (1986). Comparison of PET measurement of local brain glucose metabolism and CAT measurement of brain atrophy in chronic schizophrenia and depression. *American Journal of Psychiatry, 143,* 175–180.

Kluver, H., & Bucy, P. C. (1939). Preliminary analysis of the functions of the temporal lobes in monkeys. *Archives of Neurology, 42,* 979–1000.

★Knable, M. B., Hyde, T. M., Herman, M. M., Carter, J. M., Bigelow, L., & Kleinman, J. E. (1994). Quantitative autoradiography of dopamine-D1 receptors, D2 receptors, and dopamine uptake sites in postmortem striatal specimans from schizophrenic patients. *Biological Psychiatry, 36,* 827–835.

★Knight, R. A., Elliott, D. S., & Freedman, E. G. (1985). Short-term visual memory in schizophrenics. *Journal of Abnormal Psychology, 94,* 427–442.

★Knott, V., Mahoney, C., Labelle, A., Ripley, C., Cavazzoni, P., & Jones, B. (1999). Event-related potentials in schizophrenic patients during a degraded stimulus version of the visual continuous performance task. *Schizophrenia Research, 35,* 263–278.

Kobatake, K., Yoshii, F., Shinohara, Y., Nomura, K., & Takagi, S. (1983). Impairment of smooth pursuit eye movement in chronic alcoholics. *European Neurology, 22,* 392–396.

★Kolb, B., & Whishaw, I. Q. (1983). Performance of schizophrenic patients on tests sensitive to left or right frontal, temporal, or parietal function in neurological patients. *Journal of Nervous and Mental Disease, 171,* 435–443.

Kolb, B., & Wishaw, I. Q. (1996). *Fundamentals of human neuropsychology* (4th ed.). New York: Freeman.

Kornhuber, J., Riederer, P., & Beckmann, H. (1990). The dopaminergic and glutamatergic systems in schizophrenia. In W. E. Bunney, Jr., H. Hippius, G. Laakmann, & M. Schmaus (Eds.), *Neuropsychopharmacology 2* (pp. 714–720). Berlin: Springer Verlag.

★Kornhuber, J., Riederer, P., Reynolds, G. P., Beckmann, H., Jellinger, K., & Gabriel, E. (1989). 3H-spiperone binding sites in post-mortem brains from schizophrenic patients: Relationship to neuroleptic drug treatment, abnormal movements, and positive symptoms. *Journal of Neural Transmission, 75,* 1–10.

★Korpi, E. R., Kleinman, J. E., Goodman, S. I., & Wyatt, R. J. (1987). Neurotransmitter amino acids in post-mortem brains of chronic schizophrenic patients. *Psychiatry Research, 22,* 291–301.

★Kouzmenko, A. P., Hayes, W. L., Pereira, A. M., Dean, B., Burnet, P. W., & Harrison, P. J. (1997). 5–HT2A receptor polymorphism and steady state receptor expression in schizophrenia. *Lancet, 349,* 1815.

★Kovelman, J.A., & Scheibel, A.B. (1984). A neurohistological correlate of schizophrenia. *Biological Psychiatry, 19,* 1601–1621.

Kraepelin, E. (1896). *Psychiatrie: Ein Lehrbuch für Studierende und Aerzte* (5th ed). Leipzig: Barth.

Kraepelin, E. (1919). *Dementia praecox and paraphrenia* (R. M. Barclay, Trans., G. M. Robertson, Ed.), (pp. 1–331). Edinburgh: E. & S. Livingstone.

Kuhn, T. S. (1962). *The structure of scientific revolutions.* Chicago: University of Chicago Press.

Kuhn, T. S. (1977). *The essential tension: Selected studies in scientific tradition and change.* Chicago: University of Chicago Press.

★Kulynych, J. J., Vladar, K., Jones, D. W., & Weinberger, D. R. (1996). Superior temporal gyrus volume in schizophrenia: A study using MRI morphometry assisted by surface rendering. *American Journal of Psychiatry, 153,* 50–56.

★Kunugi, H., Nanko, S., Takei, N., Saito, K., Murray, R. M., & Hirose, T. (1996). Perinatal complications and schizophrenia: Data from the Maternal and Child Health Handbook in Japan. *Journal of Nervous and Mental Disease, 184,* 542–546.

★Kunugi, H., Takei, N., Murray, R. M., Saito, K., & Nanko, S. (1996). Small head circumference at birth in schizophrenia. *Schizophrenia Research, 20,* 165–170.

★Kuperberg, G. R., McGuire, P. K. & David, A. S. (1998). Reduced sensitivity to linguistic context in schizophrenic thought disorder: Evidence from on-line monitoring for words in liguistically anomalous sentences. *Journal of Abnormal Psychology, 107,* 423–434.

★Kutcher, S. P., Blackwood, D. H., St. Clair, D., Gaskell, D. F., & Muir, W. J. (1987). Auditory P300 in borderline personality disorder and schizophrenia. *Archives of General Psychiatry, 44,* 645–650.

Kwapil, T. R., Hegley, D. C., Chapman, L. J., & Chapman, J. P. (1990). Facilitation of word recognition by semantic priming in schizophrenia. *Journal of Abnormal Psychology, 99,* 215–221.

★Kwon, J. S., McCarley, R. W., Hirayasu, Y., Anderson, J. E., Fischer, I. A., Kikinis, R., Jolesz, F. A., & Shenton, M. E. (1999). Left planum temporale volume reduction in schizophrenia. *Archives of General Psychiatry, 56,* 142–148.

Laborit, H. (1950). *Physiologie et biologie du système nerveux végétif au service de la chirurgie.* Paris: G. Doin.

Lahti, R. A., Roberts, R. C., Cochrane, E. V., Primus, R. J., Gallager, D. W., Conley, R. R., & Tamminga, C. A. (1998). Direct determination of dopamine D4 receptors in normal and schizophrenic postmortem brain tissue: a [3H]NGD-94–1 study. *Molecular Psychiatry, 3,* 528–533.

Laing, R. D., & Esterson, A. (1964). *Sanity, madness, and the family.* London: Tavistock.

Lamb, M. E., & Bornstein, M. H. (1987). *Development in infancy. An introduction* (2nd. ed.). New York: Random House.

Landmark, J., Merskey, H., Cernovsky, Z., & Helmes, E. (1990). The positive triad of schizophrenic symptoms: Its statistical properties and its relationship to 13 traditional diagnostic systems. *British Journal of Psychiatry, 156,* 388–394.

Landre, N. A., Taylor, M. A., & Kearns, K. P. (1992). Language functioning in schizophrenic and aphasic patients. *Neuropsychiatry, Neuropsychology and Behavioral Neurology, 5,* 7–14

★Laruelle, M., Abi-Dargham, A., Casanova, M. F., Toti, R., Weinberger, D. R., & Kleinman, J. E. (1993). Selective abnormalities of prefrontal serotonergic receptors in schizophrenia: A postmortem study. *Archives of General Psychiatry, 50,* 810–818.

Lassen, N. A., Ingvar, D. H., & Skinhoj, E. (1978). Brain function and blood flow. *Scientific American, 239,* 62–71.

*Lawrie, S. M., Whalley, H., Kestelman, J. N., Abukmeil, S. S., Byrne, M., Hodges, A., Rimmington, J. E., Best, J. J., Owens, D. G., & Johnstone, E. C. (1999). Magnetic resonance imaging of brain in people at high risk of developing schizophrenia. *Lancet, 353*, 30–33.

LeDoux, J. E. (1995). Emotion: Clues from the brain. *Annual Review of Psychology, 46,* 209–235.

LeDoux, J. E. (1996). *The emotional brain: The mysterious underpinnings of emotional life.* New York: Simon & Schuster.

Lee, T. (1988). Postmortem studies of dopamine receptors in schizophrenia. In A. K. Sen & T. Lee (Eds.), *Receptors and ligands in psychiatry* (pp. 11–28). Cambridge, UK: Cambridge University Press.

*Lee, T., & Seeman, P. (1980). Elevation of brain neuroleptic/dopamine receptors in schizophrenia. *American Journal of Psychiatry, 137,* 191–197.

Lehmann, H. E., & Hanrahan, G. E. (1954). Chlorpromazine: New inhibiting agent for psychomotor excitement and manic states. *Archives of Neurology and Psychiatry, 71,* 227–237.

Lesch, A., & Bogerts, B. (1984). The diencephalon in schizophrenia: Evidence for reduced thickness of the periventricular grey matter. *European Archives of Psychiatry and Neurological Science, 234,* 212–219.

*Leudar, I., Thomas, P., & Johnston, M. (1992). Self-repair in dialogues of schizophrenics: Effects of hallucinations and negative symptoms. *Brain and Language, 43,* 487–511.

*Leudar, I., Thomas, P., & Johnston, M. (1994). Self-monitoring in speech production: Effects of verbal hallucinations and negative symptoms. *Psychological Medicine, 24,* 749–761.

Levin, S., Yurgelun-Todd, D., & Craft, S. (1989). Contributions of clinical neuropsychology to the study of schizophrenia. *Journal of Abnormal Psychology, 98,* 341–356.

Levy, D. L., Holzman, P. S., Matthysse, S., & Mendell, N. R. (1993). Eye tracking dysfunction and schizophrenia: A critical perspective. *Schizophrenia Bulletin, 19,* 461–536.

Levy, D. L., Holzman, P. S., Matthysse, S., & Mendell, N. R. (1994). Eye tracking and schizophrenia: A selective review. *Schizophrenia Bulletin, 20,* 47–62.

Levy, R., & Goldman-Rakic, P. S. (2000). Segregation of working memory functions within the dorsolateral prefontal cortex. *Experimental Brain Research, 133,* 23–32.

Lewandowsky, M., & Stadelmann, E. (1908). Über einen bemerkenswerten Fall von Hirnblutung und über Rechenstörungen bei Herderkrankung des Gehirns. *Journal of Psychology and Neurology, 11,* 249–265.

*Lewine, R. R., Risch, S. C., Risby, E., Stipetic, M., Jewart, R. D., Eccard, M., Caudle, J., & Pollard, W. (1991). Lateral ventricle-brain ratio and balance between CSF HVA and 5–HIAA in schizophrenia. *American Journal of Psychiatry, 148,* 1189–1194.

Lewis, M., & Volkmar, F. R. (1990). *Clinical aspects of child and adolescent development: An introductory synthesis of developmental concepts and clinical experience* (3rd ed.). Philadelphia: Lea & Febiger.

*Lewis, R., Kapur, S., Jones, C., DaSilva, J., Brown, G. M., Wilson, A.A., Houle, S., & Zipursky, R. B. (1999). Serotonin 5–HT2 receptors in schizophrenia: a PET study using [18F]setoperone in neuroleptic-naïve patients and normal subjects. *American Journal of Psychiatry, 156,* 72−78.

Lezak, M.D. (1995). *Neuropsychological assessment* (3rd ed.). New York: Oxford University Press.

Liddle, P. F. (1987). The symptoms of chronic schizophrenia. A re-examination of the positive−negative dichotomy. *British Journal of Psychiatry, 151,* 145−151.

Liddle, P.F. (1994). Volition and schizophrenia. In A.S. David & J.C. Cutting (Eds.), *The neuropsychology of schizophrenia* (pp. 39−49). Hove, UK: Erlbaum.

Liddle, P. F. (1996). Functional imaging—schizophrenia. *British Medical Bulletin, 52,* 486−494.

Liddle, P. F., Friston, K. J., Frith, C. D., Hirsch, S. R., Jones, T., & Frackowiak, R. S. (1992). Patterns of cerebral blood flow in schizophrenia. *British Journal of Psychiatry, 160,* 179−186.

Liddle, P. F., & Morris, D. L. (1991). Schizophrenic syndromes and frontal lobe performance. *British Journal of Psychiatry, 158,* 340−345.

Lidsky, T. I. (1995). Re-evaluation of mesolimbic hypothesis of antipsychotic drug action. *Schizophrenia Bulletin, 21,* 67−74.

*Lieb, K., Denz, E., Hess, R., Schuttler, R., Kornhuber, H. H., & Schreiber, H. (1996). Preattentive information processing as measured by backward masking and texton detection tasks in adolescents at high genetic risk for schizophrenia. *Schizophrenia Research, 21,* 171−182.

Lieberman, J. A., & Koreen, A. R. (1993). Neurochemistry and neuroendocrinology of schizophrenia: A selective review. *Schizophrenia Bulletin, 19,* 371−429.

*Lieh-Mak, F., & Lee, P. W. (1997). Cognitive deficit measures in schizophrenia: Factor structure and clinical correlates. *American Journal of Psychiatry, 154* (suppl. 6), 39−46.

Light, R. J., & Smith, P. V. (1971). Accumulating evidence: Procedures for resolving contradictions among different research studies. *Harvard Educational Review, 41,* 429−471.

*Lim, K. O., Sullivan, E. V., Zipursky, R. B., & Pfefferbaum, A. (1996). Cortical gray matter volume deficits in schizophrenia: A replication. *Schizophrenia Research, 20,* 157−164.

Lindemann, J .E., & Matarazzo, J. D. (1984). Intellectual assessment of adults. In A. P. Goldstein & L. Krasner (Series Eds.) & G. Goldstein & N. Hersen (Vol. Eds.), Pergamon general psychology series: Vol. 131. *Handbook of psychological assessment* (2nd ed., pp. 77−99). New York: Pergamon Press.

Lindenmayer, J. P. (1994). Risperidone: Efficacy and side effects. *Journal of Clinical Psychiatry Monograph Series, 12,* 53−60.

*Lindstrom, L. H. (1985). Low HVA and normal 5HIAA CSF levels in drug-free schizophrenic patients compared to healthy volunteers: Correlations to symptomatology and family history. *Psychiatry Research, 14,* 265−273.

Lindstrom, L. H., Gefert, O., Hagberg, G., Lundberg, T., Bergstrom, M., Hartvig, P., & Langstrom, B. (1999). Increased dopamine synthesis rate in medial prefrontal cortex and striatum in schizophrenia indicated by L-(beta-11C) DOPA and PET. *Biological Psychiatry, 46,* 681−688.

*Lindstrom, L. H., Wieselgren, I. M., Klockhoff, I., & Svedberg, A. (1990). Relationship between abnormal brainstem auditory-evoked potentials and subnormal CSF levels of HVA and 5–HIAA in first-episode schizophrenic patients. *Biological Psychiatry, 28,* 435–442.

Lipsey, M. W., & Wilson, D. B. (1993). The efficacy of psychological, educational, and behavioral treatment: Confirmation from meta-analysis. *American Psychologist, 48,* 1181–1209.

Lipska, B. K., & Weinberger, D. R. (2000). To model a psychiatric disorder in animals. Schizophrenia as a reality test. *Neuropsychopharmacology, 23,* 223–239.

*Litman, R. E., Hommer, D. W., Clem, T., Ornsteen, M. L., Ollo, C., & Pickar, D. (1991). Correlation of Wisconsin Card Sorting performance with eye tracking in schizophrenia. *American Journal of Psychiatry, 148,* 1580–1582.

*Litman, R. E., Hommer, D. W., Clem, T., Rapaport, M. H., Pato, C. N., & Pickar, D. (1989). Smooth pursuit eye movements in schizophrenia: Effects of neuroleptic treatment and caffeine. *Psychopharmacology Bulletin, 25,* 473–478.

*Litman, R. E., Hommer, D. W., Radant, A., Clem, T., & Pickar, D. (1994). Quantitative effects of typical and atypical neuroleptics on smooth pursuit eye tracking in schizophrenia. *Schizophrenia Research, 12,* 107–120.

Luria, A. R. (1973). *The working brain: An introduction to neuropsychology.* New York: Basic Books.

Luria, A. R. (1978). The localization of function in the brain. *Biological Psychiatry, 13,* 633–635.

*Luts, A., Jonsson, S. A., Guldberg-Kjaer, N., & Brun, A. (1998). Uniform abnormalities in the hippocampus of five chronic schizophrenic men compared with age-matched controls. *Acta Psychiatrica Scandinavica, 98,* 60–64.

Lynn, D.D., & Donovan, J.M. (1980). Medical vs surgical treatment of coronary artery disease. *Evaluation in Education, 4,* 98–99.

Lyon, H. M., Kaney, S., & Bentall, R. P. (1994). The defensive function of persecutory delusions: Evidence from attribution tasks. *British Journal of Psychiatry, 164,* 637–646.

Lyon, M., & Barr, C. E. (1991). Possible interactions of obstetrical complications and abnormal fetal brain development in schizophrenia. In S. A. Mednick & T. Cannon (Eds.), *Fetal neural development and adult schizophrenia* (pp. 134–150). Cambridge, UK: Cambridge University Press.

*Maas, J. W., Bowden, C. L., Miller, A. L., Javors, M. A., Funderburg, L. G., Berman, N., & Weintraub, S. T. (1997). Schizophrenia, psychosis and cerebral spinal fluid homovanillic acid concentrations. *Schizophrenia Bulletin, 23,* 147–154.

*Maas, J. W., Contreras, S. A., Miller, A. L., Berman, N., Bowden, C. L., Javors, M. A., Seleshi, E., & Weintraub, S. (1993). Studies of catecholamine metabolism in schizophrenia/psychosis: I. *Neuropsychopharmacology, 8,* 97–109.

*Mackay, A. V., Iversen, L. L., Rossor, M., Spokes, E., Bird, E., Arregui, A., Creese, I., & Snyder, S. H. (1982). Increased brain dopamine and dopamine receptors in schizophrenia. *Archives of General Psychiatry, 39,* 991–997.

MacLennan, A. J., Atmadja, S., Lee, N., & Fibiger, H. C. (1988). Chronic haloperidol administration increases the density of D2 dopamine receptors in the medial prefrontal cortex of the rat. *Psychopharmacology, 95,* 255–257.

MacLeod, C. M. (1991). Half a century of research on the Stroop effect: An integrative review. *Psychological Bulletin, 109,* 163–203.

Maher, B. A. (1974). Delusional thinking and perceptual disorder. *Journal of Individual Psychology, 30,* 98–113.

*Mahurin, R. K., Velligan, D. I. & Miller, A. L. (1998). Executive frontal lobe cognitive dysfunction in schizophrenia: A symptom subtype analysis. *Psychiatry Research, 79,* 139–149.

*Maier, W., Franke, P., Hain, C., Kopp, B., & Rist, F. (1992). Neuropsychological indicators of the vulnerability to schizophrenia. *Progress in Neuropsychopharmacology and Biological Psychiatry, 16,* 703–715.

*Makikyro, T., Sauvola, A., Moring, J., Veijola, J., Nieminen, P., Jarvelin, M. R., & Isohanni, M. (1998). Hospital-treated psychiatric disorders in adults with a single-parent and two-parent family background: A 28-year follow-up of the 1966 Northern Finland Birth Cohort. *Family Process, 37,* 335–44.

Mallet, L., Mazoyer, B., & Martinot, J. L. (1998). Functional connectivity in depressive, obsessive-compulsive, and schizophrenic disorders: An explorative correlational analysis of regional cerebral metabolism. *Psychiatry Research, 82,* 83–93.

*Manschreck, T. C., Maher, B., Milavetz, J. J., Ames, S., Weisstein, C. C., & Schneyer, M.L. (1988). Semantic priming in thought disordered schizophrenic patients. *Schizophrenia Research, 1,* 61–66.

Manschreck, T. C., Maher, B. A., Rosenthal, J. E., & Berner, J. (1991). Reduced primacy and related features in schizophrenia. *Schizophrenia Research, 5,* 35–41.

*Marcus, J., Hans, S. L., Lewow, E., Wilkinson, L., & Burack, C. M. (1985). Neurological findings in high-risk children: Childhood assessment and 5-year follow-up. *Schizophrenia Bulletin, 11,* 85–100.

*Marcus, J., Hans, S. L., Mednick, S. A., Schulsinger, F., & Michelsen, N. (1985). Neurological dysfunctioning in offspring of schizophrenics in Israel and Denmark: A replication analysis. *Archives of General Psychiatry, 42,* 753–761.

*Marsh, L., Harris, D., Lim, K. O., Beal, M., Hoff, A. L., Minn, K., Csernansky, J. G., DeMent, S., Faustman, W. O., Sullivan, E. V., & Pfefferbaum, A. (1997). Structural magnetic resonance imaging abnormalities in men with severe chronic schizophrenia and an early age at clinical onset. *Archives of General Psychiatry, 54,* 1104–1112.

*Marsh, L., Suddath, R. L., Higgins, N., & Weinberger, D. R. (1994). Medial temporal lobe structures in schizophrenia: Relationship of size to duration of illness. *Schizophrenia Research, 11,* 225–238.

*Martinot, J. L., Paillere-Martinot, M. L., Loc'h, C., Hardy, P., Poirier, M. F., Mazoyer, B., Beaufils, B., Maziere, B., Allilaire, J. F., & Syrota, A. (1991). The estimated density of D2 striatal receptors in schizophrenia: A study with positron emission tomography and 76Br-bromolisuride. *British Journal of Psychiatry, 158,* 346–350.

*Martinot, J. L., Peron-Magnan, P., Huret, J. D., Mazoyer, B., Baron, J. C. Boulenger, J. P., Loc'h, C., Maziere, B., Caillard, V., Loo, H., & Syrota, A. (1990). Striatal D2 dopaminergic receptors assessed with positron emission tomography and [76Br] bromospiperone in untreated schizophrenic patients. *American Journal of Psychiatry, 147,* 44–50.

*Marzella, P. L., Hill, C., Keks, N., Singh, B., & Copolov, D. (1997). The binding of both

[3H]nemonapride and [3H] raclopride is increased in schizophrenia. *Biological Psychiatry, 42,* 648–654.

Matarazzo, J. D. (1990). Psychological assessment versus psychological testing: Validation from Binet to the school, clinic, and courtroom. *American Psychologist, 45,* 999–1017.

★Mather, J. A., & Putchat, C. (1982). Motor control of schizophrenics: I. Oculomotor control of schizophrenics: A deficit in sensory processing, not strictly in motor control. *Journal of Psychiatric Research, 17,* 343–360.

★Matsue, Y., Okuma, T., Saito, H., Aneha, S., Ueno, T., Chiba, H., & Matsuoka, H. (1986). Saccadic eye movements in tracking, fixation, and rest in schizophrenic and normal subjects. *Biological Psychiatry, 21,* 382–389.

Mattes, J. A. (1997). Risperidone: How good is the evidence for efficacy? *Schizophrenia Bulletin, 23,* 155–161.

Matthysse, S., Holzman, P. S., & Lange, K. (1986). The genetic transmission of schizophrenia: Application of Mendelian latent structure analysis to eye tracking dysfunctions in schizophrenia and affective disorder. *Journal of Psychiatric Research, 20,* 57–67.

McCarley, R. W., Hsiao, J. K., Freedman, R., Pfefferbaum, A., & Donchin, E. (1996). Neuroimaging and the cognitive neuroscience of schizophrenia. *Schizophrenia Bulletin, 22,* 703–725.

★McCarley, R. W., Shenton, M. E., O'Donnell, B. F., Faux, S. F., Kikinis, R., Nestor, P. G., & Jolesz, F. A. (1993). Auditory P300 abnormalities and left posterior superior temporal gyrus volume reduction in schizophrenia. *Archives of General Psychiatry, 50,* 190–197.

McClelland, J. L., & Rumelhart, D. E., (Eds.). (1986). *Psychological and biological models: Vol. 2. Parallel distributed processing explorations in the microstructure of cognition.* Cambridge: MIT Press.

★McConaghy, N., Catts, S. V., Michie, P. T., Fox, A., Ward, P. B., & Shelley, A. (1993). P300 indexes thought disorder in schizophrenics, but allusive thinking in normal subjects. *Journal of Nervous and Mental Disease, 181,* 176–182.

★McCreadie, R. G., Hall, D. J., Berry, I. J., Robertson, L. J., Ewing, J. I., & Geals, M. F. (1992). The Nithsdale Schizophrenia Surveys: X. Obstetric complications, family history and abnormal movements. *British Journal of Psychiatry, 160,* 799–805.

★McCreadie, R. G., Williamson, D. J., Athawes, R. W., Connolly, M. A., & Tilak-Singh, D. (1994). The Nithsdale Schizophrenia Surveys: XIII. Parental rearing patterns, current symptomatology and relatives' expressed emotion. *British Journal of Psychiatry, 165,* 347–352.

McGlashan, T. H., & Fenton, W. S. (1991). Classical subtypes for schizophrenia: Literature review for DSM-IV. *Schizophrenia Bulletin, 17,* 609–632.

McGlashan, T. H. & Hoffman, R. E. (2000). Schizophrenia as a disorder of developmentally reduced synaptic connectivity. *Archives of General Psychiatry, 57,* 637–648.

★McGrath, J., Welham, J., & Pemberton, M. (1995). Month of birth, hemisphere of birth and schizophrenia. *British Journal of Psychiatry, 167,* 783–785.

McGuffin, P., Owen, M. J., O'Donovan, M. C., Thapar, A., & Gottesman, I. I. (1994). *Seminars in psychiatric genetics.* London: Gaskell.

*McNeil, T. F., Cantor-Graae, E., & Sjöstrom, K. (1994). Obstetric complications as antecedents of schizophrenia: Empirical effects of using different obstetric complication scales. *Journal of Psychiatric Research, 28,* 519–530.

*McNeil, T. F., Cantor-Graae, E., Torrey, E. F., Sjöstrom, K., Bowler, A., Taylor, E., Rawlings, R., & Higgins, E. S. (1994). Obstetric complications in histories of monozygotic twins discordant and concordant for schizophrenia. *Acta Psychiatrica Scandinavica, 89,* 196–204.

Mednick, S. A., Machon, R. A., Huttunen, M. O., & Bonnett, D. (1988). Adult schizophrenia following prenatal exposure to an influenza epidemic. *Archives of General Psychiatry, 45,* 189–192.

Meehl, P. E. (1962). Schizotaxia, schizotypy, schizophrenia. *American Psychologist, 17,* 827–838.

Meehl, P. E. (1978). Theoretical risks and tabular asterisks: Sir Karl, Sir Ronald and the slow progress of soft psychology. *Journal of Consulting and Clinical Psychology, 46,* 806–834.

Meehl, P. E. (1986). Diagnostic taxa as open concepts: Meta theoretical and statistical questions about reliability and construct validity in the grand strategy of nosological revision. In T. Millon & G.L. Klerman (Eds.), *Contemporary directions in psychopathology: Toward the DSM-IV* (pp. 215–231). New York: Guilford Press.

Meehl, P. E. (1990a). Appraising and amending theories: The strategy of Lakatosian defense and two principles that warrant it. *Psychological Inquiry, 1,* 108–141.

Meehl, P. E. (1990b). Toward an integrated theory of schizotaxia, schizotypy, and schizophrenia. *Journal of Personality Disorders, 4,* 1–99.

Meltzer, H. Y. (1993). New drugs for the treatment of schizophrenia. *Psychiatric Clinics of North America, 16,* 365–385.

*Merrin, E. L., & Floyd, T. C. (1994). P300 responses to novel auditory stimuli in hospitalized schizophrenic patients. *Biological Psychiatry, 36,* 527–542.

Mesulam, M. M. (1990). Schizophrenia and the brain. *New England Journal of Medicine, 322,* 842–845.

*Mialet, J. P., & Pichot, P. (1981). Eye-tracking patterns in schizophrenia: An analysis based on the incidence of saccades. *Archives of General Psychiatry, 38,* 183–186.

*Michie, P. T., Fox, A. M., Ward, P. B., Catts, S. V., McConaghy, N. (1990). Event-related potential indices of selective attention and cortical lateralization in schizophrenia. *Psychophysiology, 27,* 209–227.

Miller, M. B., Chapman, J. P., Chapman, L. J., & Collins, J. (1995). Task difficulty and cognitive deficits in schizophrenia. *Journal of Abnormal Psychology, 104,* 251–258.

Milner, B. (1963). Effects of different brain lesions on card sorting. *Archives of Neurology, 9,* 90–100.

Milner, B. (1964). Some effects of frontal lobectomy in man. In J. M. Warren & K. Akert (Eds.), *The frontal granular cortex and behavior* (pp. 313–331). New York: McGraw-Hill.

Milner, B., Corkin, S., & Teuber, H. L. (1968). Further analysis of the hippocampal amnesic syndrome: 14 year follow-up study of H. M. *Neuropsychologia, 6,* 215–234.

Milner, B., Corsi, P., & Leonard, G. (1991). Frontal-lobe contribution to recency judgments. *Neuropsychologia, 29,* 601–618.

*Minami, E., Tsuru, N., & Okita, T. (1992). Effect of subject's family name on visual event-related potential in schizophrenia. *Biological Psychiatry, 31,* 681–689.

*Mirsky, A. F., Ingraham, L. J., & Kugelmass, S. (1995). Neuropsychological assessment of attention and its pathology in the Israeli cohort. *Schizophrenia bulletin, 21,* 193–204.

*Mita, T., Hanada, S., Nishino, N., Kuno, T., Nakai, H., Yamadori, T., Mizoi, Y., & Tanaka, C. (1986). Decreased serotonin S2 and increased dopamine D2 receptors in chronic schizophrenics. *Biological Psychiatry, 21,* 1407–1414.

*Mjörndal, T., & Winblad, B. (1986). Alteration of dopamine receptors in the caudate nucleus and the putamen in schizophrenic brain. *Medical Biology, 64,* 351–354.

*Mohamed, S., Paulsen, J. S., O'Leary, D., Arndt, S., & Andreasen, N. (1999). Generalized cognitive deficits in schizophrenia: A study of first episode patients. *Archives of General Psychiatry, 56,* 749–754.

Moises, H. W., & Gottesman, I. I. (2000). Genetics, risk factors and personality factors. In H. Helmchen, F. Henn, H. Lauter, & N. Sartorius (Eds.), *Contemporary psychiatry* (Vol. 3), pp. 47–59. New York: Springer.

Möller, H. J., & Von Zerssen, D. (1995). Course and outcome of schizophrenia. In S. R. Hirsch & D. R. Weinberger (Eds.), *Schizophrenia* (pp. 106–127). Oxford: Blackwell Science.

Morice, R. (1986). Beyond language: Speculations on the prefrontal cortex and schizophrenia. *Australian and New Zealand Journal of Psychiatry, 20,* 7–10.

Morice, R., & Delahunty, A. (1996). Frontal/executive impairments in schizophrenia. *Schizophrenia Bulletin, 22,* 125–137.

*Morris, R. G., Downes, J. J., Sahakian, B. J., Evenden, J. L., Heald, A., & Robbins, T. W. (1988). Planning and spatial working memory in Parkinson's disease. *Journal of Neurology, Neurosurgery and Psychiatry, 51,* 757–766.

*Morris, S. K., Granholm, E., Sarkin, A. J. & Jeste, D. V. (1997). Effects of schizophrenia and aging on pupillographic measures of working memory. *Schizophrenia Research, 27,* 119–128.

Morrison, A. P., & Haddock, G. (1997). Cognitive factors in source monitoring and auditory hallucinations. *Psychological Medicine, 27,* 669–679.

*Muck-Seler, D., Pivac, N., & Jakoljevic, M. (1999). Sex differences, season of birth and platelet 5–HT levels in schizophrenic patients. *Journal of Neural Transmission, 106,* 337–347.

Müijen, M., & Hadley, T. R. (1995). Community care: Parts and systems. In S. R. Hirsch & D. R. Weinberger (Eds.), *Schizophrenia* (pp. 649–663). Oxford: Blackwell Science.

Muir, W. J., Squire, I., Blackwood, D. H., Speight, M. D., St. Clair, D. M., Oliver, C., & Dickens, P. (1988). Auditory P300 response in the assessment of Alzheimer's disease in Down's syndrome: A 2–year follow-up study. *Journal of Mental Deficiency Research, 32,* 455–463.

*Murray, A. M., Hyde, T. M., Knable, M. B., Herman, M. M., Bigelow, L. B., Carter, J. M., Weinbeger, D. R., & Kleinman, J. E. (1995). Distribution of putative D4 dopamine receptors in postmortem striatum from patients with schizophrenia. *Journal of Neuroscience, 13,* 2186–2191.

Mussgay, L., & Hertwig, R. (1990). Signal detection indices in schizophrenics on a visual, auditory, and bimodal Continuous Performance Test. *Schizophrenia Research, 3,* 303–310.

★Nagamoto, H. T., Adler, L. E., Waldo, M. C., & Freedman, R. (1989). Sensory gating in schizophrenics and normal controls: Effects of changing stimulation interval. *Biological Psychiatry, 25,* 549–561.

★Nagamoto, H. T., Adler, L. E., Waldo, M. C., Griffith, J., & Freedman, R. (1991). Gating of auditory response in schizophrenics and normal controls: Effects of recording site and stimulation interval on the P50 wave. *Schizophrenia Research, 4,* 31–40.

Naslund, B., Persson-Blennow, I., McNeil, T., Kaij, L., & Malmquist-Larsson, A. (1984). Offspring of women with non-organic psychosis: Fear of strangers during the first year of life. *Acta Psychiatrica Scandinavica, 69,* 435–444.

★Nasrallah, H. A., Schwarzkopf, S. B., Olson, S. C., & Coffman, J. A. (1990). Gender differences in schizophrenia on MRI brain scans. *Schizophrenia Bulletin, 16,* 205–210.

National Institute of Mental Health Psychopharmacology Service Center Collaborative Study Group (1964). Phenothiazine treatment in acute schizophrenia: Effectiveness. *Archives of General Psychiatry, 10,* 246–261.

Nauta, W. J. H., & Feirtag, M. (1986). *Fundamental neuroanatomy.* New York: Freeman.

★Nestor, P. G., Faux, S. F., McCarley, R. W., Shenton, M. E., & Sands, S. F. (1990). Measurement of visual sustained attention in schizophrenia using signal detection analysis and a newly developed computerized CPT task. *Schizophrenia Research, 3,* 329–332.

★Newman, S. C., & Bland, R. C. (1988). Month of birth and schizophrenia in Alberta. *Canadian Journal of Psychiatry, 33,* 705–706.

★Noga, J. T., Hyde, T. M., Herman, M. M., Spurney, C. F., Bigelow, L. B., Weinberger, D. R., & Kleinman, J. E. (1997). Glutamate receptors in the postmortem striatum of schizophrenic, suicide, and control brains. *Synapse, 27,* 168–176.

★Nopoulos, P. C., Ceilley, J. W., Gailis, E. A., & Andreasen, N. C. (1999). An MRI study of cerebellar vermis morphology in patients with schizophrenia: Evidence in support of the cognitive dysmetria concept. *Biological Psychiatry, 46,* 703–711.

★Nopoulos, P., Flaum, M., & Andreasen, N. C. (1997). Sex differences in brain morphology in schizophrenia. *American Journal of Psychiatry, 154,* 1648–1654.

★Nopoulos, P., Swayze, V., & Andreasen, N. C. (1996). Pattern of brain morphology in patients with schizophrenia and large cavum septi pellucidi. *Journal of Neuropsychiatry and Clinical Neuroscience, 8,* 147–152.

★Nopoulos, P., Torres, I., Flaum, M., Andreasen, N. C., Ehrhardt, J. C., & Yuh, W. T. (1995). Brain morphology in first-episode schizophrenia. *American Journal of Psychiatry, 152,* 1721–1723.

★Nordahl, T. E., Kusubov, N., Carter, C., Salamat, S., Cummings, A. M., O'Shora-Celaya, L., Eberlig, J., Robertson, L., Huesman, R. H., Jagust, W., & Budinger, T. F. (1996). Temporal lobe metabolic differences in medication-free outpatients with schizophrenia via the PET-600. *Neuropsychopharmacology, 15,* 541–554.

★Nordstrom, A. L., Farde, L., Eriksson, L., Halldin, C. (1995). No elevated D2 dopamine receptors in neuroleptic-naive schizophrenic patients revealed by positron emission tomography and [11C] N-methylspiperone. *Psychiatry Research, 61,* 67–83.

Norquist, G. S., & Narrow, W. E. (2000). Schizophrenia: Epidemiology. In B. J. Sadock, &

V. A. Sadock (Eds.), *Kaplan and Sadock's comprehensive textbook of psychiatry* (Vol. 1). (7th ed., pp. 1110–1117). Philadelphia: Lippincott Williams & Wilkins.

★Nuechterlein, K. H. (1983). Signal detection in vigilance tasks and behavioral attributes among offspring of schizophrenic mothers and among hyperactive children. *Journal of Abnormal Psychology, 92,* 4–28.

Nuechterlein, K. H. (1991). Vigilance in schizophrenia and related disorders. In H. A. Nasrallah (Series Ed.) & S. R. Steinhauer & J. H. Gruzelier (Vol. Eds.), *Handbook of schizophrenia: Vol. 5. Neuropsychology, psychophysiology and information processing* (pp. 397–433). Amsterdam: Elsevier.

Ober, B. A., Vinogradov, S., & Shenaut, G. K. (1995). Semantic priming of category relations in schizophrenia. *Neuropsychology, 9,* 220–228.

★Obiols, J. E., Clos, M., Corbero, E., Garcia-Domingo, M., de Trincheria, I., & Domenech, E. (1992). Sustained attention deficit in young schizophrenic and schizotypic men. *Psychological Reports, 71,* 1131–1136.

★Obiols, J. E., Soler Bachs, J., & Masana, J. (1986). Event-related potentials in young chronic schizophrenics. *Biological Psychiatry, 21,* 856–858.

★O'Callaghan, E., Gibson, T., Colohan, H. A., Buckley, P., Walshe, D. G., Larkin, C., & Waddington, J. L. (1992). Risk of schizophrenia in adults born after obstetric complications and their association with early onset of illness: A controlled study. *British Medical Journal, 305,* 1256–1259.

★O'Callaghan, E., Gibson, T., Colohan, H. A., Walshe, D., Buckley, P., Larkin, C., & Waddington, J. L. (1991). Season of birth in schizophrenia: Evidence for confinement of an excess of winter births to patients without a family history of mental disorder. *British Journal of Psychiatry, 158,* 764–769.

★O'Donnell, B. F., Faux, S. F., McCarley, R. R., Kimble, M. O., Salisbury, D. F., Nestor, P. G., Kikinis, R., Jolesz, F. A., & Shenton, M. E. (1995). Increased rate of P300 latency prolongation with age in schizophrenia. Electrophysiological evidence for a neurodegenerative process. *Archives of General Psychiatry, 52,* 544–549.

O'Donovan, M. C., & Owen, M. J. (1992). Advances and retreats in the molecular genetics of major mental illness. *Annals of Medicine, 24,* 171–177.

O'Donovan, M. C., & Owen, M. J. (1996). The molecular genetics of schizophrenia. *Annals of Medicine, 28,* 541–546.

★O'Hare, A., Walsh, D., & Torrey, F. (1980). Seasonality of schizophrenic births in Ireland. *British Journal of Psychiatry, 137,* 74–77.

Ohuoha, D. C., Hyde, T. M., & Kleinman, J. E. (1993). The role of serotonin in schizophrenia: An overview of the nomenclature, distribution and alterations of serotonin receptors in the central nervous system. *Psychopharmacology, 112,* Suppl., S5–S15.

Ojemann, G. A., Cawthon, D. F., & Lettich, E. (1990). Localization and physiological correlates of language and verbal memory in human lateral temporoparietal cortex. In A. B. Scheibel & A. F. Wechsler (Eds.), *UCLA forum in medical sciences: No. 29. Neurobiology of higher cognitive function* (pp. 185–202). New York: Guilford Press.

★Okubo, Y., Suhara, T., Suzuki, K., Kobayashi, K., Inoue, O., Terasaki, O., Someya, Y., Sassa, T., Sudo, Y., Matsushima, E., Iyo, M., Tateno, Y., & Toru, M. (1997). Decreased prefrontal dopamine D1 receptors in schizophrenia revealed by PET. *Nature, 385,* 634–636.

*O'Leary, D. S., Andreasen, N. C., Hurtig, R. R., Kesler, M. L., Rogers, M., Arndt, S., Cizadlo, T., Watkins, G. L., Ponto, L. L., Kirchner, P. T., & Hichwa, R. D. (1996). Auditory attentional deficits in patients with schizophrenia: A positron emission tomography study. *Archives of General Psychiatry, 53,* 633–641.

*Olin, S. S., Raine, A., Cannon, T. D., Parnas, J. Schulsinger, F., & Mednick, S. A. (1997). Childhood behavior precursors of schizotypal personality disorder. *Schizophrenia Bulletin, 23,* 93–103.

Olney, J. W., Newcomer, J. W., & Farber, N. B. (1999). NMDA receptor hypofunction model of schizophrenia. *Journal of Psychiatric Research, 33,* 523–533.

*Omori, M., Pearce, J., Komoroski, R. A., Griffin, W. S., Mrak, R. E., Husain, M. M., & Karson, C. N. (1997). In vitro 1H-magnetic resonance spectroscopy of postmortem brains with schizophrenia. *Biological Psychiatry, 42,* 359–366.

Osterrieth, P. A. (1944). Le test de copie d'une figure complexe. *Archives de Psychologie, 30,* 206–356.

Owen, A. M., Roberts, A. C., Polkey, C. E., Sahakian, B. J., & Robbins, T. W. (1991). Extra-dimensional versus intra-dimensional set shifting performance following frontal lobe excisions, temporal lobe excisions or amygdalo-hippocampectomy in man. *Neuropsychologia, 29,* 993–1006.

*Owen, R., Owen, F., Poulter, M., & Crow, T. J. (1984). Dopamine D2 receptors in substantia nigra in schizophrenia. *Brain Research, 299,* 152–154.

Palacios, J. M., Waeber, C., Hoyer, D., & Mengod, G. (1990). Distribution of serotonin receptors. *Annals of the New York Academy of Science, 600,* 36–52.

*Pallanti, S., Quercioli, L., & Pazzagli, A. (1999). Basic symptoms and P300 abnormalities in young schizophrenic patients. *Comprehensive Psychiatry, 40,* 363–371.

*Pallast, E. G., Jongbloet, P. H., Straatman, H. M., & Zielhuis, G. A. (1994). Excess seasonality of births among patients with schizophrenia and seasonal ovopathy. *Schizophrenia Bulletin, 20,* 269–276.

*Pandurangi, A. K., Sax, K. W., Pelonero, A. L., & Goldberg, S. C. (1994). Sustained attention and positive formal though disorder in schizophrenia. *Schizophrenia Research, 13,* 109–116.

Pandya, D. N., & Yeterian, E. H. (1996). Comparison of prefrontal architecture and connections. *Philosophical Transactions of the Royal Society, 351,* 1423–1432.

Park, S., & Holzman, P. S. (1992). Schizophrenics show spatial working memory deficits. *Archives of General Psychiatry, 49,* 975–982.

Parnas, J., Jorgensen, A., Teasdale, T. W., Schulsinger, F. & Mednick, S. A. (1988). Temporal course of symptoms and social functioning in relapsing schizophrenics. *Comprehensive Psychiatry, 29,* 361–371.

Parnas, J., Schulsinger, F., Teasdale, T. W., Schulsinger, H., Feldman, P. M., & Mednick, S. A. (1982). Perinatal complications and clinical outcome within the schizophrenia spectrum. *British Journal of Psychiatry, 140,* 416–420.

Patterson, J. V., Jin, Y., Gierczak, M., Hetrick, W. P., Potkin, S., Bunney, W. E., Jr., & Sandman, C. A. (2000). Effects of temporal variability on P50 and the gating ratio in schizophrenia: A frequency domain adaptive filter single-trial analysis. *Archives of General Psychiatry, 57,* 57–64.

*Paulsen, J. S., Heaton, R. K., Sadek, J. R., Perry, W., Delis, D. C., Braff, D., Kuck, J.,

Zisook, S., & Jeste, D. V. (1995). The nature of learning and memory impairments in schizophrenia. *Journal of the International Neuropsychological Society, 1,* 88–99.

*Pearlson, G. D., Barta, P. E., Powers, R. E., Menon, R. R., Richards, S. S., Aylward, E. H., Federman, E. B., Chase, G. A., Petty, R. G., & Tien, A. Y. (1997). Ziskind-Somerfeld Research Award 1996. Medial and superior temporal gyral volumes and cerebral asymmetry in schizophrenia versus bipolar disorder. *Biological Psychiatry, 41,* 1–14.

Perret, E. (1974). The left frontal lobe of man and the suppression of habitual responses in verbal categorical behaviour. *Neuropsychologia, 12,* 323–330.

Perry, W., Geyer, M. A., & Braff, D. L. (1999). Sensorimotor gating and thought disturbance measured in close temporal proximity in schizophrenic patients. *Archives of General Psychiatry, 56,* 277–281.

Petrides, M. (1985). Deficits on conditional associative-learning tasks after frontal- and temporal-lobe lesions in man. *Neuropsychologia, 23,* 601–614.

Petrides, M. (1990). Nonspatial conditional learning in patients with unilateral frontal but not unilateral temporal lobe excisions. *Neuropsychologia, 28,* 137–149.

Petrides, M., Alivisatos, B., Meyer, E., & Evans, A. C. (1993). Functional activation of the human frontal cortex during the performance of verbal working memory tasks. *Proceedings of the National Acadamy of Science USA, 90,* 878–882.

*Petty, R. G., Barta, P. E., Pearlson, G. D., McGilchrist, I. K., Lewis, R. W., Tien, A. Y., Pulver, A., Vaughn, D. D., Casanova, M. F., & Powers, R. E. (1995). Reversal of asymmetry of the planum temporale in schizophrenia. *American Journal of Psychiatry, 152,* 715–721.

*Pfefferbaum, A., Ford, J. M., White, P. M., & Roth, W. T. (1989). P3 in schizophrenia is affected by stimulus modality, response requirements, medication status, and negative symptoms. *Archives of General Psychiatry, 46,* 1035–1044.

*Pickar, D., Breier, A., Hsiao, J. K., Doran, A. R., Wolkowitz, O. M., Pato, C. N., Konicki, P. E., & Potter, W. Z. (1990). Cerebrospinal fluid and plasma monoamine metabolites and their relation to psychosis: Implications for regional brain dysfunction in schizophrenia. *Archives of General Psychiatry, 47,* 641–648.

*Pimoule, C., Schoemaker, H., Reynolds, G. P., & Langer, S. Z. (1985). [3H]SCH23390 labeled D1 dopamine receptors are unchanged in schizophrenia and Parkinson's disease. *European Journal of Pharmacology, 114,* 235–237.

Pincus, J. H., & Tucker, G. J. (1985). *Behavioral neurology* (3rd ed.). New York: Oxford University Press.

Pinel, J. J. (1990). *Biopsychology.* Boston: Allyn & Bacon.

Pinker, S. (1994). *The language instinct.* New York: Morrow.

Plomin, R., Owen, M. J., & McGuffin, P. (1994). The genetic basis of complex human behaviors. *Science, 264,* 1733–1739.

Pogue-Geile, M. F., & Gottesman, I. (1999). Schizophrenia: Study of a genetically complex phenotype. In B. C. Jones & P. Mormede (Eds.), *Neurobehavioral genetics: Methods and applications* (pp. 247–264). Boca Raton, FL: CRC Press.

*Pogue-Geile, M. F., & Oltmanns, T. F. (1980). Sentence perception and distractibility in schizophrenic, manic, and depressed patients. *Journal of Abnormal Psychology, 89,* 115–124.

Polich, J., & Kok, A. (1995). Cognitive and biological determinants of P300: An integrative review. *Biological Psychology, 41,* 103–146.

Polich, J., & Squire, L. R. (1993). P300 from amnesic patients with bilateral hippocampal lesions. *Electroencephalography and Clinical Neurophysiology, 86,* 408–417.

Poppelreuter, W. (1917). *Die psychischen Schädigungen durch Kopfschuss Kriege im 1914– 1916: Die Störungen der niederen and hoheren Leistungen durch Verletzungen des Oksipitalhirns* (Vol. 1). Leipzig: Leopold Voss.

Popper, K. R., Sir. (1959). *The logic of scientific discovery* (K. Popper, J. Freed, & Lan Freed, Trans.). Toronto: University of Toronto Press.

★Porter, R. H., Eastwood, S. L. & Harrison, P. J. (1997). Distribution of kainate receptor subunit mRNAs in human hippocampus, neocortex and cerebellum, and bilateral reduction of hippocampal GluR6 and KA2 transcripts in schizophrenia. *Brain Research, 751,* 217–321.

★Post, R. M., Delisi, L. E., Holcomb, H. H., Uhde, T. W., Cohen, R., & Buchsbaum, M. S. (1987). Glucose utilization in the temporal cortex of affectively ill patients: Positron emission tomography. *Biological Psychiatry, 22,* 545–553.

★Potts, G. F., Hirayasu, Y., O'Donnell, B. F., Shenton, M. E., & McCarley, R. W. (1998). High-density recording and topographic analysis of the auditory oddball event-related potential in patients with schizophrenia. *Biological Psychiatry, 44,* 982–989.

Pritchard, W. S. (1986). Cognitive event-related potential correlates of schizophrenia. *Psychological Bulletin, 100,* 43–66.

Purdue Research Foundation (n. d.). *Purdue Pegboard Test.* Lafayette, IN: Lafayette Instrument Company.

★Radant, A. D., & Hommer, D. W. (1992). A quantitative analysis of saccades and smooth pursuit during visual pursuit tracking: A comparison of schizophrenics with normals and substance abusing controls. *Schizophrenia Research, 6,* 225–235.

★Ragland, J. D., Gur, R. C., Glahn, D. C., Censits, D. M., Smith, R. J., Lazarev, M. G., Alavi, A., & Gur, R. E. (1998). Frontotemporal cerebral blood flow change during executive and declarative memory tasks in schizophrenia: A positron emission tomography study. *Neuropsychology, 12,* 399–413.

★Raine, A., Lencz, T., Reynolds, G. P., Harrison, G., Sheard, C., Medley, I., Reynolds, L. M., & Cooper, J. E. (1992). An evaluation of structural and functional prefrontal deficits in schizophrenia: MRI and neuropsychological measures. *Psychiatry Research, 45,* 123–137.

★Rajkowska, G., Selemon, L. D., & Goldman-Rakic, P. S. (1998). Neuronal and glial somal size in the prefrontal cortex: A postmortem morphometric study of schizophrenia and Huntington disease. *Archives of General Psychiatry, 55,* 215–224.

Randolph, C., Gold, J. M., Kozora, E., Munro-Cullum, C., Hermann, B. P., & Wyler, A. R. (1994). Estimating memory function: Disparity of Wechsler Memory Scale-Revised and California Verbal Learning Test indices in clinical and normal samples. *Clinical Neuropsychologist, 8,* 99–108.

Randolph, C., Goldberg, T. E., & Weinberger, D. R. (1993). The neuropsychology of schizophrenia. In K. M. Heilman & E. Valenstein (Eds.), *Clinical neuropsychology* (3rd ed., pp. 499–522). New York: Oxford University Press.

★Rantakallio, P., Jones, P., Moring, J., & Von Wendt, L. (1997). Association between central nervous system infections during childhood and adult onset schizophrenia and other psychoses: A 28–year follow-up. *International Journal of Epidemiology, 26,* 837–843.

Rao, K. M., Ananthnarayanan, C. V., Gangadhar, B. N., & Janakiramaiah, N. (1995). Smaller auditory P300 amplitude in schizophrenics in remission. *Neuropsychobiology, 32,* 171–174.

Raz, S., & Raz, N. (1990). Structural brain abnormalities in the major psychoses: A quantitative review of the evidence from computerized imaging. *Psychological Bulletin, 108,* 93–108.

★Razi, K., Greene, K. P., Sakuma, M., Ge, S., Kushner, M., & DeLisi, L. E. (1999). Reduction of the parahippocampal gyrus and the hippocampus in patients with chronic schizophrenia. *British Journal of Psychiatry, 174,* 512–519.

★Rea, M. M., Sweeney, J. A., Solomon, C. M., Walsh, V., & Frances, A. (1989). Changes in eye tracking during clinical stabilization in schizophrenia. *Psychiatry Research, 28,* 31–39.

Reichard, S., & Tillman, C. (1950). Patterns of parent–child relationships in schizophrenia. *Psychiatry, 13,* 247–257.

Reichert, H. (1992). *Introduction to neurobiology* (G. S. Boyan, Trans.). New York: Oxford University Press.

★Reynolds, G. P., & Mason, S. L. (1994). Are striatal dopamine D4 receptors increased in schizophrenia? *Journal of Neurochemistry, 63,* 1576–1577.

Reynolds, G. P., & Mason, S. L. (1995). Absence of detectable striatal dopamine D4 receptors in drug-treated schizophrenia. *European Journal of Pharmacology, 281,* R5–R6.

★Reynolds, G. P., Riederer, P., Jellinger, K., & Gabriel, E. (1981). Dopamine receptors and schizophrenia: The neuroleptic drug problem. *Neuropharmacology, 20,* 1319–1320.

Roberts, G. W., Colter, N., Lofthouse, R., Bogerts, B., Zech, M., & Crow, T. J. (1986). Gliosis in schizophrenia: A survey. *Biological Psychiatry, 21,* 1043–1050.

Roberts, G. W., Done, D. J., Bruton, C., & Crow, T. J. (1990). A "mock up" of schizophrenia: Temporal lobe epilepsy and schizophrenia-like psychosis. *Biological Psychiatry, 28,* 127–143.

★Robertson, G., & Taylor, P. J. (1985). Some cognitive correlates of schizophrenic illnesses. *Psychological Medicine, 15,* 81–98.

Rochester, S., Harris, J., & Seeman, M. V. (1973). Sentence processing in schizophrenic listeners. *Journal of Abnormal Psychology, 82,* 350–356.

Rochester, S., & Martin, J. R. (1979). *Crazy talk: A study of the discourse of schizophrenic speakers.* New York: Plenum Press.

★Rockstroh, B., Muller, M., Wagner, M., Cohen, R., & Elbert, T. (1994). Event-related and motor responses to probes in a forewarned reaction time task in schizophrenic patients. *Schizophrenia Research, 13,* 23–24.

★Rodrigo, G., Lusiardo, M., Briggs, G., & Ulmer, A. (1992). Season of birth of schizophrenics in Mississippi, USA. *Acta Psychiatrica Scandinavica, 86,* 327–331.

★Roitman, S. E. L., Cornblatt, B. A., Bergman, A., Obuchowski, M., Mitropoulou, V., Keefe, R. S. E., Silverman, J. M., Siever, L. J. (1997). Attentional functioning in schizotypal personality disorder. *American Journal of Psychiatry, 154,* 655–660.

Rosenthal, D., Wender, P. H., Kety, S. S., Schulsinger, F., Welner, J., & Ostergaard, L. (1968). Schizophrenic's offspring reared in adoptive homes. In D. Rosenthal & S. S. Kety (Eds.), *The transmission of schizophrenia* (pp. 377–391). Oxford: Pergamon.

★Ross, D. E., Buchanan, R. W., Medoff, D., Lahti, A. C., & Thaker, G. K. (1998). Association between eye tracking disorder in schizophrenia and poor sensory integration. *American Journal of Psychiatry, 155,* 1352–1357.

★Ross, D. E., Ochs, A. L., Hill, M. R., Goldberg, S. C., Pandurangi, A. K., & Winfrey, C. J. (1988). Erratic eye tracking in schizophrenic patients as revealed by high-resolution techniques. *Biological Psychiatry, 24,* 675–688.

★Ross, D. E., Thaker, G. K., Holcomb, H. H., Cascella, N. G., Medoff, D. R., & Tamminga, C. A. (1995). Abnormal smooth pursuit eye movements in schizophrenic patients are associated with cerebral glucose metabolism in oculomotor regions. *Psychiatry Research, 58,* 53–67.

Rosselli, M., & Ardila A. (1991). Effects of age, education, and gender on the Rey-Osterreith Complex Figure. *Clinical Neuropsychologist, 5,* 370–376.

★Rossi, A., Serio, A., Stratta, P., Petruzzi, C., Schiazza, G., Mancini, F., & Casacchia, M. (1994). Planum temporale asymmetry and thought disorder in schizophrenia. *Schizophrenia Research, 12,* 1–7.

★Rossi, A., Stratta, P., D'Albenzio, L., DiMichele, V., Serio, A., Giordano, L., Petruzzi, C., & Casacchia, M. (1989). Quantitative computed tomographic study in schizophrenia: Cerebral density and ventricle measures. *Psychological Medicine, 19,* 337–342.

★Rossi, A., Stratta, P., D'Albenzio, L., Tartaro, A., Schiazza, G., di Michele, V., Bolino, F., & Casacchia, M. (1990). Reduced temporal lobe areas in schizophrenia: Preliminary evidence from a controlled multiplanar magnetic resonance imaging study. *Biological Psychiatry, 27,* 61–68.

★Rossi, A., Stratta, P., de Cataldo, S., di Michele, V., Orfanelli, G., Serio, A., Petruzzi, C., & Casacchia, M. (1988). Cortical and subcortical computed tomographic study in schizophrenia. *Journal of Psychiatric Research, 22,* 99–105.

★Rossi, A., Stratta, P., Mattei, P., Cupillari, M., Bozzao, A., Gallucci, M., & Casacchia, M. (1992). Planum temporale in schizophrenia: A magnetic resonance study. *Schizophrenia Research, 7,* 19–22.

Rosvold, H. E., Mirsky, A. F., Sarason, I., Bransome, E. D., & Beck, L. H. (1956). A continuous performance test of brain damage. *Journal of Consulting Psychology, 20,* 343–350.

★Roxborough, H., Muir, W. J., Blackwood, D. H., Walker, M. T., & Blackburn, I. M. (1993). Neuropsychological and P300 abnormalities in schizophrenics and their relatives. *Psychological Medicine, 23,* 305–314.

★Ruiz, J., Gabilondo, A. M., Meana, J. J., & Garcia-Sevilla, J. A. (1992). Increased [3H]raclopride binding sites in postmortem brains from schizophrenic violent suicide victims. *Psychopharmacology, 109,* 410–414.

Rumelhart, D. E., & McClelland, J. L., (Eds.). (1986). *Foundations: Vol. 1. Parallel distributed processing: Explorations in the microstructure of cognition.* Cambridge: MIT Press.

★Rund, B. R. (1983). The effect of distraction on focal attention in paranoid and non-paranoid schizophrenic patients compared to normals and non-psychotic psychiatric patients. *Journal of Psychiatric Research, 17,* 241–250.

*Rund, B. R. (1989). Distractibility and recall capability in schizophrenics: A 4 year longitudinal study of stability in cognitive performance. *Schizophrenia Research, 2,* 265–275.

*Rund, B. R. (1993). Backward-masking performance in chronic and non-chronic schizophrenics, affectively disturbed patients, and normal control subjects. *Journal of Abnormal Psychology, 102,* 74–81.

*Rund, B. R., Landro, N. I., & Orbeck, A. L. (1993). Stability in backward masking performance in schizophrenics, affectively disturbed patients, and normal subjects. *Journal of Nervous and Mental Disease, 181,* 233–237.

*Rund, B. R., Landro, N. I., & Orbeck, A. L. (1997). Stability in cognitive dysfunction in schizophrenic patients. *Psychiatry Research, 69,* 131–141.

Rund, B. R., Orbeck, A. L., & Landro, N. I. (1992). Vigilance deficits in schizophrenics and affectively disturbed patients. *Acta Psychiatrica Scandinavica, 86,* 207–212.

Ruppin, E., Reggia, J. A., & Horn, D. (1996). Pathogenesis of schizophrenic delusions and hallucinations: A neural nodel. *Schizophrenia Bulletin, 22,* 105–123.

*Rushe, T. M., Morris, R. G., Miotto, E. C., Feigenbaum, J. D., Woodruff, P. W. & Murray, R. M. (1999). Problem-solving and spatial working memory in patients with schizophrenia and with focal frontal and temporal lobe lesions. *Schizophrenia Research, 37,* 21–33.

*Rushe, T. M., Woodruff, P. W., Murray, R. M., & Morris, R. G. (1999). Episodic memory and learning in patients with chronic schizophrenia. *Schizophrenia Research, 35,* 85–96.

*Saccuzzo, D. P., & Schubert, D. L. (1981). Backward masking as a measure of slow processing in schizophrenia spectrum disorders. *Journal of Abnormal Psychology, 90,* 305–312.

*Saccuzzo, D. S., Cadenhead, S., & Braff, D. L. (1996). Backward versus forward visual masking deficits in schizophrenic patients: Centrally, not peripherally, mediated? *American Journal of Psychiatry, 153,* 1564–1570.

*Sacker, A., Done, D. J., Crow, T. J., & Golding, J. (1995). Antecedents of schizophrenia and affective illness: Obstetric complications. *British Journal of Psychiatry, 166,* 734–741.

Saint-Cyr, J. A., Taylor, A. E., & Lang, A. E. (1988). Procedural learning and neostriatial dysfunction in man. *Brain, 111,* 941–959.

*Salame, P., Danion, J. M., Peretti, S., & Cuervo, C. (1998). The state of functioning of working memory in schizophrenia. *Schizophrenia Research, 30,* 11–29.

*Salisbury, D. F., O'Donnell, B. F., McCarley, R. W., Nestor, P. G., Faux, S. F., & Smith, R. S. (1994). Parametric manipulations of auditory stimuli differentially affect P3 amplitude in schizophrenics and controls. *Psychophysiology, 31,* 29–36.

*Salisbury, D. F., O'Donnell, B. F., McCarley, R. W., Shenton, M. E., & Benavage, A. (1994). The N2 event-related potential reflects attention deficit in schizophrenia. *Biological Psychiatry, 39,* 1–13.

*Salisbury, D. F., Shenton, M. E., & McCarley, R. W. (1999). P300 topography differs in schizophrenia and manic psychosis. *Biological Psychiatry, 45,* 98–106.

Sanyal, S., & Van Tol, H. H. (1997). Review of the role of dopamine D4 receptors in schizophrenia and antipsychotic action. *Journal of Psychiatric Research, 31,* 219–232.

*Sarfati, Y., & Hardy-Bayle, M. C. (1999). How do people with schizophrenia explain the behaviour of others? A study of theory of mind and its relationship to thought and speech disorganization in schizophrenia. *Psychological Medicine, 29*, 613–620.

*Sarfati, Y., Hardy-Bayle, M. C., Brunet, E., & Widlocher, D. (1999). Investigating theory of mind in schizophrenia: influence of verbalization in disorganized and non-disorganized patients. *Schizophrenia Research, 37*, 183–190.

Sartorius, N., Jablensky, A., Korten, A., Ernberg, G., Anker, M., Cooper, J. E., & Day, R. (1986). Early manifestations and first-contact incidence of schizophrenia in different cultures: A preliminary report on the initial evaluation phase of the WHO Collaborative Study on determinants of outcome of severe mental disorders. *Psychological Medicine, 16*, 909–928.

Saugstad, L. F. (1989). Social class, marriage, and fertility in schizophrenia. *Schizophrenia Bulletin, 15*, 9–43.

*Schlenker, R., & Cohen, R. (1995). Smooth pursuit eye-movement dysfunction and motor control in schizophrenia: A follow up study. *European Archives of Psychiatry and Clinical Neuroscience, 245*, 125–126.

*Schlenker, R., Cohen, R., Berg, P., Hubman, W., Mohr, F., Watzl, H., & Werther, P. (1994). Smooth-pursuit eye movement dysfunction in schizophrenia: The role of attention and general psychomotor dysfunctions. *European Archives of Psychiatry and Clinical Neuroscience, 244*, 153–160.

*Schneider, F., Weiss, U., Kessler, C., Salloum, J. B., Posse, S., Grodd, W., & Muller-Gartner, H. W. (1998). Differential amygdala activation in schizophrenia during sadness. *Schizophrenia Research, 34*, 133–142.

Schneider, K. (1959). *Clinical psychopathology* (5th ed., M.W. Hamilton, Trans.). New York: Grune & Stratton.

Schofield, W., & Balian, L. (1959). A comparative study of the personal histories of schizophrenic and non-psychiatric patients. *Journal of Abnormal and Social Psychology, 59*, 216–225.

*Schreiber, H., Stolz-Born, G., Born, J., Rothmeier, J., Rothenberger, A., Jurgens, R., Becker, W., & Kornhuber, H. H. (1997). Visually-guided saccadic eye movements in adolescents at genetic risk for schizophrenia. *Schizophrenia Research, 25*, 97–109.

*Schreiber, H., Stolz-Born, G., Heinrich, H., Kornhuber, H. H., & Born, J. (1992). Attention, cognition, and motor perseveration in adolescents at genetic risk for schizophrenia and control subjects. *Psychiatry Research, 44*, 125–140.

*Schreiber, H., Stolz-Born, G., Rothmeier, J., Kornhuber, A., Kornhuber, H. H., & Born, J. (1991). Endogenous event-related brain potentials and psychometric performance in children at risk for schizophrenia. *Biological Psychiatry, 30*, 177–189.

*Schroder, J., Buchsbaum, M. S., Siegel, B. V., Geider, F. J., Lohr, J., Tang, C., Wu, J., & Potkin, S. G. (1996). Cerebral metabolic activity correlates of subsyndromes in chronic schizophrenia. *Schizophrenia Research, 19*, 41–53.

*Schroeder, J., Buchsbaum, M. S., Siegel, B. V., Geider, F. J., Haier, R. J., Lohr, J., Wu, J., & Potkin, S. G. (1994). Patterns of cortical activity in schizophrenia. *Psychological Medicine, 24*, 947–955.

*Schwartz, B. D., Winstead, D. K., & Adinoff, B. (1983). Temporal integration deficit in visual information processing by chronic schizophrenics. *Biological Psychiatry, 18,* 1311–1320.

★Schwarzkopf, S. B., Nasrallah, H. A., Olson, S. C., Bogerts, B., McLaughlin, J. A., & Mitra, T. (1991). Family history and brain morphology in schizophrenia: An MRI study. *Psychiatry Research, 40,* 49–60.

Sedvall, G. (1992). The current status of PET scanning with respect to schizophrenia. *Neuropsychopharmacology,* 7, 41–54.

Seeman, P., Bzowej, N. H., Guan, H. C., Bergeron, C., Reynolds, G. P., Bird, E. D., Riederer, P., Jellinger, K., & Tourtellotte, W. W. (1987). Human brain D1 and D2 dopamine receptors in schizophrenia, Alzheimer's, Parkinson's and Huntington's diseases. *Neuropsychopharmacology, 1,* 5–15.

Seeman, P., Chau-Wong, M., Tedesco, J., & Wong, K. (1976). Dopamine receptors in human and calf brains, using [3H] apomorphine and an antipsychotic drug. *Proceedings of the National Academy of Science USA, 73,* 4353–4358.

★Seeman, P., Guan, H. C., Nobrega, J., Jiwa, D., Markstein, R., Balk, J. H., Picetti, R., Borelli, E., & Van Tol, H. H. (1997). Dopamine D2–like sites in schizophrenia, but not in Alzheimer's, Huntington's, or control brains, for [3H] benzquinoline. *Synapse, 25,* 137–146.

★Seeman, P., Guan, H. C., & Van Tol, H. H (1993). Dopamine D4 receptors elevated in schizophrenia. *Nature, 365,* 441–445.

★Seeman, P., Guan, H. C., & Van Tol, H. H. (1995). Schizophrenia: Elevation of dopamine D4–like sites, using [3H] nemonapride and [125I] epidepride. *European Journal of Pharmacology, 286,* R3–R5.

Seeman, P., & Lee, T. (1975). Antipsychotic drugs: Direct correlation between clinical potency and presynaptic action on dopamine neurons. *Science, 188,* 1217–1219.

★Seeman, P., Ulpian, C., Bergeron, C., Riederer, P., Jellinger, K., Gabriel, E., Reynolds, G. P., & Tourtellotte, W. W. (1984). Bimodal distribution of dopamine receptor densities in brains of schizophrenics. *Science, 225,* 728–731.

★Seidman, L. J., Oscar-Berman, M., Kalinowski, A. G., Ajilore, O., Kremen, W. S., Faraone, S. V., & Tsuang, M. T. (1995). Experimental and clinical neuropsychological measures of pre-frontal dysfunction in schizophrenia. *Neuropsychology, 9,* 481–490.

★Seidman, L. J., Van Manen, K. J., Turner, W. M., Gamser, D. M., Faraone, S. V., Goldstein, J. M., & Tsuang, M. T. (1998). The effects of increasing resource demand on vigilance performance in adults with schizophrenia or developmental attentional/learning disorders: a preliminary study. *Schizophrenia Research, 34,* 101–112.

Selemon, L. D., & Goldman-Rakic, P. S. (1999). The reduced neuropil hypothesis: A circuit based model of schizophrenia. *Biological Psychiatry, 45,* 17–25.

★Selemon, L. D., Rajkowska, G., Goldman-Rakic, P. S. (1995). Abnormally high neuronal density in the schizophrenic cortex: A morphometric analysis of prefrontal area 9 and occipital area 17. *Archives of General Psychiatry, 52,* 805–818.

★Selemon, L. D., Rajkowska, G., & Goldman-Rakic, P. S. (1998). Elevated neuronal density in prefrontal area 46 in brains from schizophrenic patients: Application of a three-dimensional, stereologic counting method. *Journal of Comprehensive Neurology, 392,* 402–412.

★Selten, J. P., Brown, A. S., Moons, K. G., Slaets, J. P., Susser, E. S., & Kahn, R. S. (1999). Prenatal exposure to the 1957 influenza pandemic and non-affective psychosis in the Netherlands. *Schizophrenia Research, 38*, 85–91.

Sergent, J., Ohta, S., & MacDonald, B. (1992). Functional neuroanatomy of face and object processing: A positron emission tomography study. *Brain, 115*, 15–36.

Serper, M. R. (1993). Visual controlled information processing resources and formal thought disorder in schizophrenia and mania. *Schizophrenia Research, 9*, 59–66.

Serper, M. R., Bergman, R. L., & Harvey, P. D. (1990). Medication may be required for the development of automatic information processing in schizophrenia. *Psychiatry Research, 32*, 281–288.

Serretti, A., Lattuada, E., Cusin, C., Lilli, R., Lorenzi, C., & Smeraldi, E. (1999). Dopamine D3 receptor gene not associated with symptomatology of major psychoses. *American Journal of Medical Genetics, 88*, 476–480.

Serretti, A., Lilli, R., Bella, D. D., Bertelli, S., Nobile, M., Novelli, E., Catalano, M., & Smeraldi, E. (1999). Dopamine receptor D4 gene is not associated with major psychoses. *American Journal of Medical Genetics, 88*, 486–491.

★Shajahan, P. M., O'Carroll, R. E., Glabus, M. F., Ebmeier, K. P., & Blackwood, D. H. (1997). Correlation of auditory "oddball" P300 with verbal memory deficits in schizophrenia. *Psychological Medicine, 27*, 579–586.

Shallice, T. (1982). Specific impairments of planning. *Philosophical Transactions of the Royal Society of London, 298*, 199–209.

★Sharma, T., Lancaster, E., Lee, D., Lewis, S., Sigmundsson, T., Takei, N., Gurling, H., Barta, P., Pearlson, G., & Murray, R. (1998). Brain changes in schizophrenia: Volumetric MRI study of families multiply affected with schizophrenia—the Maudsley Family Study 5. *British Journal of Psychiatry, 173*, 132–138.

★Sharma, T., Lancaster, E., Sigmundsson, T., Lewis, S., Takei, N., Gurling, H., Barta, P., Pearlson, G., & Murray, R. (1999). Lack of normal pattern of cerebral asymmetry in familial schizophrenic patients and their relatives: The Maudsley Family Study. *Schizophrenia Research, 40*, 111–120.

★Shelley, A. M., Grochowski, S., Lieberman, J. A., & Javitt, D. C. (1996). Premature disinhibition of P3 generation in schizophrenia. *Biological Psychiatry, 39*, 714–719.

★Shenton, M. E., Kikinis, R., Jolesz, F. A., Pollak, S. D., LeMay, M., Wible, C. G., Hokama, H., Martin, J., Metcalf, D., & Coleman, M. (1992). Abnormalities of the left temporal lobe and thought disorder in schizophrenia: A quantitative magnetic resonance imaging study. *New England Journal of Medicine, 327*, 604–612.

Shorter, E. (1997). *A history of psychiatry.* New York: Wiley.

Siddle, D. A. T, Packer, J. S., Donchin, E., & Fabiani, M. (1991). Mnemonic information processing. In J.R. Jennings & M. G. H. Coles (Eds.), *Handbook of cognitive psychophysiology: Central and autonomic nervous system approaches* (pp. 449–510). Chichester, UK: Wiley.

★Siegel, B. V., Jr., Nuechterlein, K. H., Abel, L., Wu, J. C., & Buchsbaum, M. S. (1995). Glucose metabolic correlates of continuous performance test performance in adults with a history of infantile autism, schizophrenics, and controls. *Schizophrenia Research, 17*, 85–94.

★Siegel, C., Waldo, M., Mizner, G., Adler, L. E., & Freedman, R. (1984). Deficits in sensory gating in schizophrenic patients and their relatives: Evidence obtained with auditory evoked responses. *Archives of General Psychiatry, 41,* 607–612.

Siever, L. J., van Kammen, D. P., Linnoila, M., Alterman, I., Hare, T., & Murphy, D. L. (1986). Smooth pursuit eye movement disorder and its psychobiologic correlates in unmedicated schizophrenics. *Biological Psychiatry, 21,* 1167–1174.

Sigwald, J., & Bouttier, D. (1953). Le chlorhydrate de chloro-3(dimethylamino-3-propyl)-10-phenothiazine en pratique neuro-psychiatrique courante. *Annales de Medecine, 54,* 150–182.

*Silverton, L., Harrington, M. E., & Mednick, S. A. (1988). Motor impairment and antisocial behavior in adolescent males at high risk for schizophrenia. *Journal of Abnormal Child Psychology, 16,* 177–186.

*Simpson, M. D., Slater, P., & Deakin, J. F. (1998). Comparison of glutamate and gamma-aminobutyric acid uptake binding sites in frontal and temporal lobes in schizophrenia. *Biological Psychiatry, 44,* 423–427.

*Simpson, M. D., Slater, P., Royston, M. C., & Deakin, J. F. (1992). Regionally selective deficits in uptake sites for glutamate and gamma-aminobutyric acid in the basal ganglia in schizophrenia. *Psychiatry Research, 42,* 273–282.

*Skagerlind, L., Perris, C., & Eisemann, M. (1996). Perceived parental rearing behavior in patients with a schizophrenic disorder and its relationship to aspects of the course of the illness. *Acta Psychiatrica Scandinavica, 93,* 403–406.

Skinner, H. A. (1961). *The origin of medical terms* (2nd ed). Baltimore: Williams & Wilkins.

*Slaghuis, W. L., & Bakker, V. J. (1995). Forward and backward masking of contour by light in positive- and negative-symptom schizophrenia. *Journal of Abnormal Psychology, 104,* 41–54.

Smith, M. E., Halgren, E., & Sokolik, M., Baudena, P., Musolino, A., Liegeois-Chauvel, C., & Chauvel, P. (1990). The intracranial topography of the P3 event-related potential elicited during auditory oddball. *Electroencephalography and Clinical Neurophysiology, 76,* 235–248.

Smith, M. L., & Glass, G. V. (1977). Meta-analysis of psychotherapy outcome studies. *American Psychologist, 32,* 752–760.

Smith, M. L., & Milner, B. (1984). Differential effects of frontal-lobe lesions on cognitive estimation and spatial memory. *Neuropsychologia, 22,* 697–705.

Smith, M. L., & Milner, B. (1988). Estimation of frequency of occurrence of abstract designs after frontal or temporal lobectomy. *Neuropsychologia, 26,* 297–306.

*Smith, R. C., Baumgartner, R., & Calderon, M. (1987). Magnetic resonance imaging studies of the brains of schizophrenic patients. *Psychiatry Research, 20,* 33–46.

*Snitz, B. E., Curtis, C. E., Zald, D. H., Katsanis, J., & Iacono, W. G. (1999). Neuropsychological and oculomotor correlates of spatial working memory performance in schizophrenia patients and controls. *Schizophrenia Research, 38,* 37–50.

*Sokolov, B. P. (1998). Expression of NMDAR1, GluR1, GluR7, and KA1 glutamate receptor mRNAs is decreased in frontal cortex of "neuroleptic-free" schizophrenics: Evidence on reversible up-regulation by typical neuroleptics. *Journal of Neurochemistry, 71,* 2454–2464.

*Souza, V. B., Muir, W. J., Walker, M. T., Glabus, M. F., Roxborough, H. M., Sharp, C. W., Dunan, J. R., & Blackwood, D. H. (1995). Auditory P300 event-related potentials and neuropsychological performance in schizophrenia and bipolar affective disorder. *Biological Psychiatry, 37,* 300–310.

Spence, S. A., Hirsch, S. R., Brooks, D. J., & Grasby, P. M. (1998). Prefrontal cortex activity in people with schizophrenia and control subjects: Evidence from positron emission tomography for remission of "hypofrontality" with recovery from acute schizophrenia. *British Journal of Psychiatry, 172,* 316–323.

★Spiegel, D., & King, R. (1992). Hypnotizability and CSF HVA levels among psychiatric patients. *Biological Psychiatry, 31,* 95–98.

Spitzer, M. (1997). A cognitive neuroscience view of schizophrenic thought disorder. *Schizophrenia Bulletin, 23,* 29–50.

★Spitzer, M., Braun, U., Hermle, L., & Maier S. (1993). Associative semantic network dysfunction in thought-disordered schizophrenic patients: Direct evidence from indirect semantic priming. *Biological Psychiatry, 34,* 864–877.

★Spitzer, M., Weisker, I., Winter, M., Maier, S., Hermle, L., & Maher, B. A. (1994). Semantic and phonological priming in schizophrenia. *Journal of Abnormal Psychology, 103,* 485–494.

Spohn, H. E., & Strauss, M. E. (1989). Relation of neuroleptic and anticholinergic medication to cognitive functions in schizophrenia. *Journal of Abnormal Psychology, 98,* 367–380.

★St. Clair, D., Blackwood, D., & Muir, W. (1989). P300 abnormality in schizophrenic subtypes. *Journal of Psychiatric Research, 23,* 49–55.

St. Clair, D. M., Blackwood, D. H., & Christie, J. E. (1985). P3 and other long latency auditory evoked potentials in pre-senile dementia of the Alzheimer type and alcoholic Korsakoff syndrome. *British Journal of Psychiatry, 147,* 702–706.

Stanley, J. A., Williamson, P. C., Drost, D. J., Carr, T. J., Rylett, R. J., Malla, A., & Thomson, R. T. (1995). An in vivo study of the prefrontal cortex of schizophrenic patients at different stages of illness via phosphorous magnetic resonance spectroscopy. *Archives of General Psychiatry, 52,* 399–406.

Starker, S., & Jolin, A. (1982). Imagery and hallucination in schizophrenic patients. *Journal of Nervous and Mental Disease, 170,* 448–451.

Stefan, M. D., & Murray, R. M. (1997). Schizophrenia: Developmental disturbance of brain and mind? *Acta Paediatrica (Suppl.), 422,* 112–116.

★Stefanis, N., Frangou, S., Yakely, J., Sharma, T., O'Connell, P., Morgan, K., Sigmudsson, T., Taylor, M., & Murray, R. (1999). Hippocampal volume reduction in schizophrenia: Effects of genetic risk and pregnancy and birth complications. *Biological Psychiatry, 46,* 697–702.

★Stefansson, S. B., & Jonsdottir, T. J. (1996). Auditory event-related potentials, auditory digit span, and clinical symptoms in chronic schizophrenic men on neuroleptic medication. *Biological Psychiatry, 40,* 19–27.

★Stirling, J. D., Helkwell, J. S. E., & Hewitt, J. (1997). Verbal memory impairment in schizophrenia: No sparing of short term recall. *Schizophrenia Research, 25,* 85–95.

★Stone, M., Gabrieli, J. D., Stebbins, G. T., & Sullivan, E. V. (1998). Working and strategic memory deficits in schizophrenia. *Neuropsychology, 12,* 278–288.

★Strandburg, R. J., Marsh, J. T., Brown, W. S., Asarnow, R. F., Guthrie, D., Harper, R., Yee, C. M., Nuechterlein, K. H. (1997). Event-related potential correlates of linguistic information processing in schizophrenics. *Biological Psychiatry, 42,* 596–608.

*Strandburg, R. J., Marsh, J. T., Brown, W. S., Asarnow, R. F., Guthrie, D., & Higa, J. (1990). Event-related potential correlates of impaired attention in schizophrenic children. *Biological Psychiatry, 27,* 1103–1115.

Strange, P. G. (1992). *Brain biochemistry and brain disorders.* Oxford: Oxford University Press.

*Stratta, P., Daneluzzo, E., Bustini, M. M., Gasacchia, M., Rossi, A. (1998). Schizophrenic deficits in the processing of context. *Archives of General Psychiatry, 55,* 186–187.

*Stratta, P., Daneluzzo, E., Prosperini, P. Bustini, M., Mattei, P. & Rossi, A. (1997). Is Wisconsin Card Sorting Test performance related to "working memory" capacity? *Schizophrenia Research, 27,* 11–19.

Straube, E. R., & Oades, R. D. (1992). *Schizophrenia: Empirical research and findings.* San Diego: Academic Press.

Strauss, J. S., Carpenter, W. T., Jr., & Bartko, J. J. (1974). The diagnosis and understanding of schizophrenia: III. Speculations on the processes that underlie schizophrenic symptoms and signs. *Schizophrenia Bulletin, 11,* 61–69.

Streissguth, A. P., Barr, H. M., & Martin, D. C. (1984). Alcohol exposure in utero and functional deficits in children during the first four years of life. *CIBA Foundation Symposium, 105,* 176–196.

*Strik, W. K., Dierks, T., Franzek, E., Stober, G., & Maurer, K. (1994). P300 in schizophrenia: Interactions between amplitudes and topography. *Biological Psychiatry, 35,* 850–856.

Stromgren, E. (1987). Changes in the incidence of schizophrenia? *British Journal of Psychiatry, 150,* 1–7.

Stroop, J. R. (1935). Studies of interference in serial verbal reactions. *Journal of Experimental Psychology, 18,* 643–662.

Sturgeon, C. (1998). A meta-analytic review of information processing deficits in schizophrenia: Event-related potentials and eye movement indices. Unpublished master's thesis, York University, Toronto, Ontario, Canada.

Stuss, D. T., Alexander, M. P., Palumbo, C. L., Buckle, L., Sayer, L., & Pogue, J. (1994). Organizational strategies of patients with unilateral or bilateral frontal lobe injury in word learning tasks. *Neuropsychology, 8,* 355–373.

*Suddath, R. L., Casanova, M. F., Goldberg, T. E., Daniel, D. G., Kelsoe, J. R. Jr., & Weinberger, D. R. (1989). Temporal lobe pathology in schizophrenia: A quantitative magnetic resonance imaging study. *American Journal of Psychiatry, 146,* 464–472.

*Sullivan, E. V., Mathalon, D. H., Lim, K. O., Marsh, L., & Pfefferbaum, A. (1998). Patterns of regional cortical dysmorphology distinguishing schizophrenia and chronic alcoholism. *Biological Psychiatry, 43,* 118–131.

Suslow, T., & Arolt, V. (1997). Paranoid schizophrenia: Non-specificity of neuropsychological vulnerability markers. *Psychiatry Research, 72,* 103–114.

*Susser, E., Lin, S. P., Brown, A. S., Lumey, L. H., & Erlenmeyer-Kimling, L. (1994). No relation between risk of schizophrenia and prenatal exposure to influenza in Holland. *American Journal of Psychiatry, 151,* 922–924.

*Swayze, V. W., 2nd., Andreasen, N. C., Alliger, R. J., Yuh, W. T., & Ehrhardt, J. C. (1992).

Subcortical and temporal structures in affective disorder and schizophrenia: A magnetic resonance imaging study. *Biological Psychiatry, 31,* 221–240.

Swazey, J. P. (1974). *Chlorpromazine in psychiatry: A study of therapeutic innovation.* Cambridge: MIT Press.

★Sweeney, J. A., Clementz, B. A., Haas, G. L., Escobar, M. D., Drake, K., & Frances, A. J. (1994). Eye tracking dysfunction in schizophrenia: Characterization of component eye movement abnormalities, diagnostic specificity, and the role of attention. *Journal of Abnormal Psychology, 103,* 222–230.

★Szeszko, P. R., Bilder, R. M., Lencz, T., Pollack, S., Alvir, J. M., Ashtari, M. Wu, H., & Lieberman, J. A. (1999). Investigation of frontal lobe subregions in first-episode schizophrenia. *Psychiatry Research, 90,* 1–15.

Szymanski, S., Kane, J. M., & Lieberman, J. A. (1991). A selective review of biological markers in schizophrenia. *Schizophrenia Bulletin, 17,* 99–111.

Takei, N., Sham, P., O'Callaghan, E., Murray, G. K., Glover, G., & Murray, R. M. (1994). Prenatal exposure to influenza and the development of schizophrenia: Is the effect confined to females? *American Journal of Psychiatry, 151,* 117–119.

★Tam, W. C. C., & Sewell, K. W. (1995). Seasonality of birth in schizophrenia in Taiwan. *Schizophrenia Bulletin, 21,* 117–127.

★Tamminga, C. A., Burrows, G. H., Chase, T. N., Alphs, L. D., & Thaker, G. K. (1988). Dopamine neuronal tracts in schizophrenia: Their pharmacology and in vivo glucose metabolism. *Annals of the New York Academy of Science, 537,* 443–450.

★Tamminga, C. A., Thaker, G. K., Buchanan, R., Kirkpatrick, B., Alphs, L. D., Chase, T. N., & Carpenter, W. T. (1992). Limbic system abnormalities identified in schizophrenia using positron emission tomography with fluorodeoxyglucose and neocortical alterations with deficit syndrome. *Archives of General Psychiatry, 49,* 522–530.

Tanaka, Y., Hazama, H., Kawahara, R., & Kobayashi, K. (1981). Computerized tomography of the brain in schizophrenic patients: A controlled study. *Acta Psychiatrica Scandinavica, 63,* 191–197.

Tang, S. W., Helmeste, D. M., Fang, H., Li, M., Vu, R., Bunney, W., Jr., Potkin, S., & Jones, E. G. (1997). Differential labeling of dopamine and sigma sites by [3H] emonapride and [3H] raclopride in postmortem human brains. *Brain Research, 765,* 7–12.

Tausk, V. (1948). On the origin of the "influencing machine" in schizophrenia. In R. Fleiss (Ed.), *The psychoanalytic reader* (pp. 31–64). New York: International Universities Press.

★Thaker, G., Kirkpatrick, B., Buchanan, R. W., Ellsberry, R., Lanti, A., & Tamminga, C. (1989). Oculomotor abnormalities and their clinical correlates in schizophrenia. *Psychopharmacology Bulletin, 25,* 491–497.

Torrey, E. F. (1995). *Surviving schizophrenia: A family manual.* (3rd ed.) New York: Harper & Row.

Torrey, E. F., Bowler, A. E., Rawlings, R., & Terrazas, A. (1993). Seasonality of schizophrenia and stillbirths. *Schizophrenia Bulletin, 19,* 557–562.

Torrey, E. F., Bowler, A. E., Taylor, E. H. & Gottesman, I. I. (1994). *Schizophrenia and manic-depressive disorder: The biological roots of mental illness as revealed by the landmark study of identical twins.* New York: Basic Books.

*Toru, M., Watanabe, S., Shibuya, H., Nishikawa, T., Noda, K., Mitsushio, H., Ichikawa, H., Kurumaji, A., Takashima, M., & Mataga, N. (1988). Neurotransmitters, receptors and neuropeptides in postmortem brains of chronic schizophrenic patients. *Acta Psychiatrica Scandinavica, 78,* 121–137.

Tramer, M. (1929). Ueber die biologische Bedeutung des Geburtsmonates insbesondere für die Psychoseerkrankung. *Schweizer Archiv für Neurologie und Psychiatrie, 24,* 17–24.

*Trestman, R. L., Horvath, T., Kalus, O., Peterson, A. E., Coccaro, E., Mitropoulou, V., Apter, S., Davidson, M., & Siever, L. J. (1996). Event-related potential in schizotypal personality disorder. *Journal of Neuropsychiatry and Clinical Neuroscience, 8,* 33–40.

*Tsai, G., Passani, L. A., Slusher, B. S., Carter, R., Baer, L., Kleinman, J. E., & Coyle, J. T. (1995). Abnormal excitatory neurotramsmitter metabolism in schizophrenic brains. *Archives of General Psychiatry, 52,* 829–836.

Tuckwell, H. C., Koziol, J. A. (1993). A meta-analysis of homovanillic acid concentrations in schizophrenia. *International Journal of Neuroscience, 73,* 109–114.

Tulving, E., Kapur, S., Markowitsch, H. J., Craik, F. I. M., Habib, R., & Houle, S. (1994). Hemispheric encoding/retrieval asymmetry in episodic memory: Positron emission tomography findings. *Proceedings of the National Academy of Science USA, 91,* 2012–2015.

Tulving, E., Markowitsch, H. J., Craik, F. I. M., Habib, R., & Houle, S. (1996). Novelty and familiarity activation in PET studies of memory encoding and retrieval. *Cerebral Cortex, 6,* 71–79.

*Tune, L., Barta, P., Wong, D., Powers, R. E., Pearlson, G., Tien, A. Y., & Wagner, H.N. (1996). Striatal dopamine D2 receptor quantification and superior temporal gyrus: Volume determination in 14 chronic schizophrenic subjects. *Psychiatry Research, 67,* 155–158.

*Tune, L. E., Wong, D. F., Pearlson, G., Strauss, M., Young, T., Shaya, E. K., Dannals, R. F., Wilson, A. A., Ravert, H. T., & Sapp, J. (1993). Dopamine D2 receptor density estimates in schizophrenia: A positron emission tomography study with 11C-N-methylspiperone. *Psychiatry Research, 49,* 219–237.

*Turetsky, B. I., Colbath, E. A., Gur, R. E. (1998a). P300 subcomponent abnormalities in schizophrenia: II. Longitudinal stability and relationship to symptom change. *Biological Psychiatry, 43,* 31–39.

*Turetsky, B. I., Colbath, E. A., Gur, R. E. (1998b). P300 subcompnent abnormalities in schizophrenia: I. Physiological evidence for gender and subtype specific differences in regional pathology. *Biological Psychiatry, 43,* 84–96.

*Turetsky, B., Cowell, P. E., Gur, R. C., Grossman, R. I., Shtasel, D. L., & Gur, R. E. (1995). Frontal and temporal lobe brain volumes in schizophrenia: Relationship to symptoms and clinical subtype. *Archives of General Psychiatry, 52,* 1061–1070.

*Uematsu, M., & Kaiya, H. (1989). Midsagittal cortical pathomorphology of schizophrenia: A magnetic resonance imaging study. *Psychiatry Research, 30,* 11–20.

Umbricht, D., & Kane, J. M. (1995). Risperidone: Efficacy and safety. *Schizophrenia Bulletin, 21,* 593–606.

Valenstein, E. S. (1986). *Great and desperate cures: The rise and decline of psychosurgery and other radical treatments for mental illness.* New York: Basic Books.

Vallone, D., Picetti, R., & Borrelli, E. (2000). Structure and function of dopamine receptors. *Neuroscience and Biobehavioral Reviews, 24,* 125–132.

★Van den Bosch, R. J. (1984). Eye tracking impairment: Attentional and psychometric correlates in psychiatric patients. *Journal of Psychiatric Research, 18,* 277–286.

★Van den Bosch, R. J., Rombouts, R. P., van Asma, M. J. O. (1996). What determines continuous performance task performance? *Schizophrenia Bulletin, 22,* 643–651.

Van den Bosch, R. J., Rozendaal, N., & Mol, J. M. (1987). Symptom correlates of eye tracking dysfunction. *Biological Psychiatry, 22,* 919–921.

★Van den Bosch, R. J., Van Asma, M. J., Rombouts, R. & Louwerens, J. W. (1992). Coping style and cognitive dysfunction in schizophrenic patients. *British Journal of Psychiatry Supplement, 18,* 123–128.

Van der Does, A. J., Dingemans, P. M., Linszen, D. H., Nugter, M. A., & Scholte, W. F. (1993). Symptom dimensions and cognitive and social functioning in recent-onset schizophrenia. *Psychological Medicine, 23,* 745–753.

Van der Does, A. W., & Van den Bosch, R. J. (1992). What determines Wisconsin card sorting performance in schizophrenia? *Clinical Psychology Review, 12,* 567–583.

★Velakoulis, D., Pantelis, C., McGorry, P. D., Dudgeon, P., Brewer, W., Cook, M., Desmond, P., Bridle, N., Tierney, P., Murrie, V., Singh, B., & Copolov, D. (1999). Hippocampal volume in first-episode psychoses and chronic schizophrenia: A high-resolution magnetic resonance imaging study. *Archives of General Psychiatry, 56,* 133–141.

★Verdoux, H., & Bourgeois, M. (1993). A comparative study of obstetric history in schizophrenics, bipolar patients and normal subjects. *Schizophrenia Research, 9,* 67–69.

Vinogradov, S., Ober, B. A., Shenaut, G. K. (1992). Semantic priming of word pronunciation and lexical decision in schizophrenia. *Schizophrenia Research, 8,* 171–181.

★Vita, A., Dieci, M., Giobbio, G. M., Caputo, A., Ghiringhelli, L., Comuzzi, M., Garbarini, M., Mendini, A. P., Morganti, C., Tenconi, F., Cesana, B., & Invernizzi, G. (1995). Language and thought disorder in schizophrenia: Brain morphological correlates. *Schizophrenia Research, 15,* 243–251.

★Volkow, N. D., Brodie, J. D., Wolf, A. P., Gomez-Mont, F., Cancro, R., Van Gelder, P., Russell, J. A., & Overall, J. (1986). Brain organization in schizophrenia. *Journal of Cerebral Blood Flow and Metabolism, 6,* 441–446.

★Volkow, N. D., Wolf, A. P., Van Gelder, P., Brodie, J. D., Overall, J. E., Cancro, R., & Gomez-Mont, F. (1987). Phenomenological correlates of metabolic activity in 18 patients with chronic schizophrenia. *American Journal of Psychiatry, 144,* 151–158.

★Voruganti, L. N. P., Heslegrave, R. J., & Awad, A. G. (1997). Neurocognitive correlates of positive and negative syndromes in schizophrenia. *Canadian Journal of Psychiatry, 42,* 1066–1071.

★Wagner, M., Kurtz, G., & Engel, R. R. (1989). Normal P300 in acute schizophrenics during a continuous performance test. *Biological Psychiatry, 25,* 792–795.

Waldo, M. C., Adler, L. E., Franks, R., Baker, N., Siegel, C., & Freedman, R. (1986). Sensory gating and schizophrenia. *Biological Psychology, 23,* 108.

★Waldo, M. C., Adler, L. E., & Freedman, R. (1988). Defects in auditory sensory gating and their apparent compensation in relatives of schizophrenics. *Schizophrenia Research, 1,* 19–24.

*Waldo, M. C., Cawthra, E., Adler, L. E., Dubester, S., Staunton, M., Nagamoto, H., Baker, N., Madison, A., Simon, J., & Scherzinger, A. (1994). Auditory sensory gating, hippocampal volume, and catecholamine metabolism in schizophrenics and their siblings. *Schizophrenia Research, 12,* 93–106.

Walker, E. F. (1981). Attentional and neuromotor functions of schizophrenics, schizoaffectives, and patients with other affective disorders. *Archives of General Psychiatry, 38,* 1355–1358.

*Walker, E. F., Baum, K. M., & Diforio, D. (1998). Developmental changes in the behavioral expression of vulnerability for schizophrenia. In M. F. Lenzenwenger & R. H., Dworkin (Eds.), *Origins and development of schizophrenia: Advances in experimental psychopathology* (pp. 469–491). Washington, DC: American Psychological Association.

Walker, E. F., Davis, D. M., & Gottlieb, L. A. (1991). Charting the developmental trajectories to schizophrenia. In D. Cicchetti & S. L. Toth (Eds.), *Rochester symposium on developmental psychopathology: Vol. 3. Models and integrations* (pp. 185–205). Rochester, NY: University of Rochester Press.

Walker, E. F., & Diforio, D. (1997). Schizophrenia: A neural diathesis-stress model. *Psychological Review, 104,* 667–685.

Walker, E. F., Grimes, K. E., Davis, D. M., & Smith, A. J. (1993). Childhood precursors of schizophrenia: Facial expressions of emotion. *American Journal of Psychiatry, 150,* 1654–1660.

*Walker, E. F., Savoie, T., & Davis, D. (1994). Neuromotor precursors of schizophrenia. *Schizophrenia Bulletin, 20,* 441–451.

Walker, W., & Green, M. (1982). Motor proficiency and attentional-task performance by psychotic patients. *Journal of Abnormal Psychology, 91,* 261–268.

Walton, J. (1985). *Brain's diseases of the nervous system* (9th ed.). Oxford: Oxford University Press.

*Ward, P. B., Catts, S. V., Fox, A. M., Michie, P. T., & McConaghy, N. (1991). Auditory selective attention and event-related potentials in schizophrenia. *British Journal of Psychiatry, 158,* 534–539.

*Warkentin, S., Nilsson, A., Risberg, J., Karlson, S., Flekkoy, K., Franzen, G., Gustafson, L., & Rodriguez, G. (1990). Regional cerebral blood flow in schizophrenia: Repeated studies during a psychotic episode. *Psychiatry Research, 35,* 27–38.

Warkentin, S., Risberg, J., Nilsson, A., & Karlson, S. (1991). Cortical activity during speech production: A study of regional cerebral blood flow in normal subjects performing a word fluency task. *Neuropsychiatry, Neuropsychology and Behavioral Neurology, 4,* 305–316.

*Watt, N. F., Grubb, T. W., & Erlenmeyer-Kimling, L. (1982). Social, emotional, and intellectual behavior at school among children at high risk for schizophrenia. *Journal of Consulting and Clinical Psychology 50,* 171–181.

Wechsler, D. (1981). *Wechsler Adult Intelligence Scale Revised.* New York: Psychological Corporation.

Weinberger, D. R. (1987). Implications of normal brain development for the pathogenesis of schizophrenia. *Archives of General Psychiatry, 44,* 660–669.

Weinberger, D. R. (1988). Schizophrenia and the frontal lobe. *Trends in Neuroscience, 11,* 367–370.

Weinberger, D. R. (1995). Schizophrenia as a neurodevelopmental disorder: A review of the concept. In S. R. Hirsch & D. R. Weinberger (Eds.), *Schizophrenia* (pp. 293–323). London: Blackwood.

Weinberger, D. R. (1996). On the plausibility of "the neurodevelopmental hypothesis" of schizophrenia. *Neuropsychopharmacology Supplement, 14,* 1S–11S.

Weinberger, D. R. (1997). The biological basis of schizophrenia: New directions. *Journal of Clinical Psychiatry, 58,* 22–27.

Weinberger, D. R., & Berman, K. F. (1996). Prefrontal function in schizophrenia: Confounds and controversies. *Philosophical Transactions of the Royal Society, 351,* 1495–1503.

★Weinberger, D. R., Berman, K. F., & Illowsky, B. P. (1988). Physiological dysfunction of dorsolateral prefrontal cortex in schizophrenia: III. A new cohort and evidence for a monoaminergic mechanism. *Archives of General Psychiatry, 45,* 609–615.

★Weinberger, D. R., Berman, K. F., & Zec, R. F. (1986). Physiologic dysfunction of dorsolateral prefrontal cortex in schizophrenia: I. Regional cerebral blood flow evidence. *Archives of General Psychiatry, 43,* 114–214.

Weinberger, D. R., & Wyatt, R. J. (1982). Cerebral ventricular size: A biological marker for subtyping chronic schizophrenia. In E. Usdin & I. Hanin (Eds.), *Biological markers in psychiatry and neurology* (pp. 505–512). Riverside, NJ: Pergamon Press.

Weiner, N., & Molinoff, P. B. (1994). Catecholamines. In G. J. Siegel, B. W. Agranoff, R. W. Albers, & P. G. Molinoff (Eds.), *Basic neurochemistry: Molecular, cellular and medical aspects.* (5th ed., pp. 261–281). New York: Raven Press.

★Weiner, R. U., Opler, L. A., Kay, S. R., Merriam, A. E., & Papouchis, N. (1990). Visual information processing in positive, mixed, and negative schizophrenic syndromes. *Journal of Nervous and Mental Disease, 178,* 616–626.

★Weintraub, S. (1987). Risk factors in schizophrenia: The Stony Brook High-Risk Project. *Schizophrenia Bulletin, 13,* 439–450.

Weisbrod, M. Maier, S., Harig, S., Himmelsbach, U., and Spitzer, M. (1998). Lateralized semantic and indirect semantic priming effects in people with schizophrenia. *British Journal of Psychiatry, 172,* 142–146.

★Weisbrod, M., Winkler, S., Maier, S., Hill, H., Thomas, C., & Spitzer, M. (1997). Left lateralized P300 amplitude deficit in schizophrenic patients depends on pitch disparity. *Biological Psychiatry, 4,* 541–549.

★Weiss, K. M., Chapman, H. A., Strauss, M. E., & Gilmore, G. C. (1992). Visual information decoding deficits in schizophrenia. *Psychiatry Research, 44,* 203–216.

★Weiss, K. M., Vrtunski, P. B., & Simpson, D. M. (1988). Information overload disrupts digit recall performance in schizophrenics. *Schizophrenia Research, 1,* 299–303.

Wender, P. H., Rosenthal, D., Kety, S. S., Schulsinger, F., & Welner, J. (1974). Cross-fostering: A research strategy for clarifying the role of genetic and experiential factors in the etiology of schizophrenia. *Archives of General Psychiatry, 30,* 121–128.

Wernicke, K. (1874). *Der aphasiche Symptomenkomplex.* Breslau, Poland: M. Cohn & Weigert.

★Whitaker, P. M., Crow, T. J., & Ferrier, I. N. (1981). Tritiated LSD binding in frontal cortex in schizophrenia. *Archives of General Psychiatry, 38,* 278–280.

Whitehouse, P. J., Lerner, A., & Hedera, P. (1993). Dementia. In K. M. Heilman & E. Valenstein (Eds.), *Clinical neuropsychology* (3rd ed., pp. 603–645). New York: Oxford University Press.

★Whitworth, A. B., Honeder, M., Kremser, C., Kemmler, G., Felber, S., Hausmann, A., Wanko, C., Wechdorn, H., Aichner, F., Stuppaeck, C. H., & Fleischhacker, W. W. (1998). Hippocampal volume reduction in male schizophrenic patients. *Schizophrenia Research, 31,* 73–81.

★Wible, C. G., Shenton, M. E., Hokama, H., Kikinis, R., Jolesz, F. A., Metcalf, D., & McCarley, R. W. (1995). Prefrontal cortex and schizophrenia: A quantitative magnetic resonance imaging study. *Archives of General Psychiatry, 52,* 279–288.

★Wielgus, M. S., & Harvey, P. D. (1988). Dichotic listening and recall in schizophrenia and mania. *Schizophrenia Bulletin, 14,* 689–700.

★Wiesel, F. A., Wik, G., Sjogren, I., Blomqvist, G., Greitz, T., & Stone-Elander, S. (1987). Regional brain glucose metabolism in drug free schizophrenic patients and clinical correlates. *Acta Psychiatrica Scandinavica, 76,* 628–641.

★Wieselgren, I. M., & Lindstrom, L. H. (1998). CSF levels of HVA and 5–HIAA in drug-free schizophrenic patients and healthy controls: A prospective study focused on their predictive value for outcome in schizophrenia. *Psychiatry Research, 81,* 101–110.

★Wik, G., & Wiesel, F. A. (1991). Regional brain glucose metabolism: Correlations to biochemical measures and anxiety in patients with schizophrenia. *Psychiatry Research, 40,* 101–114.

Willerman, L., & Cohen, D. B. (1990). *Psychopathology.* New York: McGraw-Hill.

Wolf, F. M. (1986). *Meta-analysis: Quantitative methods for research synthesis.* Newbury Park, CA: Sage.

★Wolkin, A., Jaeger, J., Brodie, J. D., Wolf, A. P., Fowler, J., Rotrosen, J., Gomez-Mont, F., & Cancro, R. (1985). Persistence of cerebral metabolic abnormalities in chronic schizophrenia as determined by positron emission tomography. *American Journal of Psychiatry, 142,* 564–571.

★Wong, D. F., Wagner, H. N., Jr., Tune, L. E., Dannals, R. F., Pearlson, G. D., Links, J. M., Tamminga, C. A., Broussolle, E. P., Ravert, H. T., & Wilson, A. A. (1986). Positron emission tomography reveals elevated D2 dopamine receptors in drug-naive schizophrenics. *Science, 234,* 1558–1563.

★Woo, T. U., Miller, J. L., & Lewis, D. A. (1997). Schizophrenia and the parvalbumin-containing class of cortical local circuit neurons. *American Journal of Psychiatry, 154,* 1013–1015.

★Woodruff, P. W., Wright, I. C., Shuriquie, N., Russouw, H., Rushe, T., Howard, R. J., Graves, M., Bullmore, E. T., & Murray, R. M. (1997). Structural brain abnormalities in male schizophrenics reflect fronto-temporal dissociation. *Psychological Medicine, 27,* 1257–1266.

★Woods, B. T., Yurgelun-Todd, D., Goldstein, J. M., Seidman, L. J., & Tsuang, M. T. (1996). MRI brain abnormalities in chronic schizophrenia: One process or more? *Biological Psychiatry, 40,* 585–596.

World Health Organization. (1992). *The ICD-10 classification of mental and behavioral disorders.* Geneva: Author.

World Health Organization. (1973). *The international pilot study of schizophrenia* (Vol. 1). Geneva: Author.

Yamamoto, T., & Hirano, A. (1985). Nucleus raphe dorsalis in Alzheimer's disease: Neurofibrillary tangles and loss of large neurons. *Annals of Neurology, 17,* 573–577.

Yee, C. M., Nuechterlein, K. H., & Dawson, M. E. (1998). A longitudinal analysis of eye tracking dysfunction and attention in recent-onset schizophrenia. *Psychophysiology, 35,* 443–451.

★Yee, C. M., Nuechterlein, K. H., Morris, S., & White, P. (1998). P50 suppression in recent-onset schizophrenia: Clinical correlates and risperidone effects. *Journal of Abnormal Psychology, 107,* 691–698.

★Young, A. H., Blackwood, D. H., Roxborough, H., McQueen, J. K., Martin, M. J., & Kean, D. (1991). A magnetic resonance imaging study of schizophrenia: Brain structure and clinical symptoms. *British Journal of Psychiatry, 158,* 158–164.

★Young, H. F., & Bentall, R. P. (1995). Hypothesis testing in patients with persecutory delusions: Comparison with depressed and normal subjects. *British Journal of Clinical Psychology, 34,* 353–369.

★Young, H. F., & Bentall, R. P. (1997). Probabilistic reasoning in deluded, depressed and normal subjects: Effects of task difficulty and meaningful versus non-meaningful material. *Psychological Medicine, 27,* 455–465.

Young, H. F., Bentall, R. P., Slade, P. D., & Dewey, M. E. (1987). The role of brief instructions and suggestibility in the elicitation of auditory and visual hallucinations in normal and psychiatric subjects. *Journal of Nervous and Mental Disease, 175,* 41–48.

★Yuasa, S., Kurachi, M., Suzuki, M., Kadono, Y., Matsui, M., Saitoh, O., & Seto, H. (1995). Clinical symptoms and regional cerebral blood flow in schizophrenia. *European Archives of Psychiatry and Clinical Neuroscience, 246,* 7–12.

★Zaidel, D. W., Esiri, M. M. & Harrison, P. J. (1997). Size, shape and orientation of neurons in the left and right hippocampus: Investigation of normal asymmetries and alterations in schizophrenia. *American Journal of Psychiatry, 154,* 812–818.

Zakzanis, K. K. (1998). Quantitative evidence for neuroanatomic and neuropsychological markers in dementia of the Alzheimer's type. *Journal of Clinical and Experimental Neuropsychology, 20,* 259–269.

★Zakzanis, K. K., & Heinrichs, R. W. (1999). The frontal-executive hypothesis in schizophrenia: A quantitative review of the evidence. *Journal of the International Neuropsychological Society, 5,* 556–566.

Zaunbrecher, D., Himer, W., & Straube, E. (1990). Sind frühe Stufen der visuellen Informationsverarbeitung bei Schizophrenen gestört? *Der Nervenarzt, 61,* 418–425.

★Zipursky, R. B., Lim, K. O., Sullivan, E. V., Brown, B. W., & Pfefferbaum, A. (1992). Widespread cerebral gray matter volume deficits in schizophrenia. *Archives of General Psychiatry, 49,* 195–205.

★Zipursky, R. B., Marsh, L., Lim, K. O., DeMent, S., Shear, P. K., Sullivan, E. V., Murphy, G. M., Csernansky, J. G., & Pfefferbaum, A. (1994). Volumetric MRI assessment of temporal lobe structures in schizophrenia. *Biological Psychiatry, 35,* 501–516.

★Zipursky, R. B., Seeman, M. V., Bury, A., Langevin, R., Wortzman, G., & Katz, R. (1997). Deficits in gray matter volume are present in schizophrenia but not bipolar disorder. *Schizophrenia Research, 26,* 85–92.

Zuckerman, M. (1999). *Vulnerability to psychopathology.* Washington, DC: American Psychological Association.

INDEX

DATE DUE